Alternative Treatments
for Fibromyalgia and
Chronic Fatigue Syndrome

Dedication

MARI

In memory of my mother,
Vivian Skelly, 1927–2006

HELEN

To Rich, with love

Ordering

Trade bookstores in the U.S. and Canada please contact:

Publishers Group West
1700 Fourth Street, Berkeley CA 94710
Phone: (800) 788-3123   Fax: (510) 528-3444

Hunter House books are available at bulk discounts for textbook course adoptions;
to qualifying community, health-care, and government organizations;
and for special promotions and fund-raising. For details please contact:
Special Sales Department
Hunter House Inc., PO Box 2914, Alameda CA 94501-0914
Phone: (510) 865-5282   Fax: (510) 865-4295
E-mail: ordering@hunterhouse.com

Individuals can order our books from most bookstores, by calling
(800) 266-5592, or from our website at **www.hunterhouse.com**

Alternative Treatments for Fibromyalgia & Chronic Fatigue Syndrome

Second Edition

Mari Skelly and Helen Walker

Hunter House
PUBLISHERS

Hunter House Inc., Publishers
PO Box 2914
Alameda CA 94501-0914

Library of Congress Cataloging-in-Publication Data

Skelly, Mari.
Alternative treatments for fibromyalgia and chronic fatigue syndrome /
Mari Skelly and Helen Walker. — 2nd ed.
p. cm.
Includes bibliographical references and index.
ISBN-13: 978-0-89793-472-5
ISBN-10: 0-89793-472-5
1. Fibromyalgia—Alternative treatment. 2. Chronic fatigue syndrome—
Alternative treatment. I. Walker, Helen, 1968– II. Title.
RC927.3.S54 2006
616.7'4—dc22   2006020902

Project Credits

Cover Design: Peri Poloni, Jinni Fontana	Book Production: John McKercher
Developmental and Copy Editor: Ann Roberts	Proofreader: John David Marion
Indexer: Nancy D. Peterson	Acquisitions Editor: Jeanne Brondino
Editor: Alexandra Mummery	Senior Marketing Associate: Reina Santana
Customer Service Manager: Christina Sverdrup	Order Fulfillment: Washul Lakdhon
Administrator: Theresa Nelson	Computer Support: Peter Eichelberger
Publisher: Kiran S. Rana	

Printed and Bound by Transcontinental Printing

Printed in Canada

9 8 7 6 5 4 3 2 1   Second Edition   07 08 09 10 11

Contents

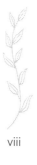

**Throughout this book, the ends of contributions
are indicated by the following symbol:** ✦✦✦

Important Note

The material in this book is intended to provide a review of information regarding fibromyalgia and chronic fatigue syndrome. Every effort has been made to provide accurate and dependable information. The contents of this book have been compiled through research and in consultation with medical professionals. However, health-care professionals have differing opinions, and advances in medical and scientific research are made very quickly, so some of the information may be disputed or become outdated.

Therefore, the publisher, authors, and editors, as well as the professionals and patients quoted in the book cannot be held responsible for any error, omission, or dated material. The authors and publisher assume no responsibility for any outcome of applying the information in this book in a program of self-care or under the care of a licensed practitioner. The information contained in this book should not be used as a substitute for the care of a medical doctor. If you think that you have some of the symptoms discussed in this book, check with a licensed physician. Always consult your physician before making any changes to your current treatment plan.

Foreword

We have come to know Mari Skelly through our work on articles for the first edition of this book in 1999, and for her second book, *Women Living with Fibromyalgia*, published in 2002. Both books provide an invaluable resource for patients struggling to understand these invisible illnesses.

In this completely revised edition of *Alternative Treatments for Fibromyalgia and Chronic Fatigue Syndrome*, Mari Skelly, and her new writing partner Helen Walker, have compiled an exhaustive manual, full of essential information and advice for the FM and/or CFS patient.

❖ ❖ ❖

A significant body of research is providing further evidence that chronic fatigue syndrome (CFS) is "a nasty mix of immunological, neurological, and hormonal abnormalities," as stated in a September 2005 *Boston Globe* article. Brain scans of CFS patients have found different patterns of blood flow to certain regions of the brain. Other studies have documented that many patients with CFS have serious cognitive problems, including difficulty in thinking and in processing information. Dr. Anthony Komaroff, a CFS expert and editor-in-chief of Harvard Health Publications, commented in the *Globe* article that "There are objective brain abnormalities in many patients with CFS that are consistent with the symptoms patients describe." In 2006 the nonprofit National CFIDS Foundation (NCF) announced that they had confirmed evidence of a previously undetected viral infection in patients with CFS. Independent research funded by the NCF uncovered a strain of Parainfluenza Virus-5 (PIV-5), which the NCF described as playing "a predominant and primary role in the development of CFS." It's promising for patients to see that medical science is finally acknowledging the biology of CFS, and is coming around to the same conclusion we, the patients, have known too well, too long: Our symptoms are real and debilitating, not imagined or fictitious.

We also have scientific proof that the *pain* of fibromyalgia (FM) is very real. Using fMRI (functional magnetic resonance imaging) to show the brain activity of FM patients versus "normal" controls in a 2002 clinical investigation, Daniel Clauw, M.D., and his fellow researchers were able to show

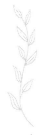

that FM patients actually experience amplified pain (described as cortical or subcortical augmentation of pain processing). Further published fMRI studies have provided additional evidence for a physiological explanation of FM pain. Now we can treat the pain of FM better than ever before, using both Eastern and Western medical approaches.

— Rich Carson and Dennis Schoen
ProHealth, Inc.
Santa Barbara, CA

Rich Carson was diagnosed with CFS in his early twenties and went on to found ProHealth, Inc., a major vitamin and supplement retailer and resource for patients with FM and CFS. ProHealth provides two websites, immunesupport.com and fibromyalgiasupport.com, and the newsletter *Healthwatch*. The company has grown to become the largest retailer of specialty FM and CFS-focused products in the United States, including dietary supplements, the *Cuddle Ewe* line of wool batting bed accessories, and other health products. **Dennis Schoen** is the CEO of ProHealth. Carson and Schoen raise money for research, and their company has funded FM and CFS studies and provided community support.

Acknowledgments

We deeply thank all the practitioners who gave so much of their time and patience to help us get this important information into the hands of FM and CFS patients. And, of course, we thank our respondents, who shared so candidly their stories of life with FM and CFS.

A special thank you to Shakeel Bandali, BSc Pharm, and Jeff Huebner, M.D., who ensured that our medical information was correct. Thanks to ProHealth, The Arthritis Foundation, and the Seattle and Eastside support groups who publicized our call for respondents. Also, thanks to LeeAnn Stiff at ProHealth for her invaluable assistance. And to our friends, Elaine Dondoyano, Erin Pearson, Diane Kerner, and David Redick for all of their help and encouragement.

Finally, we would like to thank our publisher Hunter House for giving us the opportunity to write a new edition of this book.

♣ Mari

I would like to thank my healing team. Without your constant good care, love, and support, I would still be dreaming about writing this book. Every patient deserves a team of professionals they can trust, and I'm glad to say, I have found mine. A special thank-you goes to Polly Abbott, R.N., for all of her kindness and help. My love and thanks go to Richard and Gayline Skelly and to JoAnn McMillen. A book is never a solo project, and my family and friends made my writing time possible and so much easier. My deepest gratitude goes to my spiritual family, David Redick, Maureen Brennan, Summer Cranford, and George Rohrer. And to Clay Terry for his belief in me.

Most of all I would like to thank my writing partner Helen Walker for the countless hours we spent together working on this project. We had an agreement from the beginning that our friendship would weather any concern we had about putting this book together—we managed to finish it and easily remain trusted friends, and we had a great time too! Helen, I thank you for your daily good cheer. My thanks also go to Rich Green for his patience and generosity, as he allowed me to take up so much of Helen's time. Some mornings I was the first face he saw, and some evenings the last; that had to be hard.

❧ Helen

I would like to thank my husband, Rich, who gave up so much of our time together, while I was working away furiously on this book. Thank you for encouraging me to follow my dreams. And thanks to Harry, Sally, Brother Tom, and Aretha, who sat on my laptop, pulled out my F8 key with their claws, and constantly begged to go in and out through the window. You were the best office assistants I could hope for, and without you I'm convinced this book would have been finished three months earlier.

But most of all, I would like to thank my good friend, neighbor, and writing partner, Mari Skelly, for casually asking one day, "Would you like to write a book with me?"

Chapter 1

Beginnings

As individuals, we experience life in all different dimensions, so we really want to treat each individual as a whole person, not just an arm or a leg or a tender point.

— Dennis C. Turk, Ph.D.
Director of the University of Washington
Fibromyalgia Research Center

❖ Mari's Story

IN EVERY BOOK, there's a story behind the story—this one is no exception. When I think back, 1993 was a good news/bad news kind of year for me. I had finally found a job I loved, working as a florist and shop manager in the thriving Seattle neighborhood of Queen Anne. My partner and I had bought our first house that spring, and we were excited to be creating a real home for ourselves, starting a bigger pet family, and beginning work on our garden.

The bad news: An old foot injury had returned—now both my feet hurt constantly, and the pain wasn't going away. In fact, it was getting worse. My feet were swollen and tingling, and there was stabbing pain that seemed to get worse the longer I stood, especially if I stood in one place for more than a few minutes. That's a real problem when you're working as a florist. I went to the doctor and then got a second opinion and another. Early on I was told that I had sprained my foot, or that I had gout, or maybe a stress fracture. Eventually I was diagnosed with tarsal tunnel syndrome by a podiatrist.

Time passed and I found myself living with constant pain. After several years of this agony, surgery seemed an option to consider. Back then, surgery for tarsal tunnel syndrome was considered by many to be a "cure," but like carpal tunnel surgery it didn't always bring complete relief.

Within the year, I underwent the surgery, but the pain in my feet never resolved. This pattern is typical of many people with FM and CFS who undergo unnecessary surgeries out of desperation, chasing the pain. I could not afford to take more than one month off, and soon returned to my job, where I was on my feet for eight hours a day.

Gradually I developed other symptoms. I became overcome with profound fatigue and there was pain in my back, hips, and knees. I felt frantic—I wanted to know what was happening to me. I had headaches every day. I wanted to sleep all the time, but I didn't feel refreshed when I woke up in the morning. With the mortgage to think about, it was an awful time to quit working, especially since I couldn't predict when I might be able to work again. But finally I made the decision to leave my job. I felt very scared about the future and isolated because all my friends were working. When I told people I had to leave my job because my feet hurt, it sounded so trite.

About four months after leaving my job, I consulted another doctor. I was fed up with anti-inflammatories, constantly icing my feet in five-gallon buckets of ice water (which hurt), and elevating them every moment I could. Amazingly, the new doctor was a colleague of a rheumatologist who specialized in fibromyalgia. I will never forget the day when I met the rheumatologist and was diagnosed with fibromyalgia. It began to sink in that this whole ordeal wasn't just the inability to heal after surgery, and it hadn't happened because I was a little out of shape. Most likely the stress of living with pain for so many years, coupled with my predisposition to FM, had brought me to this point. The diagnosis changed my life; I was a different person after hearing the words, "You have fibromyalgia."

Just a few months after getting the news that I had FM, I was diagnosed with CFS.

As tough as this was, I believe I had a little luck on my side. My good fortune was being diagnosed after just a few years and after only a couple of doctors, because I soon found out that many people with FM or CFS see as many as ten doctors (or more) over a decade (or longer) before being diagnosed. It was around this time that I read the amazing book *Running on Empty* by Katrina Berne. I could see myself in that book; at that point I realized I was not alone.

Aside from the pain and fatigue of FM and CFS, and all of the other symptoms that range from nagging to excruciating, it was the loss of my everyday life that I grieved the most. No more 12-hour workdays, no more spontaneous walks with my dogs, in fact, no more spontaneity.

It took me a few years to learn the steps I needed to cope with FM and CFS, which is what this book is all about:

- A great team of doctors and practitioners
- A pain-management program
- Healthy food
- Good friends for support
- Regular exercise
- Learning to pace one's self in all aspects of life

These approaches can help immensely. Once these habits become en-grained in your life, when you have a flare-up you'll still have your life skills to support you through it.

In 1998, I began work on my first book (the first edition of this book). Writing about FM and CFS helped me to accept my new life. Just knowing there were people like me, ready and willing to talk about their illnesses for the benefit of others, was a gratifying and humbling experience.

I found the contributors locally through word of mouth and doctors' offices. I interviewed them over the phone, had the tapes transcribed, and began the process of writing and rewriting until all the stories and factual information gelled into chapters.

For my second book, *Women Living with Fibromyalgia,* I found con-tributors over the Internet with the help of ProHealth. This time, I chatted with patients from all over the United States and even from Australia! I then worked with my friend, writer/editor Elaine Dondoyano, to condense the stories and make them easy to read.

Because I have FM and CFS too, I had to make it physically possible to write comfortably. That meant having moveable writing stations all over the house. I needed areas where I could stand and write or sit and write. It was necessary to physically cut up contributors' stories into piles marked "pain" or "doctors" or "tips" and put them in order. Since I write in long-hand, everything has to be typed for me. This is necessary because if I use a computer, I can't see what has already been typed, and I may get confused and forget what comes next. So to keep that from happening, I hung the pages of the chapters around the walls of my living room. It took an entire day to put them in order, but it was worth it! I'm sharing these writing tips and tricks with you to show you that, no matter what chronic illness you may have, you can always find a way to work around a problem and reach your goal.

Just before the end of 2004, I spoke with a writer who was beginning a book on FM. She asked me about my books and wanted advice on getting

her own book published. After chatting with her I realized, "Hey wait! There *is* more I'd like to say!" Around the same time, my friend Diane Kerner sent me a manuscript to read. It was her first book, *My Own Medicine: The Process of Recovery from Chronic Illness*—a terrific book, focusing on her recovery from CFS. The more I read through it, the more excited I became about rewriting *Alternative Treatments for Fibromyalgia and Chronic Fatigue Syndrome* and continuing our story together.

I was enthusiastic to do the book, but knew I needed a writing partner for such a big project. After all the hard work and success of *Women Living with Fibromyalgia*, I knew that to really bring *Alternative Treatments for Fibromyalgia and Chronic Fatigue Syndrome* up to date with all the new information available and even new contributors, I'd need a very special writing partner indeed. This person had to be understanding of my limits, a very quick study of all things FM and CFS, and a hardworking, easygoing, organized person, who didn't mind doing all the typing and who could put up with my brain fog and fatigue. After months of searching, my ideal writing partner moved in across the street!

Our cats met first. Helen's big, fat, orange cat Harry met my big, fat, orange cat Sunny, and a friendship, or at least a truce, was struck. "You have this half of the street up to the old rhododendron; I'll have the other half." Between us we have eight cats. Is that too many? Nah, cats are like shoes; you need them in a lot of colors.

Helen and her husband Rich both work for local television stations, and to my great luck, Helen is also a writer. We became fast friends and discovered that working together is a pleasure. The commute to work on the book took about 50 steps, and the traffic on our sleepy street is made up of cats and children.

✤ The New Book

So much has changed in the world of fibromyalgia (FM) and chronic fatigue syndrome (CFS) since the first edition of this book was published. We wanted to pull all this new information together and present it in a format that would be easy to read, and easy to use. We were also curious to see how our original respondents were faring seven years later—to catch up with the FM and CFS patients whose wisdom filled the pages of the first edition.

This time, we have the input of an international group of patients. Now that FM and CFS are recognized as real illnesses in the news media worldwide, it was not difficult to find people ready to talk openly about their illness.

In January 2005, with the help of immunesupport.com, arthritis.org, the Seattle FM and CFS Support Group, and the Eastside FM and CFS Support Group, we put out a request for patients to contact us if they were interested in telling their stories. Within a week we were buried under a virtual pile of e-mails from all over the world. We heard from more than 200 people—all with frank, honest insights into their illness and plenty of tips to share.

Reading the patients' stories was by the far the best part of writing this book. We received so many that we finally had to say "stop!" or we would still have our noses buried in the computer today!

Most patients told us they turned to alternative therapies, after first struggling to get help with their symptoms using conventional medicine alone. Those who get better—and there really are people who recover from FM and CFS—all seem to be on a similar path. Once they fully understood their illness, they added alternative and complementary treatments. When they cleaned up their diet, began exercising properly, and found a pain-management plan, many patients reported that they began to see positive results.

The American College of Rheumatology states that approximately seven million people in the United States have been diagnosed with FM and/or CFS. The majority of these people are women aged 30–45 years. Women are seven times more likely than men to be diagnosed with FM and CFS, but this does not necessarily mean that women are more susceptible to these illnesses. Many of the practitioners we talked with told us that men seem reluctant to report the symptoms of FM and CFS to their doctor, and therefore receive the diagnosis less frequently. Our respondents were a microcosm of the FM and CFS population, overwhelmingly women between the ages of 30 and 45, but also many men, people over 60, and college students. FM and CFS can strike anyone, at any time of life.

❖ Sound Advice

We sought experts in the field of FM and CFS and experienced practitioners of alternative therapies. They brought their knowledge, integrity, and enthusiasm to this project, because they believe, as we do, that you have the power and ability to live well with FM and CFS.

❧ How to Use This Book

In this book, we take a holistic view of medicine; we look at how to treat the whole person—body, mind, and spirit. You'll find many therapies to choose from, so you can gain a sense of what works for you and begin to build your own individual treatment plan. We can't wait to try some of the treatments in this book ourselves.

If you want to learn more about a particular treatment, turn to our Resources section for information on organizations, websites, and publications. It's organized by topic and is easy to navigate. You'll also find a bibliography, which lists every book and article we mention, plus books written by our featured providers (and some patients too).

Talk to your primary-care physician if you would like to try some of these alternative treatments. You may want to take this book with you to your next appointment and share some of the information you have found with your doctor. Feel free to scribble notes on all the pages.

Sharing this book with your family and friends is a great way to help your loved ones make sense of your illness. Reading others' stories and experiences may help them to understand what is happening to their loved one—you.

❖ ❖ ❖

We look forward to writing other books and articles. If you would like to e-mail us (and perhaps send us your answers to our questionnaire), please do so at fmcfsbook@yahoo.com—we would love to hear your story.

We thank you for your support over the years, especially since the release of *Women Living with Fibromyalgia* in 2002. Remember, you are never alone in the fight against FM and CFS—we wish you good luck and hope you enjoy meeting these amazing people as much as we have.

Many of our respondents told us they found it cathartic to really think about the way in which FM and CFS has impacted their lives. You may find it helpful to complete a questionnaire yourself.

❧ The Questionnaire

DIAGNOSIS

1. When were you first diagnosed? What made you see a doctor?
2. How long do you think you had FM and/or CFS before you were diagnosed?

3. How long did it take you to get a final diagnosis of FM and/or CFS? Along the way, were you treated with respect, and did medical professionals take your symptoms seriously?

4. Prior to your illness, were you exposed to chemicals or pesticides? Did you experience trauma (either physical or mental), surgeries, or viral illnesses?

5. Do you have any other illness or condition commonly associated with FM and/or CFS? For example:
   – Temporomandibular joint dysfunction (TMJ)
   – Irritable bowel syndrome (IBS)
   – Celiac disease
   – Thyroid disorder
   – Multiple chemical sensitivities (MCS)

6. How did you feel when you were first told you had FM and/or CFS?

7. How does your life now compare to your life before FM and/or CFS?

TREATMENT

8. Do you take medications and/or supplements for FM and/or CFS? If so, what kind do you take and do they help?

9. Have you tried any of the following therapies to relieve your symptoms of FM and/or CFS?
   – Acupuncture   – Chiropractic
   – Osteopathy   – Naturopathy
   – Physical therapy   – Yoga
   – Movement therapy   – Massage
   – Exercise   – Tai chi
   – Qigong   – Craniosacral therapy

   Tell us about your experiences with these therapies. Did they help? What about them works best for you? What didn't help?

10. Whom do you rely upon most for your primary care? How did you find this person, and are you happy with the service they provide?

11. If you have been diagnosed with CFS, what are your thoughts on the name of your illness? Does "chronic fatigue syndrome" accurately describe it? The term "Myalgic Encephalomyelitis" (ME) is commonly used in some countries, and the term "Chronic Fatigue

and Immune Dysfunction Syndrome" (CFIDS) has also been suggested as an alternative. Do either of these terms better describe CFS to you? Do you have another suggestion?

LIVING WITH FM AND/OR CFS

12. How do you cope with having FM and/or CFS? Do you have any everyday tips you would like to share with other patients?

13. Do your family and friends treat you with respect in regard to your FM and/or CFS? Do you have what you consider to be a good support network?

14. Are you able to take care of yourself? If not, who is helping you?

15. Has FM and/or CFS effected your relationship with your romantic partner?

16. Have you identified your personal life-stressors and are you actively dealing with them?

17. Please talk about your emotions regarding FM and/or CFS. Are you angry or scared; do you feel alone?

18. Do you see a mental health professional for stress directly caused by your FM and/or CFS? If so, in what ways does this help you deal with your illness?

19. Tell us about your career and the impact FM and/or CFS has had on it. Did you lose your job because of FM and/or CFS? Has it affected your job performance? Has it changed your workplace relationships?

20. Are you receiving social security benefits and/or private disability benefits because of your FM and/or CFS? If so, how long did it take to qualify for these benefits?

21. Have you taken legal action regarding your FM and/or CFS? For example, to gain social security benefits or compensation following an accident.

22. What financial challenges have you faced as a result of having FM and/or CFS?

23. Do you find there are societal pressures on people who are chronically ill? If so, how do you deal with them?

24. Compare the goals you had before your illness with the ones you have established since your diagnosis.

25. How has having FM and/or CFS changed your outlook on life?

26. What drives you forward every day? What are your rewards in life?

27. Do you talk about your illness with your friends, your family, local support groups, or online support groups? If so, which do you find the most helpful?

28. Have you researched your illness? Have you been keeping up with FM and/or CFS periodicals and the medical literature available online?

29. If you do keep up with medical advances, which new or forthcoming treatments for FM and/or CFS seem to offer the most promise? Where do you go to find information on new treatments for FM and/or CFS?

30. Do you try to think positively about your illness? Has this helped? If so, how has this "positive thinking" been beneficial to you?

31. Do you practice any of the following: meditation, guided imagery, Reiki? If so, in what ways has the practice helped you?

32. Do you keep a journal? If so, does journaling help you to cope with your illness?

33. Has having FM and/or CFS affected your spirituality or religious beliefs? If so, in what ways?

Chapter 2

Understanding Fibromyalgia

Those who have learned by experience what physical and emotional pain and anguish mean are a community all over the world. They are united by a secret bond. One and all, they know the horrors of suffering to which mankind can be subjected. One and all, they know the longing to be free from pain.

— Albert Schweitzer

T HE FIRST QUESTION on most newly diagnosed FM patients' minds is "What is fibromyalgia?" The answer is continually evolving as we learn more about this mysterious illness. In this chapter we explore the etiology of FM—what FM is, what causes it, its symptoms, and its diagnosis.

✤ What Is Fibromyalgia?

Defining FM is not a simple task. It's like working on a jigsaw puzzle, with pieces constantly being added and taken away—we're beginning to see the whole picture, but not all pieces of the puzzle are in place. A recent edition of *Time* magazine described FM as a "musculoskeletal disorder." But FM is not just a musculoskeletal disorder, or even a form of arthritis. And FM is definitely not a psychiatric condition.

CENTRAL SENSITIZATION

FM is characterized by extreme sensitization of the central nervous system (the brain and spinal cord), which then amplifies pain signals to the body. Devin J. Starlanyl, author of *The Fibromyalgia Advocate*, describes FM as a state of "central sensitization." The term *central sensitization* means that the entire central nervous system has become overly sensitive. All the senses can be affected—bright lights, loud sounds, spicy food, heavy perfume, or even the light touch of a child can be perceived as painful. Tracy G. from Portland, Oregon, says, "When my two-year-old put her hand on my thigh, it felt like a big bruise."

Not only does the FM patient feel intense pain from something that shouldn't hurt at all, but also their body amplifies normal pain situations. Banging one's funny bone on the table is painful for everybody—but for an FM patient it can result in intense, long-lasting pain. Central sensitization is not only a distorted sensory experience—an FM patient's body chemistry over-reacts too. A knock on the elbow, which wouldn't leave a scratch normally, can result in bruising, soreness, and stiffness if you have FM.

FM is body-wide, with most patients reporting a "flu-like" aching all over. "You can't have FM in your hands or back or neck," says Starlanyl. "If there is specific pain radiating down your hip, across your back or in your hands or your head, it is caused by something else. FM only amplifies the pain and other sensations."

This heightened perception of pain may be caused by an imbalance of neurochemicals (the messengers of the central nervous system). FM patients have high levels of a neurochemical called "Substance P," which transmits pain signals all over the body. When a person is injured, Substance P is released into the spinal cord—if Substance P is overproduced, the brain believes the body is in more pain than it really is.

Roland Staud, M.D., gives us some insight into how the central nervous system becomes overly sensitized. Staud and his team at the University of Florida observed the overstimulation caused by a phenomenon called "wind up" in FM patients. After a person experiences an initial pain stimulus and response, a second similar pain stimulus results in a response that is far greater and lasts longer. Like tossing a pebble into water, each stimulus results in more ripples of pain.

"PRIMARY" AND "SECONDARY" FIBROMYALGIA

FM is divided into "primary" and "secondary" diagnoses:

* "Primary FM" develops over time, triggered by stress, illness, or emotional trauma.

* "Secondary FM" (also known as "post-traumatic FM") appears after physical trauma, such as a traffic accident, fall, or injury.

11

❖ What Causes Fibromyalgia?

Many doctors, and patients too, have observed that FM tends to run in families. Dr. Christopher Lawrence, a neurologist with a special interest in FM, says, "I believe there is a genetic predisposition to FM. If you are born with certain chemical tendencies, any stress, whether physical or emotional, can trigger the illness."

THE GENETICS OF FM

Dr. Mark J. Pellegrino, a physician who is also an FM patient, believes that genetic vulnerability plays a key role in determining whether a person will develop posttraumatic FM. In his book *Fibromyalgia: Managing the Pain*, Pellegrino says, "The vulnerable person may not have any symptoms of FM whatsoever [prior to a trauma], even though the muscles are susceptible to this condition. The susceptible muscles and soft tissues are functioning adequately and are not painful. Once the soft tissues are traumatized, however, the altered pain response is triggered and the previous pain-free balance is forever disrupted, resulting in a permanently altered balance that is now painful. The muscles were pushed over the edge, so to speak."

Potential Triggers of FM in the Genetically Vulnerable Person

Stress to the central nervous system (brain and spinal cord)	Infections	Metabolic factors
Physical trauma (for example, neck injuries due to a fall, an auto accident, or surgery)	Viruses (for example, influenza or mononucleosis)	Exposure to heavy metals (such as mercury, arsenic, or lead)
Posttraumatic stress disorder	Bacterial infections such as Lyme disease (tick-borne)	Toxic chemical exposure (such as pesticides)

❖ Formal Diagnosis and Treatment

BY DR. PHILIP MEASE

Dr. Mease is a rheumatologist in private practice with Seattle Rheumatology Associates. He is also a clinical professor at the University of Washington and is the director of rheumatology clinical research at Swedish Medical Center in Seattle. He conducts research, writes, and lectures

extensively on conditions such as fibromyalgia, rheumatoid and psoriatic arthritis, ankylosing spondylitis, lupus, osteoarthritis, and osteoporosis. His research focuses on outcome measures of rheumatic diseases and emerging therapies. His practice emphasizes integration of rheumatic disease care amongst a team of providers, including nurse practitioners/physician assistants, physical and occupational therapists, behavioral medicine therapists, and complementary medicine providers such as acupuncturists.

The formal definition of FM, according to the American College of Rheumatology, is simple: a history of chronic, generalized aching and the finding, during a physical exam, of at least 11 out of 18 pre-defined tender points. Tender points, when pressed, are more painful than other points in the body; why these specific 18 sites are more tender is unclear, but it does seem to help differentiate patients with FM from those without this syndrome.

Other symptoms that are often present in someone with FM include:

❖ Fatigue

❖ Sleep disturbance

❖ Headaches

❖ Irritable bowel syndrome (IBS)—characterized by crampy abdominal pain and constipation or diarrhea (or both), alternating with normal bowel function

❖ Irritable bladder syndrome (also known as interstitial cystitis, a condition in which a person has frequent or painful urination without any evidence of infection in the urine)

❖ Restless legs syndrome (uncontrollable movement of the legs just before sleep, and/or during sleep

❖ Varying forms of mood disturbance

Although these are some of the frequent accompanying signs and symptoms that can be present in someone with FM, they are not a formal part of the definition of the condition.

FM can be present on its own—without any other diagnosis being made—or it can accompany another condition. Often, another chronic pain condition such as osteoarthritis, rheumatoid arthritis, lupus, or other types of chronic musculoskeletal pain is present. FM can be seen in con-

junction with endocrine conditions, such as hypothyroidism (under-active thyroid), or infectious diseases, such as Lyme disease (a type of bacterial infection). Often, FM emerges in someone who is experiencing physical or emotional stress.

It has been noted that people with FM have disturbances in various phases of sleep, particularly, stage IV, the deepest, most restorative phase of sleep. There is some correlation between sleep disturbance and altered nervous system function. Thus, if doctors and FM patients work toward restoring normal sleep physiology, they can often achieve improvement in the pain levels that patients experience.

Research is now pointing to a disturbance of normal neurochemical function in the pain pathways of the central nervous system (central sensitization) as the fundamental problem causing FM. A variety of factors that affect the central nervous system can lead to this disturbance and a variety of treatment approaches can improve it.

Once a diagnosis has been made, it is important to initiate treatment in order to break the cycle of pain and associated symptoms. We have also found that we get much better results by approaching treatment in a multidisciplinary way, utilizing the services of a variety of health-care practitioners, including physical therapists, acupuncturists, psychologists, and others who are knowledgeable about FM and who are able to work closely with physician and nurse caregivers. This approach, along with self-directed aerobic conditioning, stretching exercises, and other physical techniques, can significantly improve upon the benefits achieved by medications alone.

Another important aspect of treatment is the development of an emotional support system. Once a diagnosis is made, it is important for the patient to have people to talk to, someone to empathize with them and be supportive. Family members, spouses, boyfriends or girlfriends, relatives, friends, support groups, therapy groups, friends at the swimming pool or at church—this kind of human exchange is a vital part of the care of a person with any chronic illness.

Thus, one can see that there is a broad and varied approach to the treatment of FM and no single method that is optimal. There are emerging medications and drug therapies that have been found to be effective, with fewer side effects than some of the medicines traditionally used. These developments, coupled with a "team" approach to care, hold the promise of better outcomes for FM patients. ✦ ✦ ✦

❖ Symptoms

Having FM feels like you have been running a marathon in the hot sun. Your muscles hurt and you are alternately hot and cold. Your head aches and the sun hurts your eyes. You're exhausted but you can't sleep or get comfortable in any position. After eventually getting to sleep, you awake only to still feel fatigued and stiff. It takes a long time to wake up and it's difficult to think. This imaginary race becomes your life.

If you have FM, the following symptoms will be all too familiar to you; you'll probably even recognize a little of yourself in the patients who talk so openly about their experiences. Don't be shy about talking to your doctor about these seemingly unrelated symptoms. Fibromyalgia is a syndrome, a collection of symptoms—when looked at as part of the bigger FM picture, symptoms such as dizziness, vision problems, and skin sensitivities make sense. It's an "Ah-Ha" moment, when everything comes together.

NONRESTORATIVE SLEEP AND MORNING STIFFNESS

Restful sleep is hard to come by. FM patients often wake up feeling as if they haven't slept at all. This indicates that they have not achieved enough level IV sleep. Sleep deprivation affects us both physically and mentally. A sleep-deprived person can't think clearly; we feel groggy, depressed, and our perception of pain is heightened.

"Sleep is a real treat," says Tom O. from Renton, Washington. "Most of the time I'm up three or four times a night. I'll go for a month or so where I sleep like a rock. And then, for no reason that I can tell, I'll sleep for two hours and then wake up. Sometimes I lie there for hours before I can get back to sleep."

Many patients feel at their worst when they first wake up. Your body has been inactive most of the night, and your limbs become rigid and sometimes painful. You may feel like your brain has difficulty getting your body into gear: You send the message, but your arms and legs just don't respond.

PAIN

Untreated FM pain is debilitating—it increases fatigue and exacerbates the other symptoms of FM. Each person's perception of FM pain is different, but certain areas of the body show a pattern of particular tenderness. These areas are known as "tender points," and can be seen in the diagram on the next page.

15

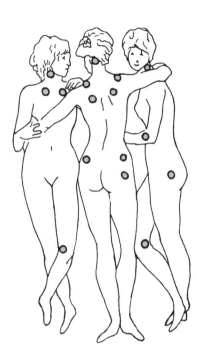

The 18 tender point locations for FM on "The Three Graces" masterpiece.
Credit: Adapted from the journal *Arthritis and Rheumatism,* with the kind permission of John Wiley & Sons, Inc.

As you can see, each tender point occurs in a pair, with one on each side of the body. These include the region just behind the ear, the lower cervical area in the neck, the shoulder blades, the upper back, the area around the third rib, the elbows, the tops of the thighs, the buttocks, and the knees.

FM pain and tenderness can be aggravated by changes in barometric pressure, precipitation, and temperature, with cold, damp weather being particularly aggravating. In Seattle (where it's often damp), rheumatologist Dr. Andrew J. Holman says, "Every October the phone calls would roll in with the first storms, 'You've got to see me!'"

FATIGUE

A certain level of fatigue is always present if you have FM. Sometimes it takes everything you have to get out of bed in the morning. For some patients, maintaining a regular sleep schedule will be all you need to alleviate your fatigue, or it can be a matter of taking a nap every day. During a flare-up fatigue can become debilitating and a patient may not be able to take care of themselves on their own. The fatigue level in FM fluctuates depending upon the time of the year, changes in the weather, your schedule,

diet, and stress level. By recognizing your fatigue and taking the time to rest, you give yourself the best possible chance to function well, despite your illness.

BODY TEMPERATURE CHANGES

An FM patient may experience changes in their body's thermal regulation system. For example, you may begin to perspire right after putting on a sweater in a cold room. Being unable to maintain your body temperature over large areas such as the thighs, back, and buttocks is called "spasticity," and it is caused by tightness and constriction in blood vessels.

BRAIN FOG

"It is ironic that my 8-year-old grandson has to keep track of me," says Carla B., from Jacksonville, Florida. For Carla, as for most FM patients, the most frustrating symptom is "brain fog" (also referred to as "fibro fog"). For anyone who has ever tried to lock their car with a cell phone, use their television remote to answer the phone, found their iron in the refrigerator, or our favorite—thrown their brand new toothbrush in the garbage after using it only once, this is a story for you:

Mari S. got lost driving on the freeway right by her house. The first time it happened, she was confused because she didn't recognize where she was. She knew she was close to home but the road and houses didn't look right. After a minute or so, her confusion passed and everything looked familiar again. Her heart was pounding and she had that funny feeling that comes over a person after a good scare—her skin was crawling. After that first time, she can recognize an episode of brain fog when it happens and does not panic anymore.

Susie S. says, "My family makes fun of my brain fog. But then, so do I. I have really done some funny things. Like shut the bird in the dishwasher. Thank goodness I didn't start it."

Another irritating aspect of brain fog is being unable to find the word you're searching for. If you're holding a Granny Smith apple in your hand, the question that comes out might be, "Do you want this green pepper?" People with FM use the word "thing" constantly.

Other cognitive problems, including short-term memory loss and the inability to concentrate, are frustrating symptoms of FM. Difficulty following a movie plot, reading a magazine, or sometimes even holding up your end of a conversation, can be unwelcome facts-of-life for people living with FM.

17

Hannah D. of Hanlontown, Iowa, used to be an excellent writer but now has trouble writing a paragraph. "I have forgotten how to spell a lot of words I didn't even think twice about spelling before," says Hannah. "My husband always attends medical appointments with me because I will not remember what the doctor said. I hesitate to call repair people out of fear I will not understand what they are telling me. Most days I don't even remember my own phone number or address."

NEUROLOGICAL SYMPTOMS

Many FM patients experience "parasthesia," a sensation of numbness, tingling, or "pins and needles," often accompanying morning stiffness. Parasthesia occurs when sustained pressure is placed on a nerve (such as when you sit with your legs crossed for too long, or fall asleep on your arm); it disappears gradually when pressure is relieved.

Other neurological symptoms of FM include tinnitus (ringing in the ears), tension and migraine headaches, and dizziness.

SENSORY OVERLOAD

Sensory overload makes shopping and socializing with groups of people hard to bear. The colors, sounds, and smells of a grocery store can be overwhelming to an FM patient. "I can smell things before anyone else can, and some smells will make me gag," says Susan M. of Odessa, Texas. Our respondents told us of the many times they have had to leave grocery or department stores because of headaches, nausea, and even fainting. In the extreme, this type of symptom can be very limiting, and as a result, many FM patients are unable to shop for themselves. Sounds are amplified and unexpected noises can actually be perceived as pain. It can feel as if an electric shock is passing through your body when a sudden loud noise catches you off guard.

FLARE-UPS

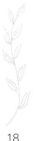

Flare-ups of your symptoms happen unexpectedly—suddenly, the pain increases and your fatigue becomes much harder to bear. Something as minor as staying up too late, eating a meal that upsets your stomach, or working too hard can trigger a flare-up. Stressful events also tend to cause flare-ups, even if it's a happy occasion—parties, weddings (especially if you are paying for them), and public speaking are prime examples. In Chapter 17, you'll find lots of advice for avoiding flare-ups and coping with them when they happen.

✤ The Challenges of Obtaining a Diagnosis

Accurately diagnosing FM is often a challenge for practitioners. The symptoms are similar to those of a number of other illnesses and can lead doctors off track. It is only when the symptoms are present together, over a period of time, that a pattern emerges indicating FM.

Most physicians end up referring their patients to a doctor who specializes in FM—usually a rheumatologist. Your specialist can rule out other conditions, such as rheumatoid arthritis or lupus, and start you on a treatment program that addresses your symptoms.

As awareness and understanding of FM increases, physicians are coming to look at the patient more as a whole, and they are therefore much less likely to miss the diagnosis. Patient advocacy has supported increased public awareness and education.

Dr. James Robinson of the University of Washington Pain Clinic says:

In the 1980s, every fibromyalgia patient I evaluated had multiple scars on his or her body from surgery. It was as though everybody was looking at one little piece of the person. If they happened to show up to a hand surgeon, they'd have carpal tunnel releases. If they showed up at a spine surgeon's office, they'd get spine surgery. There were vigorous attempts to treat the problem with aggressive treatment, based on the notion that there was a single structure causing the problem, seemingly without the surgeon being aware that there was a much, much, bigger problem going on.

Many respondents told us they were relieved to get a diagnosis and finally be able to put a name to what they were experiencing. As Danaease G. of Aylett, Virginia, explains, "I felt validated. I had been researching FM for some time and thought this was my problem. When I was told it was, it came as a relief. I felt that now that I knew what I had, I would be able to treat the illness and start to feel better."

It took 28 years for Thomas G. to be diagnosed with posttraumatic FM. Tom, a 54-year-old former Marine from Endicott, New York, says:

I was treated like a malingerer from day one. Every doctor I saw was overwhelmed because I had three or more symptoms and they all believed it was in my head. Many of them just doodled on their paper while I tried to explain my situation. I was told I was the healthiest sick man they had ever seen. Some said my depression was

19

causing my problems, but I knew my body and knew my symptoms were the cause of my depression. In 1998 the VA clinic finally started to believe in me. FM and CFS were becoming known medical issues, and I was then treated with respect, cooperation, and a diagnosis.

For Djamilla Z., a 28-year-old from Doorn, in the Netherlands, the diagnosis of FM only brought more problems. She says, "It took me seven years to get the final diagnosis. My doctor never took me seriously, actually denied on several occasions that FM existed. Although the rheumatologist did give me a diagnosis of FM, I was not really happy with her comment: 'Live with it,' after she handed me a small brochure of the FM-patient organization in the Netherlands."

Many patients reported thinking that they were going crazy because no one could find what was wrong with them. "After waiting three months for an appointment with a rheumatologist, I was eating Advil like it was candy," confided Regina L, a 51-year-old former teacher from Kenosha, Wisconsin. "I called the doctor's office and told them that if they didn't get me in by the next day I was going to sign myself into a mental ward at the hospital because the pain was all over me and was almost unbearable. They got me in right away, got me on pain medication, and sent me directly to a psychiatrist who worked closely with the rheumatologist on FM cases. These two doctors were the first to treat me with respect and take my symptoms seriously."

✤ A Patient's Story: Monique B.

Monique is a 47-year-old immunologist from Paris, France. She has two daughters. Monique had difficulty obtaining a diagnosis of FM. Here she recounts what appears to be a classic case of a person who was predisposed to developing FM, which was then triggered by physical trauma following a viral infection. Monique also tells us about the way FM is perceived and treated in France.

It took nine years for me to get a proper diagnosis. I went from doctor to doctor without any relief. It all started a few months after my second baby was born in August 1989. I started to have recurrent tonsillitis, bronchitis, irritable bowel syndrome, and endometriosis. Then, in June 1990, I fell into a severe fatigue, which completely disabled me. I was diagnosed with mononucleosis, and was still sick with mono when, two months later, I had a car accident resulting in multiple fractures and head trauma. The accident immobilized me for six months, and I developed sleep disturbances; from there I started the waltz of painkillers and sleeping pills.

After the accident and the bout with mono, I tried to maintain my shape with sports, but my muscles remained weak and I could not exercise as I did before. A year later, I began experiencing other symptoms—hypothyroidism, tachycardia, abdominal cramps, sweating, memory loss, and concentration problems. Now I can't stand cold, heat, or noise. I have also developed severe depression, behavioral problems, and agoraphobia.

I had difficulty finding anyone who specialized in this illness; I had to teach my generalist [general practitioner] about it. The French medical attitude is still oriented toward viewing FM as a depressive syndrome, and the medication allowed in France is quite limited. I began to believe the doctors who said that everything was "in my head." Anti-inflammatory pills, acupuncture, and physiotherapy had no effect. Painkillers (codeine, and then morphine) provided the only relief I could obtain. But I had to endure all the side effects you expect from these drugs.

My FM specialist in Paris prescribes minalcipran (a European antidepressant), tramadol, and paracetamol (acetaminophen); these worked at first but now seem to be ineffective. Regarding the fatigue, nothing is working, and I am planning to go to the United States to buy supplements and see a specialist.

In 1989, I was a healthy and happy woman, with two children, a nice husband, and an interesting job; now, the only reason for me to live is my two children. I have lost my job, and my husband decided to stop investing himself in our relationship. Although I have tried not to change anything in my life, everything has changed. I have tried to keep working like other people, but I had too many flare-ups of FM. People tend to exclude you from their lives—it is difficult to make someone comprehend that you have a real illness rather than a ghost illness no one understands.

Although there are many FM and CFS patients in France, there is no gathering or any willingness to share one's experiences. It is crucial that all of us go down into the streets, even in a wheelchair, proclaim our illness loudly, and ask for recognition.

I try to work from home. I go out and laugh as much as possible. I feel alone, but I have a strong inside life, I read a lot; I like to watch movies, and I listen to music. I still continue to fight for my dignity. ❖❖❖

❧ Dispatches from the FM Frontlines

BY PAUL B. BROWN, M.D., PH.D.

Dr. Brown is a rheumatologist and a fibromyalgia treatment specialist in private practice in Seattle, Washington. He is a clinical associate professor at the University of Washington, and he lectures at conferences on the West Coast.

Fibromyalgia syndrome: Why describe this condition as a "syndrome" and not a "disease"? A syndrome is a group of symptoms that do not fulfill the criteria for a disease. Does this make it less legitimate, less symptomatic, or in some cases less disabling? Absolutely not! But it does make it more difficult to evaluate and treat.

For this reason it is important to visit a knowledgeable practitioner, usually a rheumatologist. It is essential to have an accurate diagnosis. Ten years ago, FM was not often diagnosed. Today, it is overdiagnosed by well-meaning practitioners who identify every unexplained, painful disorder as FM. A knowledgeable practitioner will know that some patients who have FM will have all 18 tender points present, but also that a secure diagnosis may be established in some patients with fewer than 11 tender points, on exam.

In addition, most rheumatologists will understand how FM interacts with other diseases. For example, many patients with FM have ankylosing spondylitis, sleep apnea, thyroid dysfunction, carpal tunnel syndrome, mechanical neck and back problems, tendonitis, or other maladies. These conditions deserve and require careful evaluation and treatment, but in the face of active FM, they are often ignored and not diagnosed.

Patients with FM require the same careful approach as other patients with such complicated diseases as multiple sclerosis or lupus. A thorough history, physical, and laboratory evaluation is mandatory. This workup may include scans, sleep studies, needle testing (an electro-diagnostic test performed by a physiatrist), or appropriate consultations. Once this workup has been accomplished, the patient can be reassured and educated. The patient's level of fitness can be established and referrals for physical therapy, acupuncture, biofeedback, counseling, massage, or chiropractic care can be considered.

Medical therapy should be individualized since patients' response and sensitivity to medicines may vary. Appropriate medications may include analgesics, muscle relaxants, antidepressants, anti-seizure medicines, anti-anxiety remedies, or occasional use of a sleep aid. These medications need to be provided in conjunction with a graded exercise program and other treatments.

Fibromyalgia can certainly be a painful, disabling condition. But it doesn't have to be. With appropriate evaluation and treatment, most people improve significantly and lead full, good, useful lives. ❖❖❖

❖ Sleep Deprivation and the Stress Response

In 1975, Harvey Moldofsky, M.D., was able to recreate the symptoms of FM in students at the University of Toronto. Moldofsky did this by interrupting their stage IV sleep, the deep sleep level at which we produce hormones and heal. He used a loud noise played at a volume that didn't actually wake the subjects—but interrupted their sleep. By depriving his subjects of stage IV deep sleep, Moldofsky essentially caused the symptoms of FM.

Moldofsky repeated the experiment, this time depriving his subjects of REM sleep (the sleep stage in which we dream), but this didn't produce the same fibromyalgia-like effect. Moldofsky and his team went on to study stage IV sleep in ROTC candidates, and each time, the results were the same. Disruption of REM dream sleep had no effect, but disruption of stage IV deep sleep produced symptoms like those of FM in all his subjects.

"Moldofsky was right," says Dr. Andrew J. Holman, a rheumatologist conducting FM research. "Fibromyalgia is the predictable consequence of stage IV sleep deprivation." Holman pinpoints autonomic arousal in the brainstem as the reason for FM patients' inability to achieve uninterrupted stage IV sleep. He believes that continually elevated levels of adrenaline overactivate the stress response. "That's how an alarm clock works," says Holman. "It turns on the autonomic arousal in your brain stem, the fight-or-flight response, but it doesn't do anything to your sleep center. It's your brainstem that wakes you up, like smelling smoke or hearing a baby cry."

During the day, the overactive fight-or-flight response can be expressed as anxiety, muscle tension, abnormal sweating, increased heart rate, higher blood pressure, and bowel or bladder dysfunction—responses that are hardwired into the autonomic nervous system. But at night the heightened autonomic arousal is expressed as racing thoughts, disruptive dreams, restless legs syndrome, and teeth grinding (bruxism)—activities that disrupt stage IV sleep, just like Moldofsky's noise.

Holman believes that the overactive flight-or-fight response is due to depleted stores of dopamine—the neurotransmitter responsible for coordinating our motor movements and controlling the flow of information in the brain. Dopamine plays an important role in attention, memory, and problem solving—which also suggests its involvement in FM.

23

"The premise here is not to treat fibromyalgia as a psychiatric disease, not to treat it as just a pain syndrome, or as only a sleep disorder," says Holman, "but to understand it as the arousal that fragments sleep [arousal by the autonomic nervous system]. So we're peeling the onion just a little bit further. The idea here is not to *make* you sleep, it's to *let* you sleep." (See Chapter 14 for more information on Dr. Holman's research and treatment protocol.)

✤ A Patient's Story: Tom O.

Tom O. is a 53-year-old telephone lineman. He's been married for 33 years and is a father and grandfather. After years of dealing with mysterious symptoms, Tom was eventually diagnosed with FM. He lives with his family in Renton, Washington.

It all started back in 1992. I just felt like hell all the time, like somebody stuck me in a sack, threw me down, and walked on my body. All my joints hurt, all my muscles hurt, tendons, ligaments; everything hurt.

My job involves a lot of climbing poles, fixing poles, replacing poles, and wiring buildings as they're being constructed so that people can have telephone service. It's heavy, physical work, so I thought maybe that had something to do with it. I was tired, tired of it all.

So I went to my family doctor, but it took a long time to come up with the diagnosis of FM, almost two years. I went back two or three times to tell him that what he'd given me wasn't helping me; there was still something wrong, more than just the regular pain of getting up every day. It's frustrating—sometimes you pay for all these fancy, expensive tests and they come back normal. And yet you know there's something going on.

I eventually read an article about FM and asked my doctor, "Do I have FM?" He said, "You're a strong candidate for it." They did more tests on the tender points, and he said, "We're about 112 percent positive that's what it is."

I didn't know a heck of a lot about it before I got diagnosed. I thought, "Well, fine, they know what it is now." How naive I was. I thought, "I can deal with this." I had been dealing with it for a year or two before I even knew what it was. The only difference was that now I had a name for it.

I once could do anything, any time, all day long, and not hurt. Baseball, football, hiking, walking, fishing, lifting, pushing, shoving, anything; it did not matter. I could wrestle around with the kids. I could cut firewood all day, stack it, then get up the next day and everything would be just hunky-dory.

But those days are very rare now. I'm not as quick as I used to be, not as flexible. I wonder sometimes how much longer I can continue my job and what comes after that. I enjoy my work. It keeps me active and mentally engaged. I need that structure to keep me getting up each day to do it all over again.

I've disappointed my brother once or twice when we've been all set to go on a hike, and then I felt extremely bad and had to call it off. My family is very understanding, luckily. My wife is my greatest support; she understands my aches and pains, and why I take a lot of naps.

I do get angry at times because I know I should not feel as bad as I do. There is so much I want to do, but I have started to limit myself and that bothers me. I have always had the physical ability to do what I want and not worry about the pains, but as I age it really seems to get more intense. I am a firm believer in the "use it or lose it" school of thought. I have been as physically active as possible all my life, and I notice that I feel the absolute worst when I have been too lazy. At the gym I don't go for the mammoth muscles and good-looking physique, I go just to work all the parts and keep them mobile and agile. Sometimes I will go climb a climbing wall just to add a bit of adventure to things and change the routine. I took up kayaking because it is something different and it is a good workout. It is easy and relatively safe (safer than the drive to where I am going to kayak!).

I have a list of things I hope to attain in my life before I check out. This list has been adjusted as I age, due to more realistic expectations. More of the physical goals are beginning to go by the wayside, such as hiking all around Mt. Rainier. My major goal is to keep active, some way, some how. I still hike around the boondocks, but I am much slower and becoming much less motivated.

I had my large intestine removed in July 2001. This was the result of ulcerative colitis, and the surgery was the only sure cure. I was diagnosed with this in 1998 and limped along with the symptoms of bloating and frequent bloody stools. I eventually had to subject myself to a whole laundry list of drugs to try to keep myself in some control. Finally I came to the conclusion that I couldn't continue like this for the rest of my life and decided to accept fate and have the surgery.

I do feel getting rid of that diseased organ helped out on a few other things. I feel that though I still have FM, it has decreased in severity. When it hits me, it doesn't seem to be as harsh, but then I try harder to ameliorate the symptoms (through exercise, etc.). I think all these things are related, but I don't know how; neither do the docs, evidently. But I am doing well, keeping on keeping on. Or as a friend puts it, I'm "upright and taking nourishment." ✦✦✦

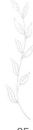

Chapter 3

Understanding Chronic Fatigue Syndrome

MOST PEOPLE WHO LIVE with CFS know the exact date they became sick. They can tell you the day and year they first felt the cold or flu that didn't go away. Often, it is the combination of illness and stress that is the last straw. Leslie C. of Peterborough, New Hampshire, says, "My mother passed away, three days later my best friend passed away, and about two weeks after that I had to have my dog put to sleep—it was traumatic. I think what finally triggered the CFS was a viral illness—I had three bouts of bronchitis, one right after the other, and I just felt like I never really recovered from that. I was so fatigued I couldn't function."

❖ What Is Chronic Fatigue Syndrome?

There is so much more to chronic fatigue syndrome than the name suggests. CFS is characterized by severe, persistent fatigue, and it is often associated with difficulties in sleep and concentration, aching muscles and joints, pain, headaches, a sore throat, and depression.

Dr. Dedra Buchwald, director of the University of Washington Chronic Fatigue Clinic, describes the daily reality that many patients experience: "Commonly, CFS takes the form of a chronic, recurring, 'flu-like' illness; for most patients, some degree of fatigue is present every day. Virtually all patients perceive themselves to be impaired in some way, some severely so. They find that the fatigue, difficulty in concentrating, and pain limit their ability to participate fully in normal life activities. Many patients are depressed or anxious, but generally they feel that the depression and anxiety have followed and been caused by the illness."

A BRIEF HISTORY OF CFS

The first documented outbreak of the illness that came to be known as chronic fatigue syndrome occurred in 1934 at the Los Angeles County General Hospital. Other outbreaks followed, in London, Florida, Nevada, and New York.

Drs. Daniel Peterson and Paul Cheney run one of the busiest CFS clinics in the country. Back in the early 1980s, their lives were changed when several people in their small community of Incline Village, Nevada, began to complain of intense fatigue. Peterson and Cheney, who struggled to understand and treat the unidentified illness, contacted the Centers for Disease Control and Prevention (CDC) for assistance. The result of the CDC's investigation was to saddle the mystery illness with a name that would forever cause it to be misunderstood by much of the medical community and the general public alike, "chronic fatigue syndrome."

Dr. David S. Bell dedicated his practice to CFS, after an outbreak in his small town of Lyndonville, New York in 1985. In his book *The Faces of CFS*, Bell tells the story of the outbreak:

> One of my young patients in town fell ill with the flu. Shortly afterward, her two sisters and a few neighbors came down what with seemed to be the same bug. Nothing much, I remember thinking. At least, it looked like a standard flu.
>
> One of the sick children had an enlarged spleen, so I ran a test for mononucleosis, one of the infectious illnesses that can cause swelling of the spleen. The results were negative. I confess that, initially, I paid little attention to the matter because these were tough kids and I was confident they would get better. Except they didn't.
>
> Several months passed without improvement in any of my young patients. They had fevers, malaise (that sick, achy-like tiredness), pain in their joints, and headaches. In time, my adult patients began to come in with the same constellation of symptoms. When the large spleen I had felt in the first child began to return to normal, I rejoiced. But her lymph nodes remained swollen, and stayed that way for nearly a year. A constant in each patient was their profound exhaustion, a fact that I ignored at first, since

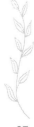

27

everyone with the flu feels exhausted. But this exhaustion lingered, and eventually, began to dominate the other symptoms. The children were unable to attend school that year, nor could the adults return to work. The patients were, in effect, completely disabled. Something was terribly wrong.

❖ What Causes Chronic Fatigue Syndrome?

The search for a cause and cure for CFS reads like a detective mystery—it has proven to be a brainteaser for even the most accomplished doctors and researchers. Although many of the symptoms of CFS tend to be similar among all patients, there appear to be a number of different underlying causes. Renowned CFS researcher and clinician Dr. Jacob Teitlebaum evaluated 64 patients with CFS. He found that 30 had low thyroid, 39 had underactive adrenal function, 23 had fungal overgrowth, 26 had low vitamin B_{12} levels, 7 had parasitic infection, and 12 had chronic depression or anxiety. Of the 64 patients, 44 also had symptoms of fibromyalgia.

DIFFERENT TYPES OF CFS?

"Someday, I believe that we will identify different types of CFS, just as we currently identify different types of diabetes," says Dr. Martin Ross of Seattle. "For instance, we might identify Type I CFS as a condition of burnout/adrenal exhaustion (hypothalamic-pituitary axis dysfunction) and Type II CFS as a condition of intracellular infection (caused by viral infections or by bacteria). Regardless of the cause, most people with CFS have immune system dysfunction, hormonal imbalances, nutrient deficits, and sleep disturbances, all of which need to be addressed."

THE NAME GAME

It is very difficult having an invisible illness, especially one in which the main symptom is fatigue. It doesn't help that CFS is known by different names in different parts of the world. In some countries it's called myalgic encephalomyelitis (ME); others call it chronic fatigue and immune deficiency syndrome (CFIDS). Most of our respondents agree—they dislike the name "chronic fatigue syndrome." Brian T. of Polperro, England, says, "I think anything with 'fatigue' in it is bad, as healthy people always say, 'Oh I get fatigued, too. Does that mean I've got it?'" Sally L. of Euless, Texas, sums it up, "If this were a condition that affected mostly men instead of women, it would be called something like *catastrophic total body dysfunction.*"

SPECIFIC CAUSES

Although the mechanism of CFS is unknown, several specific factors are thought to trigger the illness by causing changes in the body's immune system, sleep patterns, and hormone production. Long after the trigger or cause is gone, the illness continues.

Examples of Causes or Contributing Factors

Persistent infection	Toxic exposure	Genetic abnormalities	Metabolic abnormalities
Viral infection (for example, mono-nucleosis or influenza)	Heavy metal exposure (such as mercury, arsenic, or lead)	In white blood cells	Burnout (severe depletion of nutrients)
Mycoplasma (virus-like bacteria)	Exposure to toxic chemicals (such as pesticides)	In energy production within the body's cells	Hormonal imbalance (for example, low cortisol, DHEA, or thyroid)
Parasitic infections	Exposure to environmental toxins (such as "black mold")	In elevated levels of a protein associated with Huntington's disease	Low blood pressure (hypotension)
Yeast or other fungal infections		Excess glutamine (a normally beneficial amino acid)	Deficiencies of iron, B_6, B_{12}, or other nutrients
		Internal toxins that resemble ciguatera toxins in marine life	

✣ Symptoms

If you were trying to describe your symptoms to your doctor, you might say, "I have the worst flu of my life. My throat is scratchy, the muscles in my chest ache, and I feel like I've got a fever. The weird thing is, I can't shake it; it's been going on for months, and the fatigue is terrible." This is how most of the patients we interviewed described their encounter with CFS.

"I try not to be frightened by the big relapses," says Diane K. from Seattle. "But it's posttraumatic fear, since once, long ago, I got what I thought was the flu and the symptoms didn't abate for eight years. So when I relapse hard, I have this fear that it will last for years again."

CFS has many symptoms in common with FM: cognitive difficulties; short-term memory loss; trouble concentrating; neurological symptoms (such as balance difficulties, parasthesia, altered spatial perception, and loss of equilibrium); a heightened sensitivity to sound, light, and aromas; and body-wide fatigue. But in all other respects, CFS is a unique illness, with its own distinct pattern of symptoms.

LONG-TERM FATIGUE

When you have CFS, the weight of fatigue seems to come from the very heart of you. You lack stamina, your limbs are heavy, and your head feels like it's stuffed with cotton wool.

Dennis H. from Seattle says that his worst symptom was losing his ability to do physical activities. "During the early years, it was a question of how much rest I needed—several hours of napping in the middle of the day, and I spent most of my time sitting in a chair, reading or watching television. But I was always able to get up and around and to do what I needed to take care of myself during the day. As time goes by, I have become more functional; the adverse effects have grown less and less. I can go out and work in the yard or run errands. I don't get as rundown, although things do fluctuate."

SLEEP DYSFUNCTION

People with CFS have difficulty both falling asleep and staying asleep. As if that weren't enough, it's also hard to wake up in the morning; you may feel as if you haven't slept at all. After days on end of nonrestorative sleep, the body's internal clock is disrupted and the natural sleep-wake cycle is altered. Most CFS patients find themselves falling asleep in the early evening and feeling their best late at night.

There are changes in CFS patients' sleep patterns, which can depend on external factors such as stress, diet, and whether or not you are experiencing an exacerbation or remission of your symptoms. As with FM, research indicates that CFS patients do not get enough level IV sleep, the level at which the body repairs itself.

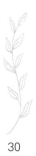

And since people with CFS are light sleepers anyway, pain, the need to urinate, night sounds, dreams, or sleep apnea can keep us awake and on guard all night. Upon awakening, the body is stiff and sore, it takes time to work out the kinks and begin the day.

MUSCLE AND JOINT PAIN

Patients living with CFS report a wide variety of aches and pains, from the allover, flu-like feeling to pain when pressure is applied to tender points. Rib and chest pain, back pain, headaches, and eye pain are also symptoms of CFS. As well as pain in the extremities. As with FM, changes in barometric pressure can cause pain to skyrocket. Stiffness can also predispose a CFS patient to injury. Be extra careful when you're having a bad time with stiffness; this is the time when your body will be most susceptible to injury.

COGNITIVE DIFFICULTIES

Many of our respondents reported cognitive difficulties to be the worst part of CFS, eclipsing both the constant fatigue and flu-like symptoms. As with FM, "brain fog" can catch you unaware—suddenly scenery in the neighborhood where you have lived for years can look unfamiliar, or you can't remember where your recycling container goes. Short-term memory is compromised. CFS patients told us that numbers and phrases seem to fly out of their heads, just moments after hearing a phone number or person's name. Memory games that used to help us remember things are useless—we can't remember the memory game itself! Equally frustrating is the difficulty CFS patients experience when trying to concentrate on tasks—it's difficult to follow a movie plot, pages of books must be read and re-read, and we often lose track of conversations. You may sometimes feel as if your hearing is failing, when it is actually a cognitive problem causing you to mishear what people are saying to you.

FLU-LIKE SYMPTOMS

The flu-like symptoms of CFS can include extreme fatigue, aching muscles and joints, a painfully tight chest, sore throat and hoarseness, cough and fever, frequent infections, chills, painful and swollen lymph nodes in the neck and armpits, night sweats, rashes, changes in eating habits, an irritable bladder and bowel, and a low-grade fever.

CHEMICAL SENSITIVITY AND SENSORY OVERLOAD

Smells of any kind, but especially chemical odors, can cause serious reactions, from headaches and nausea to severe respiratory distress. If a person

is allergic to dust or pet dander, for example, CFS can heighten the allergic response. As with FM, light and noise can be perceived as painful.

More severe symptoms of CFS can include heart palpitations, chest pain, and shortness of breath.

❖ A Patient's Story: Janet L.

Janet L. is 56 years old, and she lives with her husband and pets in Falkirk, Scotland. After many years of living with a "mystery illness," Janet was diagnosed with ME (myalgic encephalomyelitis, another term for CFS). Confronted with health-care professionals who knew little about CFS, Janet began the process of educating herself about her illness.

I became ill in 1984, but I didn't get a proper diagnosis until ten years later. In 1994, I had a serious relapse from which I have never recovered. I was told at first that I was "depressed," by a young doctor. A few months later I managed to see a GP [general practitioner] who told me it was CFS. Although my GP was sympathetic, I was told it was a mystery illness and that nothing could be done.

I was exposed to chemicals and pesticides for a long period of time, prior to becoming ill. We lived near a company that burned chemical waste from all around the world, one mile from our house as the crow flies. The cows in the farmer's field turned yellow (he took the company to court but lost), and several babies with eye defects were born nearby.

My current GP admits to not knowing much about CFS but is sensitive to my needs and agreed to read the literature I gave him lately. My previous GP was in touch with all the research on CFS, but he left the practice and moved to another town.

Before this illness, I had a career and a very good wage. I had a goal to move up one more step of the ladder, and I wanted good holidays and to help my children financially. But I had to give up work. My colleagues all thought it was "in my head," even though they had worked with me for eight years and knew I was an upbeat kind of person. I went through a bereavement process for a year when I had to give my career up, but then I accepted it.

My social life is nonexistent, I lost so-called friends, I live vicariously through my grown-up children. My husband is very supportive; he is my caregiver. He only works part-time to take care of me, and so we depend

on benefits. Our combined income has dropped from £48,000 a year to £12,000 a year [from approximately $82,000 a year to $25,000 a year]. We don't go out socially, because I can't stand noise, chitchat, bright lights, and lots of people—can't drink even a glass of wine with a meal. I'm very isolated because I don't see people very often, apart from my family. My daughter also has CFS, though it is not severe and she is able to get on with her life, so she understands. I chat online with an American chat line a few times a month.

I try to be positive; I don't dwell on the fact that I will probably never recover (a neurologist told me this, he also told me I had a "sad life," he was very cheeky and not sympathetic nor understanding). I give my husband a hard time verbally but he knows why and I try to stop doing this. It's not his fault; it's no one's fault.

My goals now are simple, I want to be able to hold my grandchildren when I get them, and I want to stay with my husband and make him happy. I'm still glad to be alive. I have my family, I have a beautiful 17-year-old cat, Rosie, I have a lovely 13-year-old dog, and I have a garden full of birds.

✤ Formal Diagnosis and Treatment

BY DR. DEDRA BUCHWALD

Dr. Buchwald is the director of the University of Washington Chronic Fatigue Clinic at Harborview Medical Center in Seattle. She is also the director of the CFS Cooperative Research Center at Harborview.

There is no single test and no simple way to make the diagnosis of CFS. The diagnosis is usually made based on symptoms alone and the absence of physician findings that indicate another disease process. On physical examination, an inflamed throat, along with swollen lymph glands in the back of the neck and under the armpit, may occasionally be seen, but these are not required to make a diagnosis. More common are points on the muscles that are very sore and tender when pressure is applied.

However, symptoms that are typical of CFS may be caused by other problems, such as thyroid disorders, anemia, infection, or depression. Because of this, the doctor needs to be sure that a patient with symptoms of CFS does not have one of these conditions, which are far more common than CFS. CFS can only be considered after other causes of chronic fatigue have been excluded.

33

CFS is characterized by a number of different clinical and laboratory features, all of which can wax and wane over time. Routine laboratory tests are usually normal. Liver function tests may be slightly elevated and occasionally autoantibody tests are positive. However, studies have shown that CFS patients differ from healthy people across many biological, social, and psychological domains. To correctly diagnose a person with CFS, physicians should use the criteria developed in 1994 by international consensus at the Centers for Disease Control. To be diagnosed with CFS, a person must meet all of the fatigue criteria listed below, and other conditions must be ruled out. In addition, four out of the eight symptom criteria must be present.

FATIGUE CRITERIA

The fatigue must

1. be of at least six months' duration
2. not be lifelong (i.e., the person can't remember ever feeling normal)
3. result in a substantial reduction of occupational, educational, social, or personal activities, as compared to the person's activities before the onset of illness
4. not be the result of ongoing exertion or be relieved by rest

SYMPTOM CRITERIA

Symptoms must have started at the same time or after the onset of fatigue and must be present simultaneously for at least six months during the illness. Patients must meet at least four of the following criteria:

1. Impairment of short-term memory or concentration that is severe enough to cause a substantial reduction in previous levels of occupational, educational, social, or personal activities
2. Sore throat
3. Tender lymph nodes in the neck or armpits
4. Muscle pain
5. Joint pain involving more than one joint, without swelling or redness
6. Headaches of a new type, pattern, or severity

7. Unrefreshing sleep

8. Malaise or fatigue lasting more than 24 hours after exertion

FACTORS TO BE RULED OUT—EXCLUSIONARY CRITERIA

The following are considered exclusionary criteria in determining a diagnosis of CFS:

1. Any other medical condition that could mimic CFS—such as a history of malignancy, chronic infection, neuromuscular disease, etc.

2. Bipolar affective disorders, psychotic or melancholic depression, schizophrenia, and dementia

3. Anorexia nervosa and bulimia

4. Alcohol or substance abuse within two years of the onset of fatigue or at any time thereafter

5. Severe obesity

Since the cause of CFS is not known, there are no specific treatments for it. However, a large number of medications have been tried, with varying degrees of success. These include anti-inflammatory agents, antiviral and immunologically active drugs, and low doses of antidepressants. The most widely used treatments are combinations of low doses of serotonin reuptake inhibitors in the morning to provide energy and tricyclic antidepressants in the evening to promote sleep. Other types of medications that interact with the serotonin and norepinephrine systems appear to help reduce pain and induce sleep. Patients are also advised to get sufficient sleep and engage in a daily, low-level exercise program—with the assistance of a physical therapist. Cognitive-behavioral therapy has proven effective in several clinical trials, and many patients are better able to cope with the illness with the help of a knowledgeable mental-health counselor. Acupuncture, massage therapy, biofeedback, and other nonpharmacological approaches have also provided benefit to some patients. Often, finding an effective treatment is a matter of trial and error. Treatment must be individualized and focused on reducing symptoms.

Although the course of CFS varies greatly, most patients do improve. Up to two-thirds of patients have moderate to complete recovery over the course of several years, though most continue to have some symptoms. Improvement is usually interrupted by relapses brought on by overexertion,

stress, or infection. Only a small percentage of patients experience progressive worsening of their illness. ❖❖❖

❖ Dispatches from the CFS Frontlines

BY MARTIN P. ROSS, M.D.

Dr. Ross is part of The Healing Arts Partnership, a private practice focusing on family medicine, acupuncture, and integrative medicine. Dr. Ross lives in Seattle, Washington.

When making the diagnosis of CFS for legal and insurance purposes, I rely upon the Centers for Disease Control definition of the illness, but I do not believe it is entirely accurate. This definition was based on the opinions of experts for research purposes, and it is too limited to accurately describe all individuals with CFS. I prefer to use the Teitelbaum definition, which defines CFS as unexplained fatigue that significantly interferes with function and is associated with any two of the following symptoms: brain fog, poor sleep, diffuse achiness, increased thirst, bowel dysfunction and/or recurrent infections, or flu-like feelings.

In 2000, I opened my practice in integrative family medicine, offering a mix of conventional medicine, herbal and nutritional medicine, and craniosacral therapy. At first I mostly treated CFS with sleep medications and pain medicines. I then began addressing thyroid problems in CFS patients, but this provided help only about 15 percent of the time. Finally, I completed my training in acupuncture and started to integrate it into my practice. Because of this, I began to attract a lot of people to my practice for pain management with acupuncture. This, too, helped, in addition to the other approaches I was already using. But I remained frustrated that I could not help more people.

At the urging of one of my patients, I explored the Teitelbaum protocol. I have offered this protocol, integrated with my other treatments, for the last two years, and I am amazed at the improvement people obtain with this approach.

ADRENAL AND HORMONE IMBALANCE (DEPLETION OR BURNOUT)

The Teitelbaum protocol is based on the theory that the cause of CFS is due to a hypothalamic and pituitary axis (HPA) dysfunction. The HPA governs the entire endocrine system, including the adrenal glands, the thyroid, and female and male hormonal systems.

In addition, the HPA helps govern sleep. When there is HPA dysfunction, deficiencies develop in the hormonal system. As a result, the immune system does not work correctly, and leaves individuals susceptible to chronic infections. Finally, because of the stress on the body, people with CFS also develop nutrient and vitamin deficiencies.

People develop HPA dysfunction due to an acute incident such as an infection, or due to chronic emotional and physical stresses to the body. In these situations the HPA exhausts its fuel supply that is provided by a cellular component called the mitochondria. In this situation, the HPA tries to correct the imbalances, but continues to exhaust its mitochondrial fuel supply.

Correcting the dysfunction requires letting the HPA rest. Under the Teitelbaum protocol, the HPA is allowed to rest by medically taking over its function through hormonal medication, sleep medication, vitamin and nutrient supplementation, and the treatment of chronic infections.

INTRACELLULAR INFECTION

In other patients, I believe the primary cause of CFS is an intracellular infection of a type of white blood cell known as a macrophage. These intracellular infections release high levels of a type of vitamin D that leads to hormonal dysregulation, inflammation, and sleep disturbances. For these people, the Marshall protocol may be helpful. Patients are prescribed a medication called Benicar, which weakens the bacteria, enabling the body's immune system to destroy it. Small doses of antibiotics are prescribed, and patients must also avoid exposure to direct sunlight, bright lights, and vitamin D. The Marshall protocol can take between three to four years to completely destroy the intracellular infection

In my practice, all patients are placed on sleep medications or nutritional or herbal supplements. For many, this is necessary in order to obtain a good night's sleep.

CANDIDA

Most CFS patients also have yeast overgrowth in their intestines, resulting in chronic candida. To treat this I either use herbal remedies, such as oregano oil, or two prescription medicines, Nystatin and Diflucan. People with CFS tend to develop chronic candida because immune system dysfunction and a history of antibiotic use causes yeast living in the intestines to overgrow. The body reacts to the yeast by producing an ongoing allergic reaction. In addition, the yeast overgrowth results in malabsorption (difficulty absorbing nutrients from food).

37

LEAKY GUT SYNDROME

In this situation, the intestinal lining literally leaks toxic biochemicals from the intestines into the body's blood stream. The leaky gut and the ongoing allergic reaction are major causes of the fatigue, muscle achiness, and brain fog that most individuals experience.

LOW THYROID LEVELS

I place all patients on thyroid medication, even if they have thyroid studies that are normal. Because of HPA dysfunction, common thyroid tests do not provide a complete picture. If a person has signs of low thyroid and the T4 thyroid hormone produced by the thyroid gland is in the normal range, I consider the person to have subclinical hypothyroidism. My preferred thyroid medication is Armour Thyroid, which is desiccated thyroid gland. I prefer it to the common synthetic medication Synthroid because it is more bioactive. It also contains the two kinds of thyroid hormone, T4 and T3, which are made by our thyroid glands.

LOW CORTISOL AND DHEA

In addition, I often place individuals on cortisol and DHEA, two hormones produced by the adrenal glands. I make the decision to use these hormones based on blood studies and the individual's symptoms. Like thyroid medication, I will place individuals on these medicines even if the blood tests are normal, when they have symptoms suggesting these deficiencies. Occasionally, based on blood tests and symptoms, I also place individuals on testosterone, progesterone, or estrogen.

NUTRITIONAL DEFICIENCIES

Finally, I assume that all CFS patients have vitamin and nutrient deficiencies, so I place my patients on a multivitamin designed for people with fatigue. I test for vitamin B_{12} and iron deficiencies, which affect about half of my patients. I also use other supplements, such as magnesium and malic acid for muscle aches, based on a person's symptoms.

In my experience, over 70 percent of the patients I treat with this protocol have marked improvement in their symptoms. Of these, 15 percent of the people actually have a cure. I treat most people on the full protocol for up to a year and then am able to start withdrawing medication. Over time, most individuals will likely require some sleep medication or herbs. In addition, they will likely continue to require a good multivitamin.

While on the protocol, I also aggressively treat a person's pain. I work with a variety of medicines and herbs, as well as acupuncture, to treat pain. For long-term control of pain I have a lot of success using a mixture of narcotics when needed, anti-seizure medications such as Neurontin, muscle relaxers such as Skelaxin, and antidepressants such as Prozac or Paxil. I also like to treat muscular pain with trigger point injections [see Chapter 8] and acupuncture [see Chapter 10]. My favorite herbal/mineral remedies for muscular pain are ginger, magnesium, and malic acid. In my experience, over a few months after the yeast syndrome is treated and the correct hormonal balance is obtained, I am able to decrease these medications or supplements.

ANXIETY OR DEPRESSION

About 20 percent of people with CFS also have mental-health issues separate from the CFS-related anxiety. Most people with CFS tend to have some degree of anxiety caused by the autonomic dysfunction that is part of this condition. Many also experience depression. The depression often is a result of the unremitting nature of the illness and the terrible psychological toll that it takes. Whether the mental-health condition is caused by an individual having CFS or whether it exists separate from the CFS, most individual's mental-health conditions improve from treating both the CFS and the mental-health issues with appropriate herbs, medications, homeopathy, vitamins, or counseling, as appropriate.

MIND-BODY INFLUENCES

I find it useful for some to look at the psycho/emotional/spiritual aspects of CFS through medical intuitive sessions. As I offer various options to my patients, I ask that they see which approach resonates best with them. I believe that each person intuitively knows what is best for him- or herself and that my role is to create the space for this to occur.

I think there is a greater acceptance of the diagnosis of CFS in the medical community now than in the past. However, I do not believe most doctors are well informed about the treatment options for this condition. For instance, most conventional medicine physicians do not realize that people with fatigue may require one or more sleep medicines or herbs at a time. Most physicians are overly concerned that individuals will become addicted to the various sleep medicines. In addition, the majority of physicians do not understand or treat the metabolic disturbances involved in this illness. This

is because many of the metabolic treatments are based on alternative medicine diagnosis and syndromes. Conventional medicine physicians still primarily use medications to treat the symptoms of CFS rather than use hormonal and infectious disease treatment approaches to create real changes and potential cures for people with CFS. ❂ ❂ ❂

❧ Additional Potential Causes

Aside from stressors such as mental or physical trauma, surgery, or chronic pain, the following conditions may also potentially trigger CFS:

NEURALLY MEDIATED HYPOTENSION

When Dr. David S. Bell investigated the Lyndonville outbreak in 1985, he found one characteristic common among his patients—a dramatic reduction in blood volume. Bell began collaborating with Dr. David Streeten, who had also been investigating low blood volumes in CFS patients. During this time, one of Bell's patients received a blood transfusion for an unrelated condition, and was left feeling wonderful—she could do the crossword puzzle again, she could play baseball with her grandchildren, and she was full of energy.

Although this "cure" didn't last, it set Bell and Streeten on the road toward understanding the link between CFS and neurally mediated hypotension (low blood pressure). "It is a little piece of the clinical expression of the illness," says Bell. "But it is an important one, and it may turn out to be *the* most important one. The reason I feel it is so important is that when Florinef [a medication used to raise blood pressure] works, it reduces all the symptoms, not just lightheadedness or near-fainting episodes.

A "GENE SIGNATURE"

In August 2005, Dr. Jonathan Kerr announced the discovery of biological markers for CFS. This "gene signature" could eventually lead to a blood test and effective treatment protocol. It also plays an important part in legitimizing the illness. Kerr's team, based at St. George's University in London, observed abnormalities in the way some genes are expressed in the white blood cells of people with CFS. The findings fit with the understanding that a virus may trigger CFS. The study also points to the possibility of exposure to organophosphates (often found in pesticides) as a potential cause of CFS.

Several of the changed genes play important roles in mitochondria, the energy factories of cells. One of the products of these genes, called EIF4G1,

is involved in protein production in mitochondria. EIF4GI is "hijacked" by some viruses, such as Epstein-Barr, so cells compensate by increasing gene expression. Other genes pinpointed by the team are involved in regulating the immune system or play important roles in nerve cells. Dr. Kerr hopes the research will "Open the door to development of pharmacological interventions."

THE HUNTINGTON'S GENE

A prior study in 2003 by the Centers for Disease Control used a similar gene expression profiling technology. The study demonstrated a clear difference between a group of CFS patients and a control group of people who did not have CFS. In every one of the CFS patients, there was evidence of a gene associated with Huntington's disease protein. This gene did not appear in any of the people who did not have CFS. Huntington's disease is a degenerative brain disorder, which causes the gradual breakdown of all motor functions and higher brain functions.

The major implication of these findings is that, like Huntington's, CFS could be a polyglutamine expansion disorder. Polyglutamine expansion stems from a problem with the patient's DNA coding, which causes an excess of the amino acid glutamine. Research is still ongoing into why this excess of glutamine leads to neurologic and cognitive impairment. In an article for the *National Forum* (a newsletter published by the National CFIDS Foundation), Alan Cocchetto postulates, "CFS patients would potentially have an 'acquired' Huntington's disease-like process occurring that is no doubt due to a yet unidentified infectious agent."

THE CIGUATERA CONNECTION

Another piece of the puzzle can be found in the odd correlation between ciguatera fish poisoning and CFS. Ciguatera is the most common form of seafood poisoning, caused by ingestion of ciguatoxins, found in large tropical and subtropical reef fish such as barracuda, grouper, and sea bass. In 2003 Dr. Yoshitsugi Hokama of the University of Hawaii found a link between ciguatoxin and CFS. Hokama tested for the ciguatera epitope in three groups of subjects (an *epitope* is a marker on the surface of an antigen, which triggers an immune response).

The first group of subjects had been diagnosed with CFS, cancer, or hepatitis. The second group had been diagnosed with ciguatera fish poisoning. The third was a control group of healthy subjects. The ciguatera epitope was found in the blood of all the CFS subjects. In fact, the subjects with CFS had some of the highest levels of the ciguatera epitope in the

41

study. These patients tested positive for the ciguatera epitope despite the fact that they had not eaten contaminated fish. Hokama's study showed that there is a toxic substance present in the bodies of people with CFS that has a molecular structure similar to that of ciguatoxin.

❖ A Patient's Story: Karin L.

Karin L. is 38 years old and lives in Seattle. She received the diagnosis of CFS in 1991 while a student in college. Karin overcame many obstacles to earn her master's degree in whole systems design. In her spare time, she enjoys gardening and weaving.

I was experiencing a lot of stress about school at the time that I first got sick. I was 23, and it was my last year in college. I was your basic over-achiever. I had very good grades; I was active; I liked to run, play soccer, swim, and ski. I had just bought my own car, but until that time I had always used my bike for transportation. The year before, I had traveled in Germany with a backpack, taking the train and doing a lot of walking. I wasn't sure what I wanted to do. I thought about going into the Peace Corps.

At first, I thought I was coming down with the flu. The Student Health Center staff were concerned that I had some sort of infection. I didn't get any worse, but I didn't get any better, and I've never felt the same since. I continue to have a sore throat, tender lymph nodes, headache, and low-grade fever. But now my main symptom is fatigue.

My mom made an appointment with a gastroenterologist, because I had had my appendix out right before I got sick. The gastroenterologist first tried to tell me it was all in my head, and he made me take a psychological test. He also did some extensive testing of my gastrointestinal system, and everything came out normal. But he did finally confirm the diagnosis of CFS. At that point, they called it "post-viral fatigue syndrome," because I hadn't been sick for six months yet. Both doctors told me that I would be well within six to ten months. So I thought, "Great, I'll just take it easy." Well, that was 15 years ago.

In a way, I was relieved when I got the diagnosis, because there was a name for my problem and we finally had an idea of what was happening. But I didn't know anyone else who had CFS, and I had never heard of it until I got sick. I was really scared, because I had read an article about it that listed all sorts of bizarre symptoms.

In 1999 I had what I call "the big crash." I had more fevers and sinus problems, my fatigue worsened significantly, and I suffered from depres-

sion. It turns out that the apartment I was living in had a serious mold problem. Moving out of the apartment stopped things from getting worse, but it's taken most of the time since then to get back to where I was when I crashed.

I finished my master's degree in December of 2003. It took me six years, but I did it! I was fortunate to attend a university that was willing to accommodate my needs. My classes were scheduled in the late afternoon and evening. On class days, I frequently rested in bed until it was time to get ready to leave. I was able to read about half of the materials before the term started. During this time, however, I had virtually no social life outside of school, because I simply had no energy left over.

As my abilities and illness shift and change, it takes a while for people to catch up. My family has mostly been very supportive, particularly as time has gone on, and I have a fabulous support network of friends. I consider myself immensely blessed to have such wonderful people around me. Most of my friends have partners and I am envious of that type of relationship. They all have jobs. I want people to understand my life. I want to be seen. There are some people in my life who do not seem very interested in the reality of my life, and that hurts.

I have learned so much since being diagnosed with CFS. Most importantly, I have to live my life—do what I need to do and ask for help if I need it. I know that health is a temporary condition. I appreciate what I am able to do in ways I never could have imagined before CFS. Having become ill at a fairly young age, I feel I have learned some life lessons that others don't learn until much later, if ever, about the tenuousness of it all, and hence the importance of being myself. It feels like I have spent my entire adult life with CFS. However, I am also happier than I was back then, and I have developed a deep sense of who I am.

I accept CFS as part of my life at this time and for the immediate future. What I have seen in both others and myself is that acceptance is key to moving forward in life. I am not intent on ridding my life of this illness. Instead, I am looking to live my life as fully and meaningfully as I can.

❖ ❖ ❖

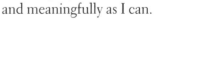

Chapter 4

Conditions That May Accompany FM and CFS

MANY CONDITIONS overlap with FM and CFS, sharing some of the same symptoms and perpetuating factors. If you recognize any of these symptoms in yourself, it's a good idea to be tested. These conditions can stimulate or aggravate FM and CFS, so it's important to address them independently to make sure that all of them are properly treated.

We begin this chapter with an in-depth look at chronic myofascial pain, a condition that is easy to confuse with FM. The rest of the chapter will review a number of other conditions often associated with FM and CFS.

❖ Chronic Myofascial Pain

BY DEVIN J. STARLANYL

Devin J. Starlanyl was trained in emergency medicine, but her life was changed by the onset of multiple chronic illnesses including fibromyalgia and chronic myofascial pain. Devin is the author of several books including *Fibromyalgia and Chronic Myofascial Pain: A Survival Manual* and *The Fibromyalgia Advocate: Getting the Support You Need to Cope with Fibromyalgia and Myofascial Pain Syndrome.* She runs an educational website for practitioners and patients, which can be accessed at www.sover.net/~devstar.

MUSCLE FASCIA

Chronic myofascial pain is often confused with FM, and people may have both conditions at the same time. FM and chronic myofascial pain are two of the three most common causes of chronic pain (the third is joint dysfunction). Both FM and myofascial pain are frequently misdiagnosed—and often go undiagnosed entirely. Typically, the patient sees as many as ten doctors and may spend ten years or longer just getting a correct diagnosis. Often patients are given many inappropriate therapies along the way. Sometimes the patient becomes totally disabled during that time.

The difference between FM and chronic myofascial pain is of critical importance. Without knowing the distinction between the two, as a care provider, you can't diagnose and treat patients completely. As a patient, you can't fully optimize your quality of life if you don't understand what you have and what is causing your symptoms.

Fascia is a type of tissue that forms a vast three-dimensional network throughout your body. Myofascia is the specific type of fascia that surrounds and permeates the muscle tissues. You can see it as the thin and, at times, translucent coating around uncooked chicken. It also lines *your* muscles and lines bundles of muscle fibers as well as the muscle fibers themselves. Myofascia is very sticky stuff; it sticks together to form tendons and ligaments at the ends of muscles.

When the body experiences pain, there is an immediate reaction (because pain signifies damage). The body goes into a self-protective stress mode. When this happens, the myofascia responds by tightening to form a sort of "splint," trying to minimize the pain by restricting movement. This "guarding" is part of the body's survival mechanism and is helpful on a short-term basis.

TRIGGER POINTS

When pain becomes chronic and guarding persists, this muscle tightness inhibits the delivery of fuel and oxygen to the cells, as well as the removal of waste—and an area of extreme sensitivity can develop. This is called a "myofascial trigger point." Myofascial trigger points are not the same as the "tender points" found in FM. A myofascial trigger point is an area that is very painful when pressed and can refer pain and other symptoms in specific patterns throughout the body. When a muscle has trigger points, it becomes weakened and shorter and cannot stretch or do its normal job. Trigger points cause pain at the end of your range of motion, so you begin to restrict your movements. They can cause you to drop things because your

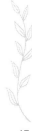

45

grip is weakened. They can also cause dizziness, buckling knees and ankles, abdominal pain, and even impotence—the symptom list seems endless.

With chronic myofascial pain, the muscle can become as hard as a rock. Yet often the trigger points can't be felt. Everything is very, very tight, and people may feel like they are wearing a wet suit that is several sizes too small. Even the sensation of tightness can be painful.

If there are perpetuating factors that are not brought under control (conditions that prevent the muscles from relaxing), the myofascial trigger points can develop throughout the body. When a muscle is weakened by trigger points, another muscle will try to overcompensate. The overworked muscle can also develop trigger points, which are called secondary trigger points. In addition, trigger points can develop in the muscles inside the referred pain pattern area. These are called satellite trigger points. Single trigger points are relatively easy to treat. However, once multiple satellite and secondary trigger points develop, it becomes increasingly difficult to bring these under control, especially if there are several perpetuating factors.

CHRONIC PAIN CONDITIONS

Perpetuating factors that can aggravate myofascial pain or FM include lack of sleep, pain conditions, or certain body movements or positions. Because these problems often accompany FM, people with FM are at greater risk of developing chronic myofascial pain. In some people, chronic myofascial pain may be experienced throughout the entire body—head-to-toe—but the pain is actually being caused by individual, overlapping trigger point referral patterns. There may be a trigger point in the middle of a referral pattern, on the side of the pattern, or even outside the pattern. Each trigger point has a specific pain pattern, which is recognizable from patient to patient.

FM amplifies myofascial trigger point symptoms, and myofascial pain can perpetuate FM. Most patients with FM have myofascial trigger points. Individual trigger points must be treated promptly, and soft tissue injuries must be treated aggressively to prevent the development of chronic pain throughout the body (central sensitization) and chronic myofascial pain.

This means educating care providers in the trenches. Primary-care physicians, emergency-room workers, and specialists such as gynecologists, urologists, and gastroenterologists can largely prevent chronic FM and chronic myofascial pain syndromes from developing, *if* they are trained. We need more preventative care and more options for symptom control. We also need a reality check when it comes to pain control. The pain from even one trigger point can be very difficult to endure. The pain from 100

46

trigger points—when amplified by FM—can be overwhelming. Pain is a major perpetuating factor, and there are a lot of ways to control it. We need to start using all of them to prevent central sensitization.

Diagnosing trigger points is a problem only if the doctor is not familiar with specific trigger point referral patterns. The situation may be further complicated if the patient has symptoms other than pain that are caused by the trigger points. For example, people may stagger and walk into walls, or their vision may be blurred. There are many other bizarre symptoms associated with trigger points—such as the inability to perceive the amount of weight you have in your hand. All of these symptoms may make getting a correct diagnosis more difficult.

SLEEP DISORDERS

People with FM often have sleep disorders, which can contribute to the development of chronic myofascial pain. When the body and the brain talk to each other, they use neurotransmitters and other informational substances (electrobiochemicals that transport messages between the brain and the body). In the case of FM, these neurochemicals don't work properly and get out of balance. This starts a neurotransmitter cascade, because every neurotransmitter is balanced by another, and hormones and other important biochemicals are regulated by neurotransmitters.

Neurotransmitters are regulated in deep sleep (level IV delta sleep), and people with FM often don't get enough of it. People may be jolted awake or experience shallow sleep due to the intrusion of alpha waves (awake brain waves). As a result, they either wake up many times during the night or sleep very shallowly. These people wake up feeling like they've been hit by a truck —they ache all over and feel stiff—because the cellular repair and neurotransmitter balancing that the body needs hasn't happened.

So sleep deprivation is a major handicap for people with FM, and it is a perpetuating factor that needs to be addressed as soon as possible. (Incidentally, sleep deprivation was used in World War II as a form of torture.) Sleep deprivation causes a lot of what we call "brain fog" and cognitive deficit memory problems. So it's critical for the FM patient to get restorative sleep.

TOXICITY

Another problem is that people with FM can become very toxic because they can't get rid of wastes in their bodies. There is growing evidence that certain biochemicals, such as hyaluronic acid, quinolinic acid, and phosphoric acid, are higher in people with FM. Many of these substances are

irritants. As pollution of the body increases, people become more suscep-tible to myofascial trigger points.

FM AND MYOFASCIAL PAIN

The hypersensitized tender points in FM patients can cause all-over achi-ness. Myofascial trigger points, however, usually cause localized pain. FM also gives you the flu-like feeling that never seems to let up. When a person has multiple trigger points and a genetic predisposition to FM, it appears that FM will develop unless both conditions are promptly treated. When FM and chronic myofascial pain occur in the same patient, it can be more than double trouble. In FM, the nervous system is like a stereo stuck on high. Everything becomes intensified, including the pain, dizziness, and other sensations caused by the myofascial trigger points.

We now have a clearer picture of the mechanisms involved in the for-mation of myofascial trigger points. I've watched a high-resolution ultra-sound video of a trigger-point twitch response. We have research that has isolated more than 30 sensitizing biochemicals produced during a trigger-point twitch. All of this gives us clues to the development of new forms of treatment. We are also learning how the system-wide pain that occurs in FM (central sensitization) can *amplify* the pain and other symptoms of myofascial trigger points, and how myofascial trigger points can perpetuate central sensitization because they are pain *generators*.

FM and chronic myofascial pain are time-consuming conditions, but your goals should focus on self-maintenance and attaining the highest quality of life possible. Although there is currently no cure for FM, many of its symptoms can be reversed. Myofascial trigger points can also be reversed by identifying and thoroughly dealing with perpetuating factors. You can improve your life situation and function very well, and many therapeutic techniques are available. You just have to find the combination that works for you. ❖❖❖

❖ Conditions Associated with FM and CFS

ADRENAL STRESS

Adrenal stress is triggered by high levels of cortisol, one of the hormones produced by the adrenal glands. Cortisol and DHEA (dehydroepiandro-sterone) control the way our bodies respond to both physical and emotional stress, instantly increasing our heart rate and blood pressure, and releasing energy stores for immediate use. This "fight-or-flight" response takes priority over all other functions in the body. It's supposed to be a temporary response to danger, but today we are surrounded by stress, constantly triggering our "fight-or-flight" response. This puts us at risk of adrenal exhaustion.

Symptoms of too much adrenal stress include a lack of energy during the day, difficulty achieving restful sleep, mood swings, and trouble losing excess weight despite dieting. In addition, too much cortisol can deteriorate healthy muscle and bone. It can also slow down healing and cell replacement, inhibit metabolism, and compromise the immune system.

Adrenal stress can be treated through lifestyle changes, by cutting out caffeine and unhealthy carbohydrates, reducing stress, increasing exercise, and getting plenty of rest.

ANKYLOSING SPONDYLITIS

Dr. Paul Brown tells us he always screens his male FM and CFS patients for ankylosing spondylitis, a condition that often mimics FM and CFS in men. Ankylosing spondylitis is a form of arthritis that causes the joints and ligaments in the spine to become inflamed, and in acute cases the vertebrae may fuse together. The disease can also progress into the upper spine, rib cage, and neck. In the most severe cases, ribs may fuse together, impairing the patient's ability to breathe. Other joints may also become inflamed, including the hips, knees, or ankles.

Unlike most forms of arthritis, ankylosing spondylitis occurs at a relatively young age, with onset usually between ages 17 and 35. It primarily affects men, and when it occurs in women, it is usually mild.

Treatment typically begins with NSAIDS (nonsteroidal anti-inflammatory drugs), which address pain and stiffness. Exercise and posture management can also help alleviate the symptoms.

ARTHRITIS

There are two main types of arthritis: osteoarthritis (a degenerative joint disease) and rheumatoid arthritis (an autoimmune disease).

In osteoarthritis, cartilage begins to break down (cartilage is the part of the joint that cushions the bones from one another). When the cartilage is damaged, the bones may rub against each other, causing pain and inhibiting movement. Osteoarthritis particularly affects the hands, knees, hips, feet, or back.

Rheumatoid arthritis is a chronic disease in which the lining of the joints (the synovium) becomes inflamed. It's estimated that 15–25 percent of FM and CFS patients have rheumatoid arthritis. In the earliest stage, inflamma-

49

tion of the synovium causes redness, swelling, stiffness, and pain around the joint. Later, the synovium thickens and eventually enzymes are released that break down bone and cartilage. This causes the joint to lose its shape and alignment, leading to severe pain and loss of movement. Early diagnosis is critical, because rheumatoid arthritis can spread to other organs in the body, including the skin, heart, and lungs. Treatment includes drugs, exercise, joint-protection techniques, and self-management programs. If diagnosed early and treated aggressively, rheumatoid arthritis can be well managed and patients can lead healthy, active lives.

BIPOLAR DISORDER

Bipolar disorder (also known as manic depressive illness) describes 10–15 percent of all patients with major depression. People living with bipolar disorder experience manic episodes, the hallmarks of which may include a decreased need for sleep, feelings of grandiosity, nonstop rapid talking, engaging in promiscuous sexual behavior, or going on seemingly outrageous shopping sprees. Bipolar disorder is more severe than major depression because patients can experience hallucinations, delusions, and psychotic behavior. People with bipolar disorder have a higher rate of suicide and hospitalization than people with major depression. It is important for the doctor not to miss bipolar disorder when making the diagnosis of depression, since many antidepressants may trigger a manic episode in bipolar patients.

There are two categories of bipolar disorder: bipolar I, in which the patient cycles between manic episodes and severe depression, and bipolar II, in which the patient cycles between elevated moods and severe depression. The distinction between bipolar I and bipolar II is important. Bipolar II patients do not experience the psychotic level of mania that bipolar I patients experience.

CANDIDA

Candida albicans is a kind of yeast that is present in most people's bodies. A healthy immune system will control the level of candida and it will not cause any harm. However, many FM and CFS patients experience an overgrowth of candida, which can build up in the body, infecting the mouth, skin, intestines, or vagina. Factors that can lead to an overgrowth of candida include high sugar consumption, prolonged use of antibiotics, use of birth control pills, diabetes, or high levels of mercury or other toxins in the body. Symptoms include fatigue and sugar or carbohydrate cravings. (See Appendix B for information on a simple candida test you can do at home.)

CARPAL TUNNEL SYNDROME

The carpal tunnel is a passageway of bone and ligament located in your wrist. It controls the sensations in the fingers, thumb, and some of the hand muscles. Carpal tunnel syndrome is the narrowing of the carpal tunnel. It's generally associated with repetitive stress injury, caused by tasks such as writing or using a computer mouse. Symptoms include tingling, numbness, pain, and a weakened grip. The extent to which the carpal tunnel has narrowed can be determined by a physiatrist in a "nerve conduction study," during which electrified needles are placed on the nerves and the response is monitored. Treatment for carpal tunnel syndrome can include wearing a wrist splint, using a wrist support when working at the computer, chiropractic care, or acupuncture. In severe cases, carpal tunnel release surgery can relieve pain and pressure.

CELIAC DISEASE

Patients with celiac disease are unable to fight the food-grain antigens contained in gluten (a derivative of grain products). The antigens in the gluten irritate the lining of the small intestine where digestion occurs, resulting in serious damage to the digestive tract and impairing proper absorption of nutrients. The mechanism of this disease has not been conclusively defined—it may be a missing intestinal enzyme, or an autoimmune process.

For patients suffering from celiac disease, specific foods that should be avoided include wheat, rye, barley, spelt, and oats, but gluten can also be found in food additives such as modified food starch (ongoing research suggests that oats may only be a risk for some celiac patients). The common symptoms of celiac disease include diarrhea or constipation, weight loss, and bloating. In some cases, celiac disease can lead to fatigue, headaches, joint pain, osteoporosis, acid reflux, or infertility.

Most FM and CFS patients have food sensitivities, so it is important to ask your doctor to check for celiac disease. By cutting out wheat and gluten, patients can alleviate many of the stomach and bowel problems associated with FM and CFS.

DEPRESSION

It's estimated that depression affects up to 25 percent of FM and CFS patients. Like FM and CFS, depression is a syndrome—a collection of symptoms. It is believed to be caused by low levels of the neurochemicals serotonin and norepinephrine. The American Psychiatric Society describes the main symptoms of depression as changes in appetite that result in

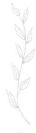

weight loss; insomnia or oversleeping; loss of energy or increased fatigue; restlessness or irritability; feelings of worthlessness or inappropriate guilt; difficulty thinking, concentrating, and decision making; thoughts of death or suicide; or attempts at suicide. Depression tends to run in families. Environmental stressors, such as loneliness or the loss of a job, can also be triggers. If you have some of the symptoms of depression, consult your primary health-care provider. He or she can evaluate and treat your depression or refer you to a mental-health professional. Depression can be treated through antidepressant medications, counseling, cognitive-behavioral therapy, or natural therapies, such as the use of St. John's wort. Exercise and changes in diet help many people suffering from mild depression. What's important is to find the right treatment for you. If you're uneasy about taking antidepressants, you may want to try counseling and alternative treatments first. It's good to keep an open mind and consider all treatment options.

EPSTEIN-BARR VIRUS

The Epstein-Barr virus (EBV) is one of the most common human viruses. In fact, most people become infected with Epstein-Barr at sometime during their lives. While infection often results in mild flu-like symptoms, it can also cause infectious mononucleosis. FM and CFS patients are especially susceptible to "mono."

The initial symptoms of mono are fatigue, loss of appetite, and chills. Symptoms intensify to include a severe sore throat, fever from 102 to 104 degrees, and swollen lymph glands. The throat becomes reddened and tonsils may have a whitish coating. Approximately 50 percent of patients develop an enlarged or swollen spleen. A small number of patients develop a splotchy red rash all over their body. There is no treatment for mono—like many viruses, it needs to run its course. Sleep and plenty of rest are recommended. Acetaminophen can be taken to alleviate fever and body aches. Naturopathy and Eastern medicine can also be effective in treating viral conditions, such as mono. It should be noted that patients should avoid activities that may cause trauma to the spleen—in rare cases, the enlarged spleen can rupture, which could be life threatening.

HEAVY METAL POISONING

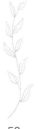

Heavy metals are inorganic elements with high molecular weights. They are toxic to living organisms and can cause damage even at relatively low concentrations. Heavy metals occur naturally in rock formations; they are also pervasive in our environment as a byproduct of mining and manufacturing. The following elements are considered heavy metals: aluminum, arsenic, barium, cadmium, chromate, chromium, cobalt, copper, gold, iron, silver, lead, manganese, mercury, nickel, selenium, uranium, and zinc. These metals do not break down and cannot be destroyed.

Since the industrial revolution, humans have harnessed the power of heavy metals. Ironically, what has brought us freedom, comfort, medical advances, better hygiene, and prolonged our life span, has also been slowly poisoning us and our planet. In 1974 the World Health Organization declared heavy metals to be one of the major causes of the world's diseases. Heavy metals are absorbed into our bodies in a number of ways, such as through food, water, and the air we breathe. Prolonged exposure to heavy metals can deplete the immune system. Metals are stored in the fatty tissues of the body and at toxic levels can lead to chronic organ damage, blood disorders, or cancer.

Robin N. was diagnosed with industrial lead poisoning. She says, "At the time I became ill, I was working for a manufacturer and thought that my exposure to acetone was causing my symptoms. It now appears that the real culprit was the metal dust that I was exposed to."

In recent years, legislation has been implemented in many countries to control the use and disposal of heavy metals. Europe and Japan have led the way in pollution-reduction initiatives. The United States banned lead from paint in 1978 and from gasoline in 1986. Recent tests have shown that American children now have blood-lead levels 90 percent lower than those of the 1970s. As a result, their IQs are at least three points higher.

HEPATITIS C

Hepatitis C is a viral infection that causes inflammation of the liver, which can result in scarring (cirrhosis), cancer of the liver, or chronic liver disease. It is caused by the hepatitis C virus (HCV). HCV is highly contagious and is spread through contaminated blood. Those most at risk include people who have received a blood transfusion, blood products, or an organ transplant prior to 1992 (when donated blood and organs began to be screened for HCV). Others at risk include individuals on long-term kidney dialysis, people who have injected illegal drugs, and health-care workers who may have accidentally come into contact with HCV-infected blood.

Babies born to HCV-positive mothers have a slight risk of developing hepatitis C. It is thought that HCV can be transmitted through sexual intercourse, but this is a rare occurrence and has not yet been scientifically proven.

HCV can lie dormant for many years: Some patients do not experience symptoms for up to 40 years or more after being infected. Many patients do

53

not develop symptoms until scarring of the liver has occurred. One of the symptoms of hepatitis C is tenderness in the right upper quadrant (the area just below your rib cage on the right side of your back). Other symptoms include diminished appetite or nausea, muscle and joint pain, and fatigue. The severity of hepatitis C varies from patient to patient; some patients experience little to no symptoms, while others will have more prominent symptoms. Some will eventually develop end-stage liver disease or liver cancer.

IRRITABLE BOWEL SYNDROME AND IRRITABLE BLADDER (INTERSTITIAL CYSTITIS)

In a 2000 article for the *Archives of Internal Medicine*, Leslie Aaron et al. reported that irritable bowel syndrome was present in 92 percent of CFS patients and 77 percent of FM patients evaluated. Irritable bowel syndrome (IBS) can cause diarrhea one day and constipation the next. Irritable bladder (also known as interstitial cystitis) causes frequent, and sometimes painful, urination. Symptoms of IBS include altered bowel habits, with diarrhea, constipation, or both, and abdominal pain, gas, and bloating. IBS is frequently treated with a high-fiber diet, regular use of psyllium (contained in Metamucil) or the Chinese herbal product DiJu (available from tummy temple.com) for the symptoms of constipation, and Bentyl (dicyclomine hydrochloride, an antispasmodic) for pain.

Early symptoms of irritable bladder include urinary frequency, with some patients having to urinate as many as 60 times a day. As the condition progresses, patients often experience an urgent need to urinate, which may become painful and eventually lead to spasms in the bladder. Pain may be present in the abdominal, urethral, and vaginal areas. In many cases hemorrhages are found on the bladder wall, and occasionally ulcers are also present, leading to a diagnosis of ulcerative interstitial cystitis. Irritable bladder is treated on a case-by-case basis. The FDA-recommended drug Rimso-50 is commonly prescribed for relief of symptoms. Patients may also benefit from low doses of tricyclic antidepressants, which have a relaxing effect on the bladder. In extreme cases, surgery may be considered.

LUPUS

Lupus is an autoimmune disease, which can affect any organ or organ system in the body but is most commonly found in the skin, joints, blood, and kidneys. The Lupus Foundation of America lists the following common symptoms of lupus: butterfly-shaped skin rashes, prolonged or extreme fatigue, achy joints, a temperature of over 100 degrees, anemia, or arthritis. Most lupus patients have a mild case, affecting one or two organs. However, when lupus becomes chronic, it can be life threatening.

There are three types of lupus: discoid, systemic, and drug-induced. Discoid lupus affects the skin only and is characterized by a rash on the face, neck, and scalp. Systemic lupus can affect any part of the body. Each case of systemic lupus is unique. One patient may have symptoms in the kidneys and lungs; another patient's skin and joints will be affected. Drug-induced lupus occurs when a patient has an allergic reaction to prescribed drugs. The drugs most commonly associated with drug-induced lupus are hydralazine (used to treat high blood-pressure) and procainamide (used to treat irregular heart rhythms). Drug-induced lupus is rare and usually clears up when the medication is discontinued.

The cause of lupus is still under investigation but scientists have pin-pointed a number of triggers, including infections, antibiotics, ultraviolet light, and hormones. Lupus has also been found to have a genetic component. According to the Lupus Foundation of America, recent studies have found a gene on chromosome 1, which appears to be associated with lupus in some families.

Lupus is diagnosed through a review of the patient's medical history, laboratory tests, and the American College of Rheumatology's diagnostic criteria. Lupus will affect each patient differently, so it is extremely important to have a thorough medical evaluation and monitor the patient's condition on a regular basis. There is no cure for lupus, but the illness can usually be managed successfully. Medications are often prescribed, depending on which organs are involved. Lupus patients are strongly encouraged to avoid drinking alcohol and smoking. An exercise program is also recommended.

LYME DISEASE

Lyme disease is an invasive infection caused by a spiral-shaped bacterium, *Borrelia burgdorferi*, which is transmitted by ticks. In the United States, two types of ticks carry the bacteria: The deer tick transmits the disease in regions of the northeast and upper midwest; the western black-legged tick transmits the disease along the Pacific coast. The hallmark of Lyme disease is a rash in the pattern of a "bull's-eye," with a pale center area surrounded by a red rim. The disease has an incubation period of several weeks. A person infected with Lyme disease usually experiences flu-like symptoms such as aches and pains in the muscles and joints, low-grade fever, or fatigue. Untreated, it can progress to affect the joints, heart, or nervous system. Lyme

55

disease is diagnosed through a medical history, a physical examination, and a blood test. Skin cultures and tests that detect the genetic material associated with the Lyme disease bacteria can also identify an active case. Treatment includes antibiotics.

MALABSORPTION

Malabsorption is often associated with irritable bowel syndrome. Patients with malabsorption have difficulty absorbing sufficient nutrients from their food. In some patients, malabsorption is specific to certain sugars, proteins, vitamins, or fats. Other patients have difficulty absorbing all nutrients. Symptoms can include diarrhea, anemia, bloating, muscle wasting, weight loss, or a distended abdomen. A slow growth rate is particularly noticeable in children with malabsorption. Untreated malabsorption can cause malnutrition and vitamin deficiencies.

Malabsorption is diagnosed through a careful medical history and is confirmed through stool and blood tests. X rays and biopsies of the small intestine may be necessary in some cases. Treatment of malabsorption is determined on an individual basis, since the cause of the disease differs from patient to patient. In the United States, cystic fibrosis is the number one cause of malabsorption. Other conditions that can lead to malabsorption include celiac disease, lactose intolerance, or Crohn's disease. Treatment is usually targeted to the underlying cause and may include dietary changes, enzyme supplements, antidiarrheal medication, or antibiotics.

MULTIPLE CHEMICAL SENSITIVITIES

Up to 30 percent of people who have FM or CFS also meet the diagnostic criteria for multiple chemical sensitivities (MCS). MCS is often described as an "environmental illness." Patients become ill when exposed to substances present in the environment, such as food, mold, pollen, or dust. Many people with MCS are particularly sensitive to man-made chemicals. MCS patients become hypersensitized to these substances, causing the immune system to overreact. These symptoms can affect any bodily system and may include headaches, nausea, fatigue, dizziness, confusion, muscle weakness, depression, anxiety, or other physical or emotional reactions.

Regina L. says, "I have trouble shopping in stores, driving in the car with the windows open, and visiting people and places for more than a short period of time. Often smog, car tires on hot pavement, gasoline, plastics, foam rubber, cigarette smoke, candles, perfumes, or alcohol in any form cause problems—such as confusion, forgetfulness, nausea, headaches, or vomit-

ing. At times I experience severe anxiety, especially around pesticides and insecticides."

Since World War II, the use of man-made products and chemicals has increased significantly. After the war, products such as herbicides, pesticides, paint, and MDF (multiple density fiberboard) became cheaper and were mass-produced; everybody could have access to them. Natural products were often considered inferior (in the 1970s people believed you couldn't get a nice green lawn without using some kind of chemical additive). At the time, we didn't realize the damage this could do to our health. Many of these products release toxic chemical gases into the air that may be toxic. Even now, most homes are full of environmental toxins.

Home hygiene is especially important for people with multiple chemical sensitivities, but it's good for everyone, too, especially patients with FM and CFS who tend to have a hypersensitivity to environmental toxins. Environmental hazards in the home include second-hand smoke, radon, and toxic mold. The chemicals in many household cleaners can be hazardous to your health. There are a wide range of products in the home that can trigger sensitivity, such as plastics, synthetic carpeting or fabrics, cosmetics, and certain food additives.

To manage MCS, patients must eliminate as many of the aggravating substances as possible from their lives, including all scented products, detergents, pesticides, and fertilizers. Nontoxic cleaning and gardening products are available in many stores. It's also best to wear only natural fiber clothing such as 100 percent cotton, linen, silk, or wool. Many patients find that keeping to a strictly organic diet makes a tremendous difference to the way they feel.

Mold

Mold is a form of fungi. It can be found outdoors in the soil, on plants, and on dead or decaying material. Mold tends to grow in warm and humid conditions. Like most fungi, mold produces microscopic cells, called spores, which become airborne. Spores spread like the seeds of a flower, forming new colonies when they come upon ideal conditions. Fungal spores are everywhere and we all breathe them in on a daily basis. However, some types of mold can be more damaging then others, and some people are more susceptible than others.

Most household mold originates outdoors. Mold needs moisture to grow, so if you have indoor moisture as a result of flooding, high humidity, or dampness, you will also have mold. Bathrooms, kitchens, and basements

57

are particularly susceptible. It's important to open windows or use extractor fans or dehumidifiers to remove moisture from these areas of your house.

"Black mold," which is actually greenish-black in color, is a particular kind of mold whose technical name is *Stachybotrys chararum.* It commonly occurs after heavy water damage. Black mold has been linked to severe health problems.

Mold should not be allowed to accumulate in large quantities because it can cause health problems, particularly in children, the elderly, or other people who are particularly sensitive to it. First, fix the source of the moisture problem, and then attack the mold. If you attack the problem the other way round, the mold will just come back. Minor mold problems can be taken care of with bleach and water (the recommended solution to kill mold is 50 percent bleach and 50 percent water); make sure to dry the area completely. Wear gloves, eye protection, and a respirator or dust mask (available from the hardware store). If you have an extensive problem with mold growth, you can contact professionals who will take care of the problem for you.

Most people do not experience negative reactions to mold. Allergic reactions similar to those of pollen are the most common adverse effects. However, mold can also aggravate asthma, and people with multiple chemical sensitivities can become very ill when in contact with mold.

Radon

Radon is the second leading cause of lung cancer in the United States. In 2005, the surgeon general issued a health advisory, warning Americans about the health risk of exposure to radon in indoor air. Radon is an extremely toxic, colorless gas. It is derived from the radioactive decay of uranium and is used in cancer treatment and radiography. Radon can leach into the home through soil and rock beneath the foundation. It may also be present in well water or building materials. Human exposure to radon occurs by breathing the gas in the air or by drinking radon in water. Radon test kits are available from many hardware stores. If you find radon in your home, you will need to find a contractor specializing in radon mitigation work. Contact your municipal water supplier if you are concerned about radon levels in your water supply.

MULTIPLE SCLEROSIS

The National Multiple Sclerosis Society reports that approximately 2.5 million people in the world today are living with multiple sclerosis (MS).

MS attacks the central nervous system, specifically, the myelin sheath (the protective insulation surrounding nerve fibers). The myelin is destroyed and replaced by sclerotic (hardened) tissue. Irrevocable damage occurs to the underlying nerve, which is no longer protected by the myelin sheath. The damage affects multiple sites within the central nervous system. The myelin sheath can be likened to the insulation around electrical wiring—when the insulation is damaged, the wires start to short out. The same thing happens in the human body: When the myelin sheath is damaged, signals to and from the brain are not processed correctly. Although the cause of MS is still being studied, many researchers believe MS to be an autoimmune disease. It is extremely difficult to diagnose, due to the erratic nature of the symptoms, which vary not only between patients but also within a single patient.

NEURALLY MEDIATED HYPOTENSION

Blood pressure is regulated by our autonomic nervous system—a reflexive action occurs between the brain and the heart, adjusting blood pressure according to the body's needs. For example, when you stand up, gravity causes blood to rush to your legs and feet, and your autonomic nervous system compensates by increasing blood flow to the brain. But in a patient with neurally mediated hypotension, an abnormal interaction occurs between the heart and the brain. When blood pressure levels are inadequate and organs do not receive needed oxygen or nutrients, the result can be extreme fatigue, lightheadedness, headaches, fainting, and mental confusion.

Peter Rowe, M.D., a pediatrician at Johns Hopkins, discovered a link between CFS and neurally mediated hypotension. In a Johns Hopkins study published in the *Journal of the American Medical Association*, 22 out of 23 patients with CFS tested positive for neurally mediated hypotension. After treatment, nine patients reported almost complete recovery from fatigue, while others noted some level of improvement.

Neurally mediated hypotension cannot be detected through routine blood pressure testing, but it can be detected through a procedure known as the "tilt table test" (see Appendix B for details on how to perform a version of the test yourself). Treatment can include a simple increase of salt and water intake or drug therapy.

POLYMYALGIA RHEUMATICA

Polymyalgia Rheumatica (PMR) is a form of arthritis that affects the muscles. PMR is characterized by pain and stiffness in at least two of the following areas: the neck, shoulders, upper arms, hips, thighs, knees, and lower back. The symptoms of PMR are usually at their worst when the patient first wakes up, and can be accompanied by fatigue or low-grade fever. PMR can also cause anemia, weight loss, or night-sweats.

PMR typically affects women in their late fifties and is usually treated with steroids, stretching routines, and low-impact exercises. The intensity of PMR varies from patient to patient; for some, PMR may be mild and disappear without treatment in one to four years. For others, PMR may be a long-lasting and disabling condition.

POST-TRAUMATIC STRESS DISORDER

Patients living with post-traumatic stress disorder (PTSD) experience mental and physical responses to past trauma, as if it were happening in the present. These flashbacks can happen at anytime, triggered by memories, thoughts, or a discussion of the trauma, whether it resulted from an abusive situation, a difficult childhood, memories of war, or a car crash. People with PTSD can witness an event that reminds them of the trauma and be transported back—it is as if the body is re-experiencing the event. These flashbacks cause an adrenaline rush (the fight-or-flight response).

PTSD can affect an individual soon after the trauma, and if properly treated, can be resolved quickly. This type of PTSD is known as "acute PTSD," and it lasts no longer than six months following a traumatic event. "Chronic PTSD" lasts far longer than six months, sometimes enduring for the patient's lifetime. It is also important to note that the onset of PTSD can be delayed. A person may feel that they have not been affected by a particular trauma, yet the effects will eventually reveal themselves in the form of delayed PTSD.

PTSD is usually treated with both counseling and drug therapy. Clinical trials have shown cognitive-behavioral therapy to be particularly effective for the treatment of PTSD, and certain acupuncture techniques can also be helpful.

RAYNAUD'S PHENOMENON

Raynaud's phenomenon is a circulatory disorder in which blood vessels constrict in response to cold temperatures or emotional stress, known as a vasospasm. When this occurs, blood flow to the affected areas of the body is restricted. Raynaud's affects the extremities, most often the fingers and toes. It can also be present in the nose, ear lobes, lips, nipples, or knees. Patients may have Raynaud's in just one part of the body, in certain areas,

or in all of these areas. During a vasospasm, the affected areas feel cold, achy, sometimes painful, and may become discolored due to a decrease in circulation and oxygen. A vasospasm can last anywhere from less than a minute to several hours.

The most common and mildest form of Raynaud's phenomenon is classified as "primary Raynaud's." This type of Raynaud's is not related to any other condition the patient may have. "Secondary Raynaud's," which can be debilitating, is caused by a connective tissue illness, such as Sjögren's syndrome or lupus.

RESTLESS LEGS SYNDROME

It is estimated that 31 percent of FM patients have restless legs syndrome (RLS). Just as it sounds, patients with RLS experience an uncontrollable urge to move their legs. The movements are not involuntary, but rather a response to a tingling sensation deep within the legs. RLS can occur in one or both legs, and it occasionally occurs in the arms or trunk. Patients experience trouble sleeping and are tired during the day due to their lack of restorative sleep. RLS has a circadian rhythm just like the human body—in most patients, RLS is worse in the evening hours, and it is especially severe when the patient is inactive. Physicians recommend RLS patients adjust to a later sleeping schedule and sleep from 2:00 A.M. to 10:00 A.M. Often, physicians prescribe dopamine medications, such as Mirapex.

SARCOIDOSIS

Sarcoidosis results from the inflammation of body tissues. It usually starts in the lungs or lymph nodes but can appear in almost any organ. Small lumps, known as "granulomas," appear in the affected tissues. The first symptoms are shortness of breath and a persistent cough. Skin rashes may also occur in the early stages of the illness. Other symptoms include inflamed eyes and red bumps on the face, arms, or shins. Sarcoidosis causes weight loss, fatigue, night sweats and fever. There is no cure at present, but physicians are very knowledgeable in the management of this illness, and most patients with sarcoidosis lead normal lives.

SJÖGREN'S SYNDROME

In Sjögren's syndrome (pronounced *show-grins*), the body's immune system attacks the moisture-producing glands—the lacrimal glands, which produce tears, and the parotid glands, which produce saliva. The most common symptoms are dry eyes and dry mouth. Other symptoms include

61

fatigue and joint pain, digestive problems, increased dental decay, dry nose and dry skin, and a change in the sense of taste and smell. Sjögren's is diagnosed through a series of blood tests. There is no cure for Sjögren's, but there is plenty you can do to manage the symptoms. The Sjögren's Syndrome Foundation recommends some over-the-counter products, including preservative-free artificial tears and saliva. Nine out of ten Sjögren's patients are women. The average age of onset is in the late 40s, although Sjögren's can occur in all age groups and both sexes.

SLEEP APNEA

Dr. Andrew J. Holman estimates that 40 percent of FM patients have sleep apnea. If you think you might be one of them, it is important to be properly diagnosed and treated, as sleep apnea can severely hinder your treatment program for FM and CFS.

Sleep apnea patients stop breathing at intermittent times during their normal sleep cycle. Each time the patient stops breathing, a "drowning" response is triggered in the brain, and the patient briefly awakens. Patients are often unaware that they are constantly waking up during the night, and they cannot understand why they are so tired during the day. Sleep apnea puts strain on the heart, since each time a person stops breathing, the heart must kick-start the respiration process. Left untreated, this condition can cause cardiovascular problems, weight gain, impotency, and headaches. The lack of restorative sleep can lead to cognitive problems, which may be dangerous, as patients are less alert during the day. One of the most distinctive symptoms of sleep apnea is excessive snoring. If you suspect you have sleep apnea, ask your physician to refer you to a sleep clinic where your sleep can be monitored and evaluated. Sleep apnea primarily affects men over the age of 40, particularly if they are overweight. However, it also runs in families and anyone can be affected, including children.

Sleep apnea can be managed through the use of a home medical device that supports breathing while one sleeps through continuous positive airway pressure therapy (CPAP). Your doctor can help you obtain a CPAP machine. For Richard G., the CPAP machine had an immediate positive effect: "I sleep much deeper and feel more rested when I wake up. I also find I don't need as much sleep as I did before because the quality of sleep I'm getting is better." Richard has taken his CPAP everywhere from the United Kingdom to Belize. "Traveling with a CPAP is easy. I've noticed other passengers with their machines, too. Getting through security was no problem, as they see quite a few CPAPs. It's best to get a note from your doctor explaining the condition, just in case."

TEMPOROMANDIBULAR JOINT SYNDROME (TMJS)

Temporomandibular joint syndrome (TMJS) is a dysfunction that causes grinding and clicking in the jaw (in the temporomandibular joint, located where the temporal bone of the skull connects to the lower jaw). TMJS can also cause pain in the ears, face, or head, as well as fatigue, soreness of the jaw muscle upon waking, and stiffness of the jaw itself. Treatment may include medical, dental, or chiropractic intervention. Physical therapy may be recommended. Various techniques are used to sedate, desensitize, or eliminate the pain caused by TMJS. Anesthetics or saline may be injected, or a dry needle may be inserted into the joint.

THYROID DISORDERS

It's estimated that 47 percent of FM and CFS patients have a dysfunctional thyroid—so if you have FM or CFS, it is best to have your thyroid hormone levels checked. Hypothyroidism (an underactive thyroid) is particularly common among women living with FM or CFS. Symptoms include weight gain, constipation, fatigue, heavy periods, and dry skin and hair. Hypothyroidism is confirmed by a simple blood test and is treated with prescribed thyroid supplements. Hashimoto's thyroiditis is one of the most common forms of hypothyroidism. It is an autoimmune disease in which the healthy tissue of the thyroid is attacked by the body's own immune system.

VITAMIN D DEFICIENCY

Vitamin D plays a vital role in the body. It's best known for promoting healthy bones by leading to the absorption of calcium, but ongoing research indicates that vitamin D can also help prevent cancer and many other disorders. The common symptoms of vitamin D deficiency are aching bones and muscle discomfort. Prolonged vitamin D deficiency can lead to osteoporosis or a softening of the bones.

The number one source of vitamin D is sunlight—it stimulates human skin to synthesize vast quantities of the vitamin. But for this process to take place, we need full sun, not simply daylight. In northern latitudes, the sunlight isn't strong enough during fall and winter to promote the production of vitamin D. In a 2003 study at the University of Maine, Sullivan et al.

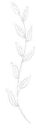

63

found that adolescent girls in Maine did not get enough sunlight for adequate vitamin D production.

Vitamin D deficiency has been linked to forms of cancer and may also be linked to diabetes and multiple sclerosis. In fact, people in higher latitudes do have greater instances of these illnesses. A 2004 study published in *Neurology* found that women who got doses of at least 400 units of vitamin D per day were 40 percent less likely to develop multiple sclerosis compared with those not taking any supplements.

Dr. Michael Holick of Boston University School of Medicine says, "Activated vitamin D is one of the most potent inhibitors of cancer cell growth. It also stimulates your pancreas to make insulin. It regulates your immune system."

In his controversial book *The UV Advantage*, Holick recommends increased exposure to sunshine. The book is controversial because it encourages people to go without sunscreen and discredits much of what we have been told about the carcinogenic effect of UV rays. However, even Holick recommends common sense and the avoidance of tanning booths. This topic is still the subject of heated debate. But one undisputed point is that sunscreen blocks the sun's rays and therefore stops the production of vitamin D. So if it's dangerous to expose our skin to the sun, how do we get enough vitamin D?

Vitamin supplements provide the best and most convenient source of vitamin D. Salmon, sardines, mackerel, and the rather unappetizing cod liver oil (now available in lemon flavor) are some of the few foods that provide vitamin D naturally. In addition, an increasing number of foods such as milk, orange juice, margarine, and cereal are now being fortified with vitamin D.

VULVODYNIA

Many women who have FM or CFS also experience vulvodynia—pain in the female genitalia. Each patient experiences the pain of vulvodynia differently; some describe it as a raw, burning, or aching pain. Others describe it as a deep stabbing pain that starts in the vulva and extends to other areas. Some women experience the pain only during intercourse, some experience the pain intermittently, and for others it is constantly present.

Myofascial trigger points may be the cause of vulvodynia. A myotherapist can locate the trigger points and stretch them. Myotherapy is a noninvasive treatment involving the application of pressure to trigger points (see Chapter 8 for more information on myotherapy). You can learn to do myo-

therapy for yourself and there are also simple exercises that help to relieve pain in the vaginal muscles.

✤ A Patient's Story: Mary R.

Mary R. is 55 years old and lives in Mount Forest, Ontario, Canada. She has multiple chemical sensitivities (MCS) and FM. Mary is an advocate for MCS in Canada.

It took at least a couple of years for me to be diagnosed with MCS. An emergency room doctor, upon prescribing prednisone, declared with disbelief that he'd never heard of anyone having breathing difficulties after exposure to smoke on someone's clothing. Even my own doctor had to be convinced—I did my research and informed her along the way. She finally noticed that I was better if I stayed away from the work environment but had no idea why that was!

I figured this out myself, rather than having a doctor pronounce what was wrong. As such, there was some relief to finally understand what I had so that I could begin to learn how to help myself. Before I became ill, I could do anything. Now I am quite limited. For example: I can no longer travel, participate in community groups, attend meetings, visit with family, or go to the movies—and I can no longer work. I used to be able to hike— now I must walk on fairly level, smooth trails, because looking down to be sure of my footing puts too much stress on my neck, shoulders, and back, thus increasing the pain. Skating, tobogganing, and cross-country skiing are also things I can no longer do.

For the past year or more it has been very difficult to visit my doctor's office since they have moved and renovated (new walls, paint, lots of wallpaper). I would become sick each time I went to see her, because of the office environment, even if I wore a mask. I am scared that if I get sick with something that requires hospitalization, the environment at the hospital will make me even worse. I've met many nurses who wear strong perfume and are completely unaware that this could be a health issue for anyone.

My family has no idea what life is like with MCS—even though I've explained it again and again, they still don't quite "get it." They seem to think that a little bit of perfume or smoke for a couple of hours is OK. My children recently refused to accommodate me so that I could be included in a family function—my suggestion that we meet in an appropriate restaurant to visit after the event, was ignored. They all met at my daughter's house,

where there were two cats, two dogs, one hamster (I have allergies to the animals), and smelly oil plug-ins.

I cannot visit my mother, my sister, or my daughter because they smoke in their homes and/or have pets. We can only visit outside during good weather. My mother and sister live in Quebec; even the restaurants there are not OK for me, since smoking is allowed in them. A neighbor thinks it's all in my head and finds ways to put me down; i.e., "If you just decided that this really didn't make you sick, wouldn't you be OK?" and "I wouldn't let that stop me from doing what I wanted." And, "Really? I don't smell anything!" (in reference to his oil plug-ins).

The social pressures arise mostly from the fact that there is no education about these chronic, invisible conditions and people generally have absolutely no understanding of what the condition is, much less an appreciation of what might be done to help or include us in community life. For example, having unscented soap in public washrooms would improve accessibility, and thus inclusion, for those of us with MCS.

Before my illness, I was a struggling single parent raising two challenging, ill children. I upgraded my credentials to qualify for a job in a new business sector. My goal was to be able to provide for myself and my children. My children are now living on their own.

My goal now is to be able to provide for myself, financially, and this has been quite a struggle. But my goal is also to take better care of myself—to rest when I need to and do what I can when I can. No more alarm clocks. No more rushing. It used to be that the only times I was able to attain peace were when we were camping as a family in the summer. Now I live in a park year-round and nature is my source of spirituality. ❖❖❖

❖ ❖ ❖

We hope these first four chapters have opened your eyes to the bigger picture of FM and CFS. These illnesses are complicated and at times confusing, but hopefully, in reading these chapters, you will have begun to think about your own symptoms and recognize yourself in some of the patients we have featured. As you begin to have a greater understanding of your illness, you can start to think about building a treatment program. In the following pages, we'll show you how to develop a treatment program that will help you live well with your illness.

Chapter 5

Healing Begins with You

It is okay, and even normal, to feel weak and helpless when you're sick. The trouble comes when you define your *self as weak and helpless, rather than your physical experience. You are still the strong and powerful person you were before the illness. This is so hard to remember. You certainly don't feel powerful! But, tell me, how can a weak and helpless person contribute anything towards their own healing?*

— Diane Kerner
From *My Own Medicine:*
The Process of Recovery from Chronic Illness

SOMETHING AMAZING has happened in the last few years—FM and CFS have come out of the closet. In 1999, when the first edition of this book was published, there weren't many books available on these conditions. Now you can find everything from cookbooks to books written by physicians who themselves are living with FM and CFS. It's also possible to find a wealth of information by visiting websites or by chatting online with other patients.

The media too are paying more attention, gradually legitimizing FM and CFS in the minds of the public. Today, it seems most people know someone who has one or both of these illnesses. This is a great thing—the more people who understand FM and CFS, the better for patients.

While the public images of FM and CFS have changed, we patients haven't changed a bit. The typical FM and/or CFS patient is still a hard-working, high-achieving person, struck down in the prime of their life by an illness that completely changes everything.

For us to live well, we must begin the healing process right where it should start—with ourselves.

❧ A State of Mind

When you look inside yourself for healing, see yourself as you were at the healthiest time of your life. Focus on how happy and healthy you were then. That is the best place to begin your healing journey.

Make the decision to live the best life possible in spite of your illness. Find inside yourself the ability to sustain a positive mind-set. Your body's natural state is one of complete health. If you do everything you can to bring about a healthy life, you will be better able to fight FM and CFS.

Mari S. says, "There are days when I just can't fight the pain of FM. Those are the days I stay home and try to keep my mind off the pain by reading or sleeping. I need several days a week to be alone and to relax by myself in order to make the best of the rest of the week. I know that keeping a positive attitude is very important—just as important as the medication I take and the exercises I do every day."

YOUR NEW LIFE

Your new life begins to take shape in the first year after your diagnosis. It is crucial to begin your treatment program right away. Studies show people with FM and CFS have the best chance for healing in the first few years after onset.

Living with a chronic illness requires organization, determination, and a whole lot of patience. Chances are, it's taken a while to get your diagnosis. Now is the time to do everything you can to better understand your illness. Decide what has top priority. Will you see a doctor of conventional medicine, a naturopathic doctor, or perhaps both? Do you want to consult a specialist? Will you consider medication, supplements, or a combination? Which alternative treatments will you use?

Dr. James Robinson of the University of Washington's Pain Clinic told us he encourages his FM patients to be good managers of their own illness. He makes an analogy with diabetes management: "Diabetes is a disorder where we as physicians can only help to a certain extent; there's an awful lot left that we can't do. The patient has to be intimately involved with their treatment and work very, very hard to mitigate the adverse effects of diabetes. I think FM is a similar thing. So I try to get the patients involved so they are devoting all of their resources to getting as well as they can with this condition."

RESEARCHING YOUR ILLNESS

Your first responsibility is to find out all there is to know about your illness. Researching your own illness is not just a smart thing to do—it could save you money, time, and in some cases even your life. If you had heart disease and were told you needed open-heart surgery, wouldn't you want to know all you could about the other treatments available? If your life were on the line, it's guaranteed you would make time for research and perhaps talk to others who had undergone the same procedure that you need. Almost all the practitioners we talked with remarked on how well informed their FM and CFS patients are. The better informed you become, the greater your sense of empowerment. It's up to you to find the best practitioners and treatments for yourself. Take a proactive stance towards your illness. This means standing up for yourself. Ultimately, you are the person who knows the most about your body, and with a little research you can also be well versed in your illness.

❖ Choosing the Right Doctor

Choosing a doctor is one of the most important decisions you will make. What qualities are you looking for in a doctor? Do you want a primary-care physician to work closely with you to find medications and treatment? Do you need a specialist? Will this specialist be seen primarily for medication?

When you find the right doctor, relax and focus on taking good care of yourself while your doctor points you in the right direction. No matter what your doctor's specialty, if you are comfortable and trust him or her, you have made a good match. One of the best ways to find a good physician is by asking for references at a support group. Often, support groups have lists of doctors who understand FM and CFS and treat their patients with care.

Dr. Martin Ross feels that the medical community is too quick to discount the experiences of people with CFS because they don't know how to diagnose or treat the condition: "Many people with CFS are very fearful of being misunderstood and dismissed by the health professionals they see. Most important for people with this condition is that they have a forum where they feel heard and supported in their experience. This requires more than the standard 10 to 15 minute visit provided by most medical professionals."

Erin P. is still looking for a primary-care provider who fits her needs. "I'm extremely motivated to do my own research and educated experimen-

69

tation," she says. "If I could find an excellent primary-care provider who would be willing and able to work collaboratively with me and act as my coach or mentor in this process, I would be so happy."

❧ The Doctor-Patient Relationship

It is important to be able to talk with your doctor easily and openly. If you feel you can't communicate with your doctor, it is time to find a new practitioner with whom you are comfortable. The doctor-patient relationship must be built on trust, respect, and confidence.

The right doctor for you is the one who listens, cares, and actively participates in your healing. Naturopath JoAnna Forwell from Bastyr University in Seattle, Washington, agrees: "I often hear my patients express relief to know that they have been heard when they come to a doctor's office to tell their story. Paying careful attention to a patient's history and getting a comprehensive picture of the case is crucial when dealing with complex conditions such as FM and CFS. It is essential that the diagnosis be as accurate as possible, because the success of the treatment depends on it."

How does one know when they've found the right doctor? Dayle R., from Lower Hutt, New Zealand, says, "Finally, I was being heard. I was being treated with dignity and respect. I was believed. And I was being helped."

Karin L.'s primary-care provider understands that there is more to her than her illness. "I am always amazed that she has the time to take a couple of minutes to talk about the nonmedical aspects of my life," says Karin. "That affects the quality of my care immensely. There have been times when her best medicine is a hug."

❧ Your Rights and Responsibilities as a Patient

YOUR RIGHTS

As a patient, you have the right to expect honesty, confidentiality, and respect from your physician and the staff at the clinic. You also have a right to be told the fee schedule, billing information, the availability of your doctor, and the hours the clinic will be staffed. You have the right to talk to your doctor for at least 15 minutes. (Some naturopathic physicians and acupuncturists provide visits of 30 minutes or longer.) This should be enough time for a follow-up appointment to discuss what has worked over the time between visits and to make any changes to your treatment plan. While you must be understanding regarding emergency situations, you have a right to be seen close to your appointment time. Most importantly, you have the right to skilled and compassionate care.

If you believe that you need more care than the doctor can give, seek a second opinion or find another physician. Legally, you have the right to request copies of all your records. As long as your account is up-to-date, you should have no problem getting copies of the paperwork or your records. If you are still making payments on your account, your new doctor can request the records.

THE RESPONSIBILITIES OF A PATIENT

In this age of managed care, doctors are busier than ever and often need to rush patients through their appointments. Doctors must see as many patients as deemed possible by the company they work for, but we have to remind ourselves that doctors don't like this situation any more than we do. So, being on time for your appointment is a good habit to get into. Respect goes both ways in the doctor-patient relationship.

Prepare for your appointment by writing out a list of concerns before you go. Be sure to bring a list of all your medications, their dosages, and schedule. If this appointment is a follow-up for a new drug or treatment, be ready to talk about any changes you have noticed in your condition since starting the regimen. If you are having side effects, discuss them with your doctor. Be prepared for your doctor to suggest changing medications or dosages, or trying an additional drug. Consider these possibilities before you get to the doctor's office; this way you can use the in-office time to come up with a plan that works for both you and your doctor.

Be as organized as you can. If your pain medication prescription needs to be written out each month, remember to give your doctor a couple of days notice. Even if you just need to pick up a sample of the medication, call ahead; the doctor's staff will appreciate you for it.

If you have an issue you wish to talk about with your doctor between visits, be prepared to leave a message or talk to your doctor's assistant. If your issue is very important, say so in the message. Remember, the more you say while leaving the message, the more complete the response will be. Be patient; it may take a day or so for the doctor to call back. In an emergency, call 911. You or someone else can notify your doctor later, after the crisis has passed.

If you are having a flare-up and need advice or additional medication, be sure to ask a friend or family member to call your doctor's office for you, particularly if you are unable to make the call. If you are living with a

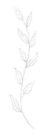

71

chronic illness, no matter your age, it is wise to choose someone to speak on your behalf, just in case you become too ill to speak for yourself. Most doctors' offices and hospitals can help you obtain the correct paperwork to authorize this and will give you information on how to complete the forms.

❖ Your Healing Team

You are the number one member of your healing team. The part you play is of the utmost importance because you will ultimately have the final decision on your treatment.

A primary-care physician, a specialist, and a chiropractor or acupuncturist form the basic core group of care providers for most of the patients we interviewed. On top of this "main team," patients added yoga teachers, Reiki practitioners, massage therapists, and more, depending on which illness they were living with, how much their insurance covered, and how much they could afford to spend out-of-pocket.

"I have a great deal of faith in my doctors—they are well educated and know how to help me take care of my body," says Regina L., an FM patient from Kenosha, Wisconsin. "I feel that they are dedicated and do their homework to keep up-to-date on what is happening with FM and CFS. Most importantly they use a holistic approach. I rely on my chiropractor, rheumatologist, and psychiatrist to all work together, so that the left hand knows what the right hand is doing."

Each practitioner on your healing team has his or her own specialty and brings that expertise to your treatment program. Your primary-care physician cares for your body, your specialist cares for your illness, and your therapist cares for your mind. Together as a whole, your team provides a strong foundation. Instead of being someone who "suffers" from FM or CFS, someone who is weighted down and debilitated by your illness, your team can help you become someone "living" with FM or CFS, finding joy and fulfillment in life.

❖ A Patient's Story: Carola M.

Carola M. is 61 years old and lives in Moonee Ponds, Australia. Carola was diagnosed with FM in 1994. Her healing team currently includes her family doctor, a chiropractor, an acupuncturist, a fitness instructor, and a massage therapist.

I had persistent pain in my upper arms at first, which then spread to my shoulders. My doctor initially thought it was some kind of arthritis that would resolve itself. I had the pain for about four months and it did not get better. I belong to the Victorian Arthritis Association, and in its quarterly newsletter there was an article on fibromyalgia—I was amazed at how many of the symptoms fit what I was experiencing.

I saw my local GP shortly after reading the article and the longer we discussed my symptoms and what he knew of FM, the more convinced we both were that we had discovered what my problem was. It hit me hard and I was very worried about what the future had in store for me.

The pain has gradually moved across my whole body, including my feet. Bushwalking [hiking] or long walks are not possible at this point—likewise, repetitive gardening activities like digging, weeding big areas, cutting lawn edges, and carrying anything heavy. I have to work in short spurts and rest in between activities. This is a very hard thing to have to adjust to, after always having been fit and strong. My husband has taken over cleaning the house, as it is too taxing for my body. It is also hard to stay positive and outwardly happy at times when the pain really hits.

I am lucky to have a family doctor who has been looking after my family since 1978; I trust him and respect him, and he has always taken my symptoms seriously. He tries very hard to think of something new that could help, but feels frustrated that he does not have the magic potion I would love for him to have.

I suffer from irritable bowel syndrome and I have chronic sleep problems. During flare-ups I get "brain fog" to the point that I am scared to drive my car because my reaction time and judgment are impaired. Restless legs trouble me at times—mainly when I am extra-tired.

I go to water aerobics once a week. This is the only exercise I can do safely without getting too sore afterwards. I have an excellent leader who makes sure the whole body gets a workout without getting overworked. I find the stretching and toning exercises very beneficial and these classes have become an important part of looking after myself.

I have been having remedial massage therapy every fortnight for many years now. I have found a very good massage therapist who has studied various techniques, and she can feel where the tension is and what needs to be treated each time. It is very painful, but it helps to relax my neck, shoulders, and back muscles, and I get worse if I stop the massages.

Acupuncture has also helped me over the years. At one stage, I had constant pain in my legs, which nearly drove me mad; a series of acupuncture treatments almost eliminated that pain. My head and neck pain is also helped by acupuncture. I am currently having a series of treatments to stabilize my mind and body; the frequency of flare-ups has decreased and I seem to be coping better even after a night of bad sleep. Again, I have found a therapist who is very caring and tries hard to work out a program for my particular problems. Recently, we have been experimenting with stimulating a couple of points in my right ear to ease the pain in my feet—and my feet have improved!

I have learned that every case of FM is different and the condition itself is up-and-down in any given individual. Some days coping is really hard; other days life is not so bad. I personally try hard to focus on the positives in my life: family (especially the joy of seeing my grandchildren grow up), having a nice home and no desperate money worries, having a stable marriage, a few good friends, and coming to terms with the fact that there will be bad days, but they will pass. ❖❖❖

❖ Really Resting

Resting is a big part of the perfect day. An afternoon nap helps you feel better and gives you the energy to get through the evening. When you live with FM or CFS, it is vital to schedule rest times and stick to them. Decide if a few catnaps make enough of a difference or if a longer nap is needed after lunch. Remember, watching television or playing video games is not resting!

Leave your worries outside your bedroom door. If you are lying comfortably in bed but letting your mind wander, mulling over every worry of the day, you are not resting.

Imagine cutting into a grapefruit, pink and full of juice. Now, what just happened? Did you get shivers down your spine and a tart, tangy feeling in your mouth? Images can seem surprisingly real. That, in a nutshell, is what happens to your body and mind when you are thinking about your daily worries. You have a physical reaction as a result of the scenario you experience in your mind. It is imperative to separate your rest time from your worrying time. Give yourself fifteen minutes a day to worry. Just worry and worry the whole time and see where it gets you. There's not one thing that comes out of worrying except tight muscles and fatigue. It does your body so much more good to rest and recuperate.

Deborah A., an FM patient from Grafton, Massachusetts, says, "The way I cope is by trying to get out and get fresh air or a walk when I least feel like it. It's so easy to stay in bed, keep your pjs on, and sip tea. Even a trip to the coffee shop or grocery store and a conversation with the clerk can make you feel like you're still part of the world. But there's always the struggle of balance—when do I need to rest and when do I need to push myself just a bit?"

SETTING BOUNDARIES

One of the hardest things to learn after being diagnosed with FM or CFS is how to establish boundaries for yourself. It is difficult to say no to friends when they want to go out at night for a movie or a drink (but you know that for you, it could take several days of rest to recover). Even little things may seem uncomfortable at first—like pointing out your limits when going for a walk with a friend. However, you need to let your friends know when you just feel up to walking a short way.

Robin N., an FM patient from Tucson, Arizona, says, "Set small goals. Focus on whatever it is you are able to do and build on it in small increments. Allow yourself time to *be*—rather than to *do*. Enjoy the solitude and sit outside in the sunshine whenever possible. Be grateful."

STRESS

Stress is a buzzword that's been around since the superbusy 1980s, when being "stressed out" was an international pastime. Think of Japanese business people being profiled as the most stressed out workers—or was it air traffic controllers? Or postal workers? (We vote for writers.)

Stress is a physiological response that affects all of us differently. Stress will exacerbate your FM or CFS symptoms tenfold. Think about it; if stress leads to fatigue in people who *don't* have a chronic illness, imagine what it can do to you.

Carola M. says, "I know that stress at work or at home makes my condition worse, so I try my hardest to minimize stress of every kind. I try not to get upset over small things and generally to keep my life as stress-free as possible."

When we relax, our heart rate and our blood pressure go down, blood travels toward internal organs, breath rate decreases, blood sugar levels balance out, and our digestion is better. The relaxation response also stimulates our immune system to promote healing. Put simply, relaxation is good for you.

75

❧ Your Energy Bank

Sometimes even the best-laid plans go awry—the importance of being organized cannot be overstated. For example, planning ahead can make or break a vacation. Even a day trip that has been carefully planned can help you stay on schedule with your medications and allow you to make good food choices. If you are traveling a long distance by car, make sure you take a break every hour or so. Get out and walk around, do a few stretching exercises, and remember to drink enough water to keep hydrated. A bag filled with another layer of clothing, a few snacks, and a day's worth of medication can be a lifesaver. A cell phone is invaluable. If by chance you get stuck somewhere and become too exhausted to drive, you can call for help or at least let your family and friends know you are taking a break and resting before continuing your journey. Make sure your traveling companions understand your illness before you leave home. It's too late once you're on the road and you find that you can't keep up with their hectic itinerary.

Monitor your energy expenditure, taking into account what you did the day before and any appointments you must fulfill the next day. This will help you decide if staying an extra hour at a friend's house or running all your errands at once is possible. If so, then by all means do it and have fun, but remember what you spend today may be a loan from tomorrow's energy bank.

Chandy W. from Shelbyville, Tennessee, says, "I am a 'giver,' so I have had to learn to say no. And now I purposefully choose what I am willing to pay the price for doing. In other words, I have learned that stress (whether it is good or bad) brings on higher pain levels and saps my strength. So I mindfully choose which activities are worth the sacrifice, knowing that the consequence is being out of commission for two to three days."

In her book *My Own Medicine*, Diane Kerner concurs, "Make whole blank days on your calendar a goal. If it's a work day, see about staying in that night. If I plan any activity for the better part of one day, I leave the next day blank so that I can be quiet and rest. Remember that you will be able to loosen up on these changes once you are better. It's just for now, for you."

❧ Driving: When Is It Time to Pull Over?

If you are sleepy, tired, or have just started a new medication, do not drive! An estimated 50 percent of all fatal accidents are caused by drivers falling asleep at the wheel. In addition, many states have a law very much like DUI

(Driving While Under the Influence of Alcohol) that says if you are caught driving under the influence of drugs (even if they are prescribed for you by your doctor), you can get a hefty fine. You have to make the decision. If there is the slightest doubt in your mind, don't drive. Call someone to come and pick you up, stay overnight at a friend's house, take a cab, or book a hotel room—but do not get behind the wheel.

❖ ❖ ❖

The impetus for living well with FM and CFS has to come from within— you need to be your own best friend. The next step is to think about your relationships with your family and friends. If you've had a hard time adjusting to life with your illness, this may be a process of reconnection for you. Many of our respondents told us they felt disconnected from their family and friends—even those they were closest to sometimes didn't seem to understand their illness. Deborah A., from Grafton, Massachusetts, says, "My best friend and I joke that many people in our families don't even know how to pronounce 'fibromyalgia,' never mind trying to understand what it is and how we struggle. We call it 'fibromyopia,' the inability to see what their loved ones are really dealing with." In our next chapter, we'll look at those exasperating, loving, caring people we call family and friends.

Chapter 6

Family and Friends

A sense of humor can be a great help—particularly a sense of humor about oneself.

— Dwight D. Eisenhower

W E ALL WANT TO FIT in and be accepted for who we are, especially when we have a chronic illness. Living with FM or CFS can bring stress to our relationships with families, friends, and coworkers. Patients often look well, making it difficult for people to understand just how debilitating FM and CFS can be. Yet inevitably, the lives of your loved ones are going to be touched by your illness.

Just talking with an understanding person can help ease the stress of a particularly bad day. It can be hard to find confidants you can trust with your worries and frustrations, especially if your life before FM or CFS revolved around your career. It is extremely important for a newly diagnosed patient to have a good support network, whether it's a group of friends to talk with when the going gets rough, family to rally round you in times of need, or coworkers to offer kind words. Checking in with someone once a day, especially during flare-ups or other difficult times, keeps you connected and reminds you that there is life beyond pain and fatigue.

✤ Your Friendship Bank

Several counselors told us they encourage their FM and CFS patients to come up with a list of at least five people who can be counted on to help weather the storm. The thought is that if you have at least five people in your "friendship bank," you won't burn out one particular friend or family member. Even the most stalwart friend can grow tired of being a sole supporter. No matter how much they care about you, no one wants to hear about your FM or CFS all of the time—besides there's so much more to you than just your illness.

You could fill your friendship bank with a number of people from different areas of your life: for example, a support group member, a close friend, someone in your family, a friend from your place of worship, and a neighbor. Having a diverse support network means you'll have friends who can help you out at different times of day and with different types of problems. Remember, you also have lots to offer, and you can be an invaluable part of others' friendship banks.

But what if you are alone and feel as though you have no one to talk to? There are many ways to connect with people who understand your illness and would like to be part of your friendship bank. An online chat group can become a lifeline. Any time, day or night, there are groups talking about FM and CFS all across the world. Jeri-Lynn K. of Long Beach, California, told us the online community of FM and CFS patients has given her the inspiration and support she needs: "I could kvetch at will, via my keyboard, and I could actually feel them nodding their heads in understanding," she says.

If you don't have a computer, you may be able to use the computers at your local library free of charge. If you don't know how to use the computer, try signing up for a computer class (you may even meet a member of your friendship bank there). Call your local hospital and inquire about FM or CFS support groups; you could join one or be the first to start one in your area.

Gaye B. from Papakura, New Zealand, says, "We have a small group of fibro folk here in Papakura that meet every few months and these meetings are so wonderful—we all understand each other and have the same limitations and pains. I think we might make these meetings monthly because they benefit us all."

It's a great idea for people with FM and CFS to get together and *talk*. Talk about what works for you and what doesn't. Get out the fear and frustration these invisible illnesses bring you. Your support group may consist of a group of FM and CFS patients who meet regularly at a local clinic. Or it could be a potluck lunch club that meets once a month to discuss new treatments and the work of local doctors. It could be a group of people who get together to discuss how to live with a chronic illness and still be a vital part of the community. Your support group can be anything you want it to

79

be. All that matters is that you find an outlet to talk about the frustrations, concerns, and difficulties of living with your illness.

✤ Helping Your Friends and Family Understand Your Illness

Before you explain your illness to your loved ones, be sure *you* understand and accept the diagnosis yourself. Learn all you can about your illness until you are comfortable talking about it with others. As Robin N. told us, "Before I got sick, I thought the solution to FM was to just push oneself to overcome it—until it happened to me, and now I know better."

No matter how close you are to your family and friends, it can be difficult to tell them you have a chronic illness—and they may not always understand. Linda M. from Edmonds, Washington, says, "My family kept expecting (or wanting) me to be the same person I was before. FM isn't always obvious, like a broken leg or a missing limb, so it's easy for others to forget we're in chronic pain—especially if we take care of our physical appearance."

It doesn't have to be so hard to tell your friends and family you have FM or CFS. After all, you've been there for them during the ups and downs of their lives. Remember, most people want to know what they can do to help when a friend or family member is confronted with such a life-altering event. Don't be afraid to open up. You and your loved-ones will both benefit from the experience.

Talk about your illness in a way that is easy to understand. You may want to invite your family and friends to your support group. Just being in the presence of others with the same illness may do wonders to help them realize what you are going through. Most support groups set aside time during their meetings to allow each member to speak. When your friends and family hear people talk about their fatigue and pain in much the same way that you do, it can be an eye-opening experience for them.

If someone has difficulty understanding and accepting your illness after all your best efforts, you may find that you just have to let go. Beth O. from Louisville, Kentucky, describes this experience: "My family has been very supportive and loving. But I had friends who had no experience with chronic illness and were unable to be supportive. These people are no longer a part of my life."

There is a saying, "Surround yourself with people who love you." This is particularly important if you are living with a chronic illness. You can't

afford to have people around you who don't understand you and have no patience. It's too draining—not just on your relationship with that person, but also on your health.

❖ Telling Your Partner

If you have been in a romantic relationship during your search for a diagnosis, chances are your partner is aware of what you have been going through. Still, it is important to set aside time to talk with him or her about the situation and decide how to go about making changes in your life together.

When one partner is healthy and the other is sick, it creates a physical and emotional imbalance in the relationship. The healthy partner may feel guilty if they go out by themselves because their partner feels too tired. The sick partner may worry about becoming a burden. The healthy partner can find it frustrating if there isn't anything they can do to help, and they may feel ineffectual. The sick partner may worry that they will be left alone.

Having FM or CFS brings with it a sense of loss, as you long for the life you had before. When talking to your partner about your illness, you must realize that he or she will also experience this loss and will miss the way things used to be. Just like you, your partner will have plenty of questions and will want answers from your doctor. Your partner too must respond to other people's remarks, such as, "Why doesn't he work?" or, "She's just being lazy." Sometimes those statements come from within the family or from people you considered friends.

Tell your partner everything that is going on. Make sure he or she understands they aren't being asked to fix this problem. Tell your partner your needs, but also tell them you will be there for them, just as you have always been.

Beth O. says, "I learned many important lessons from FM. I learned to ask my husband for help and to gracefully accept help. I became more interdependent with him, which helped us grow closer in our marriage."

Involve your partner as you educate yourself about FM and CFS. Have your partner accompany you to your doctor's appointment. Read a book or two together on FM and CFS (perhaps this one), or do some online research. You could both join a support group that includes family and friends of patients. When it comes to talking about your illness with your partner, remember that the challenges in our lives can make our relationships stronger.

❖ Having a Sexual Relationship

Being disabled or living with a chronic illness doesn't have to limit our sexuality, as long as there is love and the willingness to have a relationship. Through planning, creativity, and openness with one another, we can usually overcome any situation. However, before you can be cherished by another, you must learn to cherish yourself. You are still the same person you were before your diagnosis. You have the same wants and needs. Now you must give yourself and your partner time to understand what is happening to you.

Talking with your lover about the changes in your body can be a way of becoming intimate. Try to look at this time of learning as a way to become even closer, rather than as a list of the ways in which your body has betrayed you. Changes in your skin texture, loss of hair, and weight gain or loss can result from medication side effects. Let your partner know if you are experiencing these problems and work together to come to a place of understanding.

"There have been times when I am too tired or too achy to enjoy intimate relations," says Susan M. "But my husband has been so supportive of me and helps me through these situations. He understands the issues and makes an effort to accommodate me when we are intimate, in order to minimize the pain."

Being in pain doesn't make you feel very sexy, but there are ways to get past your symptoms and have a healthy sex life. First, consider what time of day you feel your best. Is it in the morning, when you feel most rested, or is it at night when you've had time to relax? Time your medication so that you have the least amount of pain when it's time to make love.

Making an occasion out of lovemaking can relax both of you and take your mind off your symptoms. Intimate rituals, such as lighting candles and playing "your" song, can remind you that this is your special time and place together. Make sure your sanctuary has lots of pillows for comfort and support.

Early on in your love making, stimulation and pressure can bring on pain. Remind your partner of the places that hurt. Encourage soft stimulation with a light touch. Reassure your lover that you will make it known if you are too tired to make love or if you are experiencing pain or discomfort during lovemaking—your partner will appreciate your openness. Simply discussing your needs will go a long way towards creating the bond that will get you both through this new part of your life. Remember, this is a time to slow down and be close. Put thoughts of pain and fatigue out of your mind, and enjoy sharing your love.

❖ Children of FM and CFS Patients

Tracy G. says, "Will I be so tired I can't get off the couch? Will my back hurt so much I have to almost overdose on pain meds? I used to be able to plan my days; now I have to wait and see how I feel. I tell that to my children when they ask, 'Can we go to this place on Friday?' 'We will have to wait and see how Mommy feels.' What kind of life is that? I hope they don't grow up to hate me because Mommy never felt like doing anything."

Children can get upset when you are not able to take part in an activity you had planned to do together. But it's really the quality of time together that counts with children. Your kids just want to be with you. You don't have to play rough and tumble games all the time for kids to enjoy being with you.

Be as honest as possible with your children, using simple language they can understand. For example, to a little kid, every illness is "catching." They may worry that they'll catch FM and CFS from you.

Emphasize all the things Mommy, Daddy, or Grandma *can* do and not just what you cannot do. If you have FM, try showing a child a picture of the tender points, and explain to them that those places hurt. You may be surprised at how understanding children can be.

Show them how they can help you when you're not feeling well. Kids like to help. Children can be very observant; it's best to be as honest as you can with them.

Talk with your children about FM or CFS several times during each phase of childhood. Remind them that your illness is just one part of you and that it is nobody's fault. When the kids are older they may resent the time your illness takes to manage each day and how it competes with them for your attention. This should clue you in to the fact that your kids are growing up. If they're old enough to resent your illness, they're old enough to go to a support group with you, read a book on FM and CFS, or explore some of the many excellent websites that are available (see the Resources section for some suggestions). Understanding their parent's illness is an important life lesson, and part of growing up that you can share.

Children have a huge capacity for love and understanding, and if you are honest and upfront with them, you might be amazed at the results.

✤ Your Circle of Friends

Beth O. confided to us:

> When I got sick, I often felt pressured because I was still young and was unable to go dancing with friends or stay up late anymore. I could no longer go to a late movie yet was often urged by friends to go with them, even though I told them that I was too sick to tolerate a long night out. I eventually let go of all the friendships I had before I became ill and formed new ones with people who understood my illness. I came to realize that no one can understand what it is like to be chronically ill unless one has been through it. I had to change my outlook on my abilities and expectations, even though it wasn't consistent with the attitude of my peers.

Friends come along throughout your life, loving and changing as you age. Chances are your closest friends are a variety of people with an amazing range of personalities. But you will probably find that once *you* accept your illness as part of your life, many of your friends will accept it too. After all, you are still you.

Friendships are a two-way street. Even though you are struggling with your illness, you still have to keep up your side of the friendship. Most friends do not like to always be the one to initiate times to get together and suggest activities to do. When you live with long-term pain, it changes your perspective on life—a healthy person may just want to curl up by the fire with a good book when they are having a temporary bout of pain, but when pain is a constant in your life, you simply have to decide if you are going to stay home or put yourself out in the world. If your close friends have a problem understanding and accepting your diagnosis, maybe it's not about you. Perhaps they are uncomfortable around pain and loss. Give them as much help as you can. Don't give up on them just because they seem to have difficulty at first. Give each of them time to evolve into the best friend they can be. As Susie S. explains, "I have to be the one to reach out and not be hurt because people have moved on with their lives and didn't reach *in* to me. I have to forgive people who don't understand chronic illness. I used to be one of them."

✤ A Patient's Story: Diane K.

Diane K. is 52 years old and works for Bastyr University in Seattle. She is author of the book *My Own Medicine: The Process of Recovery from*

Chronic Illness, which tells the story of her life with CFS and FM. Diane lives with her family in Seattle.

I don't think that most people who know me understand even slightly what I go through. Early in my illness I used to make an effort to explain my situation. In many cases I got the vibe that the other person figured I could just snap out of it if I really wanted to. I didn't like hearing myself complain any more than I liked some of the reactions I got, so I closed up and became more socially isolated. What I know now is that we all have to find our own way in our own time. It's been a valuable lesson and made me a better person.

My friends are my lifelines. When I need to talk about my health, I call one of several good friends who are also ill or a 'best-friend-forever' who is not ill, but who is compassionate, knowledgeable about medical issues, and who loves me absolutely unconditionally. In general, though, I try not to focus so much on being sick or talk about it too much. As the beloved George Harrison might say, "It's a drag, really."

I always have a hard time telling family and friends that I can't tolerate lengthy visits or phone calls. This alone is a big reason why people with CFS hang out with each other more than with their healthy friends. They don't need to explain as much—most of us are usually keenly aware and thoughtful of each other's limitations. How do you explain that just having a visitor in the room, no matter how much you care about them, is tiring?

My husband helps a lot when I am going through periodic rough times. During a relapse I can't even fathom being on my own. My husband does the driving and takes care of dinner. He offers companionship and relief from boredom. He is a blessing and I know I am fortunate. However, it's difficult for my husband to deal with my illness—he is always afraid I will have a severe relapse and go back to the point where I am acutely ill, like I was for the first six years or so. There are a lot of things we don't do that we might otherwise, like enjoying nightlife. But I am fortunate because we both love our home and being with our dogs.

I try not to fall back into seeing myself as a victim when I have relapses, which can feel as devastating as ever. I often remind myself not to fear relapses. I have found that the fear I add makes it much more unbearable than it would be otherwise. That, at least, I can control. Other than my attitude, which can certainly be useful as a self-help tool, my illness has remained pretty consistent (meaning inconsistent—isn't that its nature?).

Before my illness I wanted to go to college and get my degree in child play therapy. I have tried to manage school twice since becoming ill and

85

have had to drop out. I still believe that a psychology degree would have been the best fit for me. I have a job, but it is not what I would have chosen to do had I felt I had limitless options.

I was much more active physically and socially before I became ill. I had my whole life ahead of me and all options were open. I sometimes become acutely aware of how I am not like everyone else. There are many things I simply can't do now, so the thought that I can do whatever I dream of has been lost. At the same time, I think that if you can be creative and flexible enough you might be able to do many of the things you want—you just might have to approach them differently. ❖ ❖ ❖

❖ Caregivers

During Mari S.'s early years of living with FM and CFS, she relied on her partner and family to help care for her when she had a flare-up. Sometimes, it was hard for her family to see that she needed the extra help. Mari's brother says, "I'd never heard of FM before, and I didn't know how to help her." Some of us need a full-time caregiver, a role that cannot always be filled by a family member. Caring for a loved one with a chronic illness takes time, patience, dedication, and a lot of love.

SIGNS OF CAREGIVER STRESS

If you are taking care of a family member with FM or CFS, remember to watch for signs of fatigue and depression in yourself. It takes a strong person to look after a chronically ill friend or family member. It's important to take time out for yourself to exercise and keep up with your regular routines. You may want to check your local hospital for classes that teach caregivers to take good care of themselves.

How to recognize when you need some time off:

❖ **Anger and irritability:** blowing up at the person who is sick. Anger is the flipside of fear. The fear and worry about your loved one's illness can sometimes get out of perspective and overwhelm you. Occasionally, you need to take a few days off from caring for your loved one.

❖ **Anxiety:** worrying about the future ("What will happen to my friend if I can't go on caring for him?") or being anxious about spending time away from your own family.

❖ **Withdrawal:** withdrawing from your own family and friends and becoming over-involved in the patient's life.

- ❖ **Sleep problems and exhaustion:** overworking, and having trouble sleeping because you are trying to do everything for the patient and also maintain your own health and responsibilities.
- ❖ **Decline in your own health:** caring for your loved one begins to take a toll on your own health; you're too busy to eat properly and get enough sleep.
- ❖ **Lack of concentration:** you're so distracted by your role as a caregiver that you find it difficult to perform everyday tasks such as paying your bills on time or buying groceries.

Richard S. and his wife are in their seventies. Richard is his wife Vivian's main caregiver, which turned the tables on the way things had been throughout their 59 years of marriage. "I was really worried about her. She used to do everything for me," says Richard. "Since she took care of the kids and the house, just about everything, I thought, I'd better get with it and help her as much as I could, any way I could."

Remember that your illness affects everyone in your family and your close circle of friends. No one who cares about you is immune to the stress that goes along with having FM or CFS. Keep in mind the principles we have covered in this chapter:

- ❖ Develop a friendship bank you can draw on when you need it.
- ❖ Help your loved ones to understand your illness.
- ❖ Talk openly and lovingly with your partner.
- ❖ Be honest with your children and talk to them in language they can easily understand.
- ❖ Appreciate your caregiver (and if you're the caregiver, take care of yourself too!).

No matter how well you explain FM or CFS, some family members may have difficulty accepting your limits. That's just the nature of illness and the nature of family life. If you put the principles of this chapter into play, you'll probably find it fairly easy to rekindle old friendships and to feel like a member of the family again. Wouldn't you like to be thought of as a good friend and cherished family member, rather than regret the time lost by keeping your distance? You are not your diagnosis; you are still the same person you always were—and your family and friends will welcome you back.

Chapter 7

Conventional Therapies

Pain is whatever the patient says it is.

— Scott Fishman, M.D., and Lisa Berger
From *The War on Pain*

We believe controlling our patients' pain is important. For that reason we will administer medication before, during, and after your pet's medical procedure to control pain, reduce discomfort, and promote recovery.

— A sign at Lien Animal Clinic, Seattle

MANY OF OUR RESPONDENTS told us they had the greatest success treating their illness when they combined conventional and alternative treatments in their FM and CFS management programs. "My doctor has taught me to never apologize to pharmacists or anyone else for having to take some of the medications I need to take," says Gerry L., an FM patient from Lemont, Illinois. "I have learned that there is a place for both traditional and alternative, or complementary, medicine, as I like to call it."

Most doctors or specialists will begin to treat FM and CFS by focusing on the symptoms best relieved through conventional means—symptoms such as sleep disorders, thyroid dysfunction, pain, depression, and biomechanical changes (for example, myofascial trigger points or postural-issues). A conventional treatment plan is not just a pharmacological approach. In addition to medications such as painkillers, sleep aids, antidepressants, and thyroid hormone replacements, your doctor may also refer you to a physical therapist and talk about something called "sleep hygiene."

In this chapter, Dr. Christopher Lawrence explains the importance of combining the most effective medications and finding the correct dose for each patient. Doctors James Robinson and Michael P. Young talk about pain management and the role of narcotic pain medication in FM and CFS, and Dr. Kim Bennett shows us how physical therapy can bring relief to painful joints and muscles. At the end of the chapter, you'll find some wonderful tips for achieving good sleep hygiene.

Please remember that the information in this chapter is not intended to be a substitute for talking with your doctor. However, we do hope it will help you to become as informed as you can possibly be. (See Appendix A for detailed information on the medications most commonly prescribed for FM and CFS.)

MANAGING YOUR MEDS

Many FM and CFS patients cannot tolerate regular doses of traditional medicines. "It's a slow process," says Dr. Christopher Lawrence. "Patients have to start at exceptionally low levels and gradually build up." Therefore, it is important to always have one doctor who is aware of all the medications you are taking and how they work together. In most cases this will be either your primary-care provider or your specialist.

MISTAKE-PROOF MEDICATION

❖ Remember to take your medications at the same time every day.
❖ Try using a container with compartments for each day of the week. Some even have compartments that hold medication for breakfast, lunch, dinner, and evening. You can get these plastic pill containers at your pharmacy. If you don't like to use pill containers, try numbering your pill bottles and making a spreadsheet to keep track of them (or a handwritten list if you prefer).
❖ A note in the cupboard where you store your medications will help you keep up with the refill dates. Develop a list of all your prescriptions, the date you last filled them, and when they need to be refilled. Make note of any changes your doctor has made for the month ahead. Be sure to schedule your refills several days before you run out of medication; that way, you allow for any delays and will not be stuck without a particular pill.

SLEEP: A HARD DAY'S NIGHT

A lack of restorative sleep aggravates FM and CFS symptoms, making just about everything feel more painful, tiring, and confusing. That's why tackling sleep disorders is your first line of defense in the battle against FM and CFS. There are many options when it comes to sleep medication, so you should be able to find a medication suited to your situation and needs.

Many healthy people use a sleep aid for just one or two nights at a time, perhaps because they have to get up extra early in the morning, or because they want to get some sleep on a red-eye flight. But patients with chronic conditions like FM and CFS often need long-term therapy. Sleep medications work for FM and CFS patients in two ways. First, they help you achieve restorative sleep, which in turn lessens the severity of your symptoms the next day. Secondly, because of their effect on the central nervous system, they play a role in decreasing the perception of pain as you're falling asleep.

Medications that help you sleep work mostly on your central nervous system. At bedtime, neurons (nerve cells) in the central nervous system (the brain and spinal cord) signal your body to relax and calm down, relieving anxiety and initiating sleep or drowsiness. The neurotransmitter GABA (gamma amino butyric acid) is the messenger that initiates this process of relaxation and sleep. There are a number of drugs that enhance the effects of GABA, creating a relaxed state that is conducive to sleep and rest. These medications include the benzodiazepines (e.g., Ativan and Valium), Ambien, and Sonata.

Older medications such as Ativan are still being used and are beneficial to many people, but newer sleep medications such as Ambien and Sonata are more popular now. These work quickly so you can get to sleep fast and, unlike the older medications, they don't last very long in the body so you are not left feeling sleepy in the morning. Lunesta works even faster (within five to ten minutes) and has been shown to be beneficial for use for up to six months.

Most FM and CFS patients have low levels of the neurotransmitter serotonin. Serotonin is made in the brain, derived from the amino acids in the protein we eat. The link between serotonin and mood is commonly acknowledged (serotonin brightens and stabilizes our moods, and low serotonin is a major cause of depression), but less well known is the important role serotonin plays in the management of appetite, pain perception, and sleep.

In *Beyond Prozac*, Michael J. Norden, M.D., likens serotonin to the brain's surrogate parent: "Like a good parent serotonin both discourages behavior that might get us in trouble and comforts us when trouble nevertheless arrives—soothing worry, pain, and most forms of stress."

Doctors frequently prescribe the selective serotonin reuptake inhibitor (SSRI) class of antidepressant, such as Paxil and Prozac, to regulate sleep. SSRIs prevent serotonin from being absorbed by nerve-endings, leaving it in the spaces surrounding the nerve endings, where it can be most effective. SSRIs are not an instant cure for sleep problems but are very effective over time. As Dr. Christopher Lawrence explains, "All the SSRIs initially disrupt sleep but once an individual has been on them for six to eight weeks, they sleep more deeply. This occurs because SSRIs help to regulate the whole serotonin metabolism and the primitive nervous system. The real action takes place in the autonomic nervous system because that is where people deal with stress."

Your doctor may want to try another class of antidepressant, called tricyclics (such as Elavil, Tofranil, or Sinequan). Tricyclic antidepressants work by increasing the levels of both serotonin and norepinephrine, which is another major neurotransmitter that helps regulate many of the body's systems. In contrast, SSRIs as their name implies, selectively inhibit serotonin only. This major difference affects not only the efficacy of the drug but also its potential for causing side effects. Tricyclics are weaker than SSRIs and tend to have a sedative effect on the body, which makes them more suited as a nighttime sleep aid. Be sure to find out which class of antidepressants you are taking, as this will have a bearing on the time of day you should take them.

YOUR THYROID

As we mentioned in Chapter 4, hypothyroidism is one of the most common disorders accompanying FM and CFS. Fatigue, weight gain, heavy menstrual periods, dry hair, and brittle nails are just a few of the bothersome symptoms that can be alleviated by thyroid hormone replacement therapy, using supplements such as Armour Thyroid or Synthroid. Your thyroid gland is your body's clock; it regulates everything, including your heartbeat. If your thyroid isn't working properly, your FM and CFS symptoms become aggravated. If you treat your thyroid dysfunction, you win part of the battle, and you will have increased energy and stamina.

PAIN: IT'S A PAIN

Suzan B., an FM patient from Seattle, has a small pill bottle in her purse marked "PAIN" in big blue letters. "It makes me smile when I pull it out," she says. "I think everyone needs a 'PAIN' bottle. But it is just a piece of my pain-management plan, which is so important to my survival."

There are several types of pain relievers (analgesics). Over-the-counter medications such as Tylenol (acetaminophen) are the most common pain relievers. However, they do not possess any anti-inflammatory properties.

Nonsteroidal anti-inflammatory drugs (NSAIDs) are pain and inflammation relievers, and this group includes aspirin, ibuprofen, and naproxen. NSAIDS, however, do not tend to be very effective for FM and CFS patients, except as a relief for headaches. Other categories of pain medications include COX-2 inhibitors, which are selective NSAIDS, mu receptor antagonists, muscle relaxants, corticosteroids for inflammation, and narcotics for severe pain.

Together, you and your doctor can make the choice of which pain medication is right for you. If one pain medication doesn't work, your doctor may suggest another one, or a combination. For example, MS Contin is a long-acting pain medication, and Oxycodone is short acting, with its effects lasting only four to six hours. Many doctors successfully prescribe MS Contin several times a day as needed and Oxycodone for breakthrough pain.

✤ Perspectives for Pain Management

BY DR. JAMES ROBINSON, M.D.

Dr. Robinson is a clinical associate professor in the Department of Rehabilitation Medicine at the University of Washington and an attending physician at the University of Washington Pain Center. Dr. Robinson also spent 11 years in private practice, specializing in musculoskeletal pain.

I became interested in pain through my personal experiences with it—I played a lot of sports when I was younger and had many injuries. Prior to going to medical school, I got my Ph.D. in psychology, so I was used to the idea that we don't always have clear-cut, objective measures of suffering. This is always the case with depression or anxiety, for example. We, as health-care practitioners, cannot necessarily see what is going on. The challenge that many physicians have when working with pain is this lack of visibility of the experiences people report.

I went into rehabilitation medicine in large part because I felt that in order to understand and treat pain, one really has to know something about the biological basis, the medical basis of pain, as opposed to just the psychological and psychiatric basis.

We treat a wide range of pain problems at the University of Washington Pain Center. Because this is a hospital setting, there is an enormous diversity in the types of people who come here and the disorders we treat; our patients include people with very serious conditions, such as spinal cord injuries. In many instances, what we do at the pain clinic, like everyone else in the health-care field, is determined by the financial resources and insur-

ance coverage of the patients we are treating. If we have, for example, an individual who has health coverage that includes mental health benefits and they are having some struggles coping with their FM, I would involve a pain psychologist. But many folks come in and they simply don't have that coverage. So, unfortunately, our decisions are frequently not based on the clinical needs of the patient, but more on the resources that are available.

I give my new FM patients an article called *Management of Fibromyalgia Syndrome* by Don Goldenberg [see Bibliography], which is a comprehensive review of the therapeutic approaches to FM that have a research background. I say, "I want you to review this, I want you to think about which, if any, of these approaches you've been involved in, and which ones make sense, and then let's talk about it." That paper is not meant to be an editorial in any way, but it simply shows that the approaches that work the best tend to be those that really engage people—including cognitive behavioral therapy, regular exercise, and medications. But I want my patients to look carefully, to do the homework, to relate the concept in this paper to their experience and come back with a plan.

Here at the University of Washington Pain Center, we are primarily involved with helping physicians in the community to do their job as well as possible. We can, for example, start FM patients on different therapeutic regimens, but their care then transfers to the community physician. FM is a condition where you have to look at the long run. It isn't enough to say, does the person feel better because they got a massage treatment that afternoon? That's really not what we're interested in. What we're interested in is are they functioning better six months later? ❖❖❖

❖ Finding a Winning Combination for FM

BY DR. CHRISTOPHER LAWRENCE, M.D.

Dr. Lawrence is a neurologist with a special interest in fibromyalgia. He has a private practice in Seattle.

In my experience, there is no one medication that works for all the symptoms of FM. If medical studies show that a medication doesn't work for FM, in most cases, it just means that the medication was not combined appropriately, or that the dosage was not tailored specifically to the individual patient. In order to treat FM effectively, we need to find the right combination of medications that balance each other out, so people feel better and function more normally.

93

FM is a vicious cycle—when a patient's sleep becomes disrupted and they become less active physically, they lose aerobic conditioning, so they cut back further on their exercise, they sleep poorly, and on and on. The key part of treatment is to find a combination of medicines that helps to normalize the patient's neurochemistry so they can achieve restorative sleep, wake up rested, and thus be more physically active.

SLEEP

Simply knocking a person out at night, while it may induce better sleep, doesn't improve their daytime functioning and can leave them feeling sedated. For that reason, I rarely use prescription sleep aids, because they tend to leave patients feeling somewhat groggy when they wake up. Instead I often prescribe antidepressants or the muscle relaxants Flexeril and Zanaflex. However, there is one prescription sleep aid, Rozerem (ramelteon), which is showing some promise for sleep without much daytime sedation. It works on the melatonin receptor in the brain.

NECK AND JAW TENSION

Many people with FM experience neck and jaw tension, which we refer to as "clenching." The anti-anxiety drug BuSpar (buspirone) seems to work best for this, but in order to be effective BuSpar must be taken in combination with either an SSRI or tricyclic antidepressant. It is important for the dosage of these two classes of medication to be well balanced, as most antidepressants have a tendency to aggravate clenching.

The dose of BuSpar required to treat muscle clenching is often far less than that needed to treat anxiety. The typical dose for anxiety is 30 mg a day; in contrast, I find most FM patients get relief from clenching on a nighttime dose of between 2.5 mg and 5 mg (some FM patients can't even tolerate a dose that low because they experience side effects such as nightmares, agitated sleep, or a feeling of being drugged the next day). On the other hand, if the patient has a great deal of anxiety, then I increase the BuSpar to a full dose over the course of a few months. This helps the anxiety, and it also helps the antidepressant work better. Many people who suffer from muscle clenching also develop plantar fasciitis, which is inflammation of the fascia in the sole of the foot. This group of muscles also responds best to BuSpar. A calcium and a magnesium/malic acid supplement, taken in addition to BuSpar, can help with bruxism (teeth grinding), another condition that often accompanies FM.

If a patient cannot tolerate BuSpar, I recommend a medicine like Mirapex. Developed for the treatment of Parkinson's disease, Mirapex works in

FM patients to treat restless legs syndrome, and it also helps with clenching symptoms. Another medicine for the treatment of clenching is the anti-seizure drug Keppra. The only drawback with Keppra is that some patients get very tired and moody, so I don't start people on that medication unless they are taking something to counteract moodiness, such as an antidepressant. Lithium, a drug often prescribed for bipolar disorder, also works well for clenching. I prescribe 5 mg of organic lithium to be taken at night for six to eight weeks (organic lithium is made from minerals and has few side effects). Some women respond better to true pharmaceutical lithium, especially those experiencing perimenopause (the transition period preceding menopause). At one-half or one-third of the normal dose, the side effects are fairly mild.

THE MUSCLES TELL THE STORY

I can tell from a patient's pattern of muscle tightness which class of medication they need. Each type of medication seems to relax certain muscle groups better than others. For example, SSRI antidepressants tend to relax the muscle along the back of the neck, shoulders, and upper back (the upper trapezius) as well as the muscles in the calves and feet. I have found that when one group of muscles starts to relax, the others follow.

Assessing muscle tightness also helps me determine the necessary dosage for each patient. If, after six weeks of treatment, I see that a patient's forearms and anterior chest wall are still too tight, I boost the dose of the SSRI. If the jaw and the hip-flexors are still tight, I boost the dose of BuSpar. I also adjust the dose of the nighttime medicine, depending on how groggy the patient feels in the morning and how they perceive their own sleep. It is interesting to observe how the different muscles react to different classes and doses of medicines. Everyone is a little different. Some people respond to a miniscule dose, and some people need a regular or higher dose.

WEATHER SENSITIVITY

Many people with FM become weather-sensitive. We've discovered that low doses of the muscle relaxants Flexeril or Zanaflex or low doses of doxepin (an antidepressant) given at night seem to improve weather-induced stiffness. Many of my patients take this class of medication from October until about May, when it's chilly and damp here in Seattle, or even during the summer if the weather warrants it.

If all the muscles respond to the medication except the muscles in the jaw, I get a TMJ (temporomandibular joint dysfunction) practitioner involved. However, I usually don't bring in these practitioners until the rest of the muscles are looser, and we know there is nothing more we can do with medication.

PAIN MEDS

If I have to rely on pain medications, it means I haven't found the right combination of other drugs to normalize the myofascial textures and to allow the patient to exercise more extensively. I prescribe pain medications occasionally, but only as a temporary measure. It usually takes three to four months for a patient who relies on pain medication to feel better and function well.

Anti-inflammatories are not very effective in treating FM pain, and few people are happy using only narcotics in the long term, because narcotics tend to be depressants and can interfere with one's thinking process. Additionally, over the course of several months, the effectiveness of narcotics seems to decrease. However, narcotics do play a role in the treatment of FM —in combination with other medications.

In my practice, I prescribe the whole spectrum of narcotics from short-acting Vicodin to Oxycontin and methadone. The narcotic Ultram (tramadol) is unusual in that it works better if the dosage is slowly built up and then maintained at a steady level, as opposed to taking it as needed, as you would a traditional pain pill. Ultram also boosts the neurotransmitters serotonin and norepinephrine.

ANTIDEPRESSANTS

Antidepressants can be used to treat pain, sleep disturbance, and depression. If a patient is particularly fatigued, I may prescribe Prozac in a low dose. Zoloft also works well; however, many women complain about its sexual side effects. These people seem to tolerate Celexa somewhat better. With antidepressants, we often start with a small dosage and build up slowly. If the patient has a true depressive component to their illness, then they need a full dose. If they have just myofascial pain, we can usually get by with less.

Another condition sometimes associated with FM is bipolar disorder (manic-depressive illness). These patients often report "feeling strange" after taking even a small dose of an antidepressant; they feel agitated and energized, which is a side effect that is the opposite of what is typical. In such cases, I often prescribe an anti-seizure drug instead of an antidepressant. I have had pretty good results with Lamictal, a seizure medication that slightly increases one's energy. It helps with bipolar disorder by stabilizing mood, and it also helps with FM pain. The dosage of Lamictal must be slowly increased because the drug can result in a very rare, but serious reaction called Stevens Johnson Syndrome, wherein the patient develops a severe rash involving the mucous membranes and has to be hospitalized. Lamictal increases clenching quite a bit, so patients need something to counteract the clenching as well, such as BuSpar. Lamictal can be very effective if patients have reacted abnormally to antidepressants in the past. It can sometimes be a more subtle way of helping the pain and mood without causing the patient to feel too "flat" or too "hyped-up."

In FM patients, antidepressants can sometimes be replaced by aerobic exercise. An hour to an hour and a half of exercise can reduce stress and lessen sleep disruptions. If the patient is managing stress effectively and everything else is okay, they can do fairly well without the medications or use significantly less medicine.

In the future, patients' biochemical tendencies will be analyzed by DNA microanalysis of their neurotransmitters and receptors—then a more appropriate combination and dosage range will hopefully be easier to find. At present, my rule of thumb is that people should be on the medications for a period of time equal to how long they've had FM. For example, if they've had FM for five years, then they're placed on the medications for at least five years. At that point, if they are able to engage in both aerobic and stretching exercises, such as tai chi or yoga, and if they are managing the stress in their life, then we get them off the medications. However, after being on the medications for a while, there are some patients whose muscles feel normal but they still have pain, and they have a lag period of several months until their brain acknowledges that there is no pain. There are often deeper psychological stresses in these patients, which we try to address.

The main thing patients tell me about how my treatment plan has helped them is that they are able to do more, without paying for it a day or two later with severe pain that requires bed rest. Basically, I know how they are doing by the amount of aerobic activity they can tolerate. And that's how I judge success—by the kind of life my patients are living. ❖❖❖

❖ Managing Pain with Narcotics

Deciding whether or not to include narcotics as part of your pain-management program is between you and your doctor. When prescribed for people

in chronic pain, narcotics can alleviate moderate to severe pain, giving the patient a better quality of life. As a patient in chronic pain, you should be given the choice.

There are three facts every FM and CFS patient must know before considering narcotics:

1. Narcotics are potent, potentially addictive drugs.
2. Addiction is largely biologically determined, and most people with chronic pain do not become addicted to narcotics.
3. Narcotics may be the only way to relieve your chronic pain.

There are FDA regulations in place for doctors to follow when prescribing narcotics. When coming to your own decision about narcotics, you should be aware of the distinction between narcotics as chronic pain medication, and narcotics as recreational drugs. Narcotics are abused as recreational drugs because they produce a euphoric effect in some people. Oxycontin, for example, has become well known as a street drug. Easily available to drug-abusers, it creates a strong, lasting euphoric effect. Drug abusers do not take narcotics in their prescribed form. A prescription will clearly state that the particular medication should be taken either orally, through a skin patch, in liquid form, or intravenously. When used as street drugs, narcotics are chopped up and snorted through the nose, giving users a stronger, more potent concentration and a quicker effect. Patients in chronic pain rarely experience the euphoric effects of narcotics, and only a small percentage of chronic pain patients ever become addicted. Dr. Andrew J. Holman concurs: "It's interesting; most people with FM and CFS experience so many side effects to medicines. Talk about a group that doesn't want to take any pills. So the addiction questions are kind of silly."

When Sandra W. of Seattle was prescribed the narcotic methadone, she was overwhelmed with concerned family and friends who questioned her use of the drug. But, for Sandra, methadone was a stepping-stone back to her life before the pain of FM: "To wake up and not have pain in the morning, to not have to deal with that on a daily basis, was pretty amazing. It was very emotional for me. Before, I hated taking medication, and I hated the fact that my ex-husband would call me a drug addict, because he does not even take aspirin. So I had to deal with stigma, too—people making value judgments about what I was doing to my own body. The methadone has allowed me to function." As for people who would call her a drug addict, Sandra wants them to know this: "I don't get high on methadone; I get hope."

✤ Prescribing Narcotics: A Doctor's Perspective

BY DR. MICHAEL P. YOUNG, M.D.

Dr. Young specializes in urgent and immediate care. He has a private practice in Portland, Oregon.

Doctors are wary of prescribing narcotics for long-term pain for several reasons: fear of causing addiction, fear of side effects (constipation, lethargy, respiratory problems), and lack of experience in the treatment of chronic pain. A more pressing fear is, of course, loss of licensing. Relevant to this fear are the attitudes of medical disciplinary boards.

Many physicians believe that treatment of chronic nonmalignant pain with narcotics is almost never appropriate, and practitioners who continue to prescribe this form of treatment are at risk of sanctions and restrictions from their medical board. The practical effect of any restriction, which is the minimum action taken by the board, is loss of one's ability to practice. Most physicians are not willing to risk losing their license for the sake of providing pain relief.

The Oxycontin crisis caught America off guard and lead to tightening of controls on prescribing Schedule II narcotics. Similarly, the decline in the wide use of COX inhibitors such as Vioxx and Bextra, over fears that these medications increase risk of cardiovascular disease, has added to the dilemma of pain management. The Vioxx lesson seems to be that even when an effective treatment is found, fear of litigation and product liability can quickly remove access to that treatment.

Many doctors are also unwilling to risk the possibility that a patient will become addicted, although this risk is negligible in chronic-pain patients. The number of people at risk for opiate addiction in the general population is unknown, but it is certainly below 10 percent. The dilemma of treatment can be illustrated by posing the following question: Assume a 10 percent risk of addiction upon exposure to opiates for every 10 people who present with chronic intractable pain that is unresponsive to treatment other than with narcotic medications. If one of these people will become addicted to the treatment, is it ethical to withhold treatment from the other nine to avoid the risk of addicting the one? I say the answer to that question is "No," and an emphatic "NO!" when you consider that the actual risk is far below 10 percent.

Narcotic analgesics such as Oxycodone are a proven and effective treatment for chronic, nonmalignant pain. I have cared for patients who have

99

been incapacitated and unable to accomplish activities of daily life, much less hold down a job, due to chronic pain. These same patients have successfully returned to work and recovered joy in their life by taking safe doses of narcotics, and they have suffered no adverse affects. They are able to maintain scheduled doses without tolerance or addiction. We know from research that the risk of addiction in treatment of chronic pain is low. In a Boston collaborative drug study, only four out of 11,882 patients treated with opiates became addicted. In national burn centers, none of the 10,000 patients treated became addicted. Of 2,369 patients treated for migraine headaches, only three became addicted.

In the treatment of FM and CFS with narcotics, however, I do have some reservations. First, I believe alternative therapies should be tried and exhausted. Second, I believe that the diagnosis of depression should be addressed as well. Finally, I believe a written contract for the proper and safe use of opioid drugs should be made and honored. With those caveats, I believe there is a place for treatment with narcotics for patients with FM and CFS. ❖❖❖

❖ A Patient's Story: Linda M.

Linda M. is a 60-year-old author from Edmonds, Washington. She developed posttraumatic FM following a car accident in 1987. Linda's physician manages her pain with narcotics, enabling her to get the most out of life and continue to teach the art of belly dancing. Linda is author of the book *Poetry of Pain* (see Bibliography).

When I was healthy, I had so much energy! My husband once told me, "You don't just get out of bed in the morning, you erupt." I miss that energy. Now, when I wake up, I'm in pain, and I feel wiped out, not rested. I stay in bed about an hour and a half before I get up. My condition hasn't improved since I first developed FM. But I feel better now because I have a compassionate physician who helps manage my pain with prescription pain medication.

Pain management is essential for me. Without adequate pain management, I couldn't even think, much less accomplish goals. Without pain management, it would be impossible for me to teach belly dance, which gives me the physical and mental exercise I need, and the beauty I crave. So if you have chronic pain and you haven't already addressed pain management, put it at the top of your list.

Earlier in my FM, my pain was so intense that I considered suicide on more than one occasion. I had tried every treatment my physician suggested and nothing had helped, yet I was afraid to ask him for pain medication. We've all been told to "Say No" to drugs, and I was sure my doctor would think that I was a drug addict if I asked.

Now isn't that silly? To be willing to kill myself rather than ask for something to soothe my pain? Finally, my doctor almost put the words in my mouth, and I realized he had been *waiting* for me to ask!

I decided that instead of ending my life, I had to become politically active in order to change Washington state laws regarding the use of prescription opiates for the treatment of chronic pain. I joined with other pain activists to lobby the Washington State Legislature and helped write new pain-management guidelines.

My cookbooks, *Simply Salmon* and *Simply Shrimp*, were personal accomplishments, but in 1996 I wrote another type of book, *Poetry of Pain*. Although I initially wrote it for my own therapy, I wanted to share my poems with other pain sufferers who lacked the words to describe their own pain. I wanted them to be able to give a particular poem to their doctor or family member and say, "This is how I feel!" One young woman I met at a conference told me, "Your book has changed my life. I asked my friends to read certain poems, and they treat me differently now. They take care of me."

It makes me feel happy to know I've helped other pain sufferers in such an important way. I am proud of the things I've accomplished since I've had fibromyalgia. It would have been easier to hide in my bedroom, but I think I would have become bored pretty quickly.

I had been taking belly dance classes for ten years prior to my car accident, and although a physical therapist told me to stop dancing until my back pain went away, after three years, I realized that my pain might not ever go away, and I decided I would just dance anyway! I signed up for more classes, and have been dancing ever since.

Since 2001, I've taught belly dance in my home studio. Of course, there are days when my pain is out of control and I can't do much. But I have never canceled a dance class because I didn't feel well (and I teach four or five classes per week). There are times when I'm so tired I can hardly drag myself downstairs to teach, or I'm hurting so much I can hardly move, and I feel like I just *can't* do it, but I know I'll feel better once I start dancing, because *I always do!*

When I first started teaching, I didn't tell my students about my pain. Then one evening, after sitting on the floor for quite a while, I stood up to get something and I couldn't stand up straight; I had to hobble across the room. My students all looked so frightened! I explained to them that I was okay; that I have fibromyalgia and that getting stiff after sitting was one of my symptoms.

It was such a relief not to have to try to hide my symptoms anymore! Now I explain my symptoms to my students; I explain that I have short-term memory loss and that occasionally it might take me a few minutes when I'm trying to remember a word or the name of a dance step. And I explain that if I'm a little "tippy" sometimes when I'm teaching a dance step, it's because I lose my balance easily. I tell them, "If it looks like I'm falling over—I am!"

A number of students who have physical disabilities have told me they were inspired to take my dance class *because* I have FM. Several have told me, "If *you* can do it, *I* can do it too!" It makes me feel great to know I am influencing their lives in such a positive manner.

I've formed a belly dance troupe, "Troupe Levant." We perform in shows, at events, and in restaurants. I won't say I don't get frustrated when my memory blanks out during a performance. But I've learned to be kinder to myself when it happens. There's a saying in Islam, "Only Allah is perfect." All we can do is try to do our best, given what we have. ❖❖❖

❖ Physical Therapy

BY DR. KIM BENNETT, P.T., PH.D.

Dr. Bennett manages a group of physical therapists in private practice at Olympic Physical Therapy in Seattle. She also teaches gross anatomy and is a clinical assistant professor of rehabilitation medicine at the University of Washington. She is the author of two chapters on therapeutic exercise in the book *Therapeutic Exercise: Moving Toward Function,* edited by C. Hall and L. Thein-Brody.

I treat biomechanical problems, which occur when the joints aren't lining up correctly and are thus causing pain and movement issues. Much of my treatment is aimed at addressing specific physical faults that have a bio-mechanical basis. For example, I might work on a shoulder joint that is out of alignment and perhaps eliminate the discomfort that causes a person to awaken in the middle of the night. If we can eliminate that problem, it's a step toward helping the patient to sleep better.

I'm very interested in people and their backgrounds. That's probably one of the things that helps me when treating FM and CFS patients—so many factors affect these illnesses, and they in turn have an effect on so many aspects of my patients' lives. The more I understand about the lives of the people I treat, the better job I'm able to do.

Since I started working in physical therapy, I've become interested in people who have multiple problems that are typically chronic in nature. Rarely do my patients come in with just a sprained ankle. Usually, it's something that's been going on for a long time, and many parts of their body may be involved. Over the years I have also gained a great respect for how important the mind is in healing. I am a strong believer in educating patients about the nature of their problems and the things they can do for self-treatment. Some of the energy-draining anxiety that goes along with a chronic problem can be relieved when the patient gains more control over their healing.

One intervention for people with FM is exercise—but, as anyone with FM knows, exercise is a double-edged sword. If you do it right, it can be helpful. But it is easy to do it wrong, to overexert, and then it will set you back. Part of my role as a physical therapist is to help people learn how to progress with their exercise program and to convince them that holding back is often really better than "just doing it." [For FM- and CFS-friendly exercises, see Chapter 9.]

Another way that physical therapy can benefit FM and CFS patients is through hands-on work to treat specific joints or areas where the pain occurs due to biomechanical dysfunction. I see many FM and CFS patients who are sedentary, or perhaps do not always rest in good postures, so they push themselves out of alignment. I frequently see people with headaches, shoulder problems, or low-back pain; this generalized pain is often associated with a FM or CFS diagnosis. But in reality, it is a problem that a person without FM or CFS might have too, because their body is in poor alignment.

THE BODY/MIND CONNECTION

I have observed some patterns in FM and CFS patients that I find very interesting. It's common to find that people with FM or CFS are very intelligent high achievers, but they might also be hyper-vigilant worriers who feel responsible for everybody and never quite let themselves rest. They're constantly in a state of anxiety, worrying about what's coming next. In general, the autonomic nervous system of people in chronic pain is geared to avoiding an attack, just because of the pain.

I believe that stress and imbalance in the autonomic nervous system can cause some of the symptoms commonly seen in FM and CFS patients.

It is possible to "get stuck" in the fight-or-flight response (also known as the stress response, generated by the sympathetic nervous system). When this occurs, the body fails to switch back into rest, repair, and relaxation (generated by the parasympathetic system). The sympathetic part becomes way too active, and the parasympathetic part isn't active enough. Physical therapy teaches relaxation techniques and other tricks to increase the activity of the parasympathetic system and decrease sympathetic activity.

To achieve these treatment goals, I teach people progressive relaxation (a type of meditation), biofeedback techniques, and proper breathing. People with FM tend to hold their breath or be upper-chest breathers, which is an abnormal breathing pattern that can contribute to pain, as well as result from it.

LEARNING TO HELP YOURSELF

Another really important part of physical therapy is teaching people to treat themselves and to make better use of resources. Most FM and CFS patients I've met are highly informed, but occasionally I'll meet someone who is newly diagnosed or has not yet reached out into the community to see what information and support is available to them. So part of my responsibility is to help them become aware of books or other resources. We also talk a lot about pacing—not just in exercise, but also in everyday life. I teach my patients how to treat themselves using ice, heat, and electrical stimulation. Almost everything that I do to help get their joints back into alignment, I can also teach them to do for themselves with some degree of efficiency. My goal is to help patients realize that there are many different tools; we try to find the things that will work for them.

FINDING A PHYSICAL THERAPIST

Your physical therapist should specialize in treating people with FM or CFS. If I had either condition and I didn't know who to go to, I would ask my physician who they send their patients to, so that I'd know I was going to someone with experience. If you don't have that option, I would strongly recommend calling physical therapists directly and asking them to explain what they do. There are physical therapists who are so busy they wouldn't have time to do that, and I think you would want to avoid those people in general. If their priority is not patient education, you probably don't want to see them. Once you are in treatment, if you have concerns about how things are going, discuss your issues to be sure you are on the same wavelength as your physical therapist.

If you can't find someone who has experience with your specific conditions, the next best step is talking to a physical therapist who has experience working with one of the rheumatic diseases, like rheumatoid arthritis. Another option is working with someone knowledgeable about other chronic conditions in which the therapist needs to understand how joints work and also know how to be gentle. However, many orthopedic physical therapists deal primarily with sports injuries, and their expectations about levels of performance may be too high for patients with FM or CFS.

People living with FM and CFS may have some symptoms that are fixable; physical therapy can help with those symptoms. But more than that, physical therapy is an education process about how to live with a chronic physical problem. This is a discipline that teaches you tools you can use to treat yourself, and that's a good reason to go through the physical therapy process. However, when you participate in physical therapy, be sure you are allowed to be an equal team member in your treatment plan and that you are acknowledged as the one who has ultimate responsibility for taking care of your body. ❖❖❖

❖ Therapeutic Ultrasound, TENS, and CES

Physical therapists often use therapeutic ultrasound or electrical stimulation to warm muscles prior to exercise or to help a patient relax after a PT session. The following list describes some of the ways these therapies can be used:

❖ Ultrasound is best known as a diagnostic imaging device, but it is also a powerful healing tool. Therapeutic ultrasound stimulates the repair of soft-tissue injuries and reduces inflammation. It also relieves pain and helps muscles relax, increasing a patient's range of motion. During therapeutic ultrasound, high and low frequency sound waves (out of human hearing range) are targeted at problem areas of the body. These sound waves generate deep heat that draws blood into the tissues, delivering oxygen and nutrients, and removing cell waste. It can be administered to the skin directly, using a probe and 'coupling gel' or through a water medium. Patients feel a slight tingling sensation during treatment.

❖ A TENS (transcutaneous electrical nerve stimulation) device uses mild bursts of electrical impulses to block the message of pain from the nerves to the brain. Electrodes are attached to the patient's

105

skin in the area where they are experiencing pain. With guidance from your physical therapist, you can learn how to use a TENS unit yourself. Sometimes TENS can be too strong or irritating for FM patients.

✤ CES is a palm-sized device that provides cranial-electrical stimulation; this unit is better suited for home use. CES clips onto the ears, and it delivers a very mild, low-level current through the brain. CES is also useful for treating anxiety, insomnia, and depression. CES has a whole-body effect. Nancy Campbell of Therapeutic Resources tells us, "The message of pain comes from the brain. CES approaches FM and CFS from a systemic standpoint, bringing the brain back into homeostasis (balance)."

✤ Biofeedback

Can you "think" your headache away?

Biofeedback works on the principal that we can learn to exert influence on the natural functions of our bodies. Through biofeedback, we can consciously influence the autonomic nervous system, lowering our blood pressure, easing tension in our muscles, or decreasing our heart rate.

Biofeedback techniques are easy to learn in just a few sessions with a biofeedback therapist, and they are especially effective for the treatment of headaches. Using a machine that records the body's responses, the biofeedback therapist teaches the participant to control processes that are normally involuntary. Often a physical therapist can refer you to a biofeedback therapist.

There are several types of biofeedback. Each one focuses on a different system of the body, providing information such as pulse rate, muscle contractions, or skin temperature. EEG biofeedback uses an electroencephalogram to record brain wave responses. The therapist begins by attaching sensors to your scalp that measure muscle tension. The sensors send information to an electronic device that measures these signals and provides feedback via visual image such as a line graph or even through sound such as a tone. The participant learns to recognize and control facets of the stress response using visualization and breath work.

David A. describes the biofeedback process: "[I began by meditating for a little while.] When I opened my eyes, I was looking at a monitor showing the tension in the various muscles to which electrodes were attached. We

started talking a little bit and I noticed the tension gradually increasing in my neck and shoulders. And it would go up and down depending on what topic we were talking about. After another five or ten minutes of talking, the sort of meditative state I'd been in had completely worn off and I was back to feeling incredibly tense in my neck and shoulders. And that's when I first became aware of being tense, and how it applied all over my body."

✤ Good Sleep Hygiene

If you think of FM and CFS symptoms as a pie chart, sleep disorders take up about a quarter of the pie. Although sleep appears elusive for many FM and CFS patients, it is essential to find ways to obtain restorative sleep because it is during this time that your muscles repair themselves and your body heals. If you can conquer your sleep problems, you will be a long way toward feeling better, and you will be in better shape to take on the day. Before considering sleep medications, be sure you have done everything to prepare your environment for sleep. In other words, practice good sleep hygiene.

A PLACE FOR REST

First ensure that your bedroom is a tranquil retreat. Remove any items that will distract you from your main objective—getting to sleep. This does not mean sweeping the kids' toys under the bed. Ideally, do not use your bedroom as a place to socialize or as an office—this room should be a haven for relaxation, sex, and sleep.

Invest in the best mattress you can afford. If you are trying to sleep on a bumpy, uncomfortable mattress, and you can't afford a new one, try adding a mattress pad or a foam-rubber pad. Foam rubber is used in hospitals and is very comfortable to sleep on. There are no springs or hard spots pressing into your back and lower body, just foam that contours to your shape. (Note: While foam rubber is great for your back, it is a synthetic material that may not be such a good idea to use if you have multiple chemical sensitivities.) Many of our respondents recommended feather beds (fluffy, foldable mattresses, about three or four inches thick, that feel like heaven to lie on when laid over a mattress or foam pad). Spend as much as you can on your bedding—cotton or linen sheets and soft blankets with a down comforter is a perfect combination, both soft and durable. Don't pile the blankets too high. For optimal restorative sleep, your body temperature should be lower than it is during the day. So, try to keep your room cool and well ventilated.

107

"You can never have enough pillows!" says chiropractor Dr. Mick Tiegs. Pillows help to support and brace your body as you sleep. Purchase enough to support your head and neck, with one to put under your knees to take the pressure off your back. You may want to try foam contour pillows, which are wonderful for alignment and tend to improve sleep. There are also full-sized body pillows available that support your whole body.

A HEALTHY ENVIRONMENT

Make your bedroom as toxin free as possible (this is especially important if you have multiple chemical sensitivities or allergies). You can buy sheets and pillows made of hypoallergenic natural fibers (we recommend some places to buy natural products in the Resources section at the back of this book). Also consider eliminating furniture constructed with synthetic materials. Some synthetics, such as particleboard and certain kinds of paint, leak chemical vapors into the air. The best kind of furniture for a healthy environment is made with unfinished wood or older furniture that has had the time to outgas the toxins. The same is true for flooring; synthetic carpets are treated with chemicals, and they also tend to harbor all sorts of allergen-introducing bugs, germs, and dirt. Wood flooring is the healthiest option for your bedroom, but if you must have carpet, try sisal, lambswool, or natural-fiber throw rugs that can be washed frequently.

PEACE AND QUIET

It's difficult to fall asleep with irritating noises in the background, and sudden noise all too often jolts us awake. External noises can be dampened by the addition of thick rugs, heavy drapes, or extra furniture, or try placing a bookshelf crammed with books against the offending wall. You may want to generate a continuous background sound to block out noise and lull you to sleep. A fan is one possibility that provides the added benefit of cooling your room. For some, the radio, or even the sound of a television show, is a relaxing way to fall asleep. Many people who live alone feel secure with the company of a favorite radio host or late-night chat show. But do remember to set the timer so your television or radio will turn off—another show may come on that stimulates your brain and causes you to wake up. Relaxing music or sounds can also help you drift off. Some alarm clocks have a function that allows you to fall asleep to one source and wake to another (you can also set the sleep volume low, and have your wake-up volume set higher). There are reasonably priced alarm clocks available with sound generators that can be set to both soothe you to sleep and help wake you up gently. Various sound effects are available, such as rainstorms, waves breaking, or jungle wildlife. Earplugs are another option for muffling the sounds you hear. They are fairly inexpensive and can be easily molded to your ear.

NIGHTTIME

Some people like the security of a nightlight, and others cannot sleep without the light on, but most of us need darkness to fall asleep. If there is too much light coming through your windows at bedtime, you may want to consider buying blackout shades or blackout liners for your curtains (these are especially recommended if you have a daytime sleep schedule or live in Alaska). These liners are also helpful if the early morning sun frequently wakes you up.

Darkness tells our brains that it's time to sleep. Before the invention of the electric light bulb, humans went to sleep and awoke with the sun. Modern appliances such as computers, televisions, and video games interfere with our circadian rhythms and contribute to insomnia. Try limiting your light exposure in the hours leading up to bedtime. Don't sit in front of the television or surf the Internet right before you go to bed. If you like to read in bed, use a low-level reading light. Reading lights that clip onto a book are ideal, because they provide enough illumination for you to read without straining your eyes but are dim enough to signal your brain that it's time to start winding down. You may want to suggest this to your partner if he or she likes to stay up reading when you want to go to sleep. Eye masks are another possibility, although you may find it difficult to get to sleep with something covering your eyes.

If your alarm clock is illuminated, don't forget to turn it away from you (or see if it has an option to turn off the illumination). Not only can the glow from a digital clock or a luminous clock face contribute to sleepless nights, but one often also ends up watching the time tick by, which can increase anxiety and make it more difficult to get to sleep.

ELECTROMAGNETIC FIELDS

You may want to throw away (or relocate) your radio alarm clock and your TV. To create a healthy environment, many natural home specialists recommend eliminating appliances that emit electromagnetic fields (EMFs), which may cause tension and nervousness in humans. Every electrical product emits electromagnetic radiation. Certain devices emit particularly high levels of EMFs, such as traditional cathode ray computer monitors (Some people report that replacing a CRT computer monitor with an LCD flat

panel monitor can really improve their energy and focus). Research is inconclusive about whether exposure to household EMFs causes harm to humans; however, eliminating as many electrical appliances as possible certainly can't hurt and does create a beautifully relaxing environment.

NATURAL SLEEP AIDS

Introducing natural scents into the room can help lull you to sleep. Aromatherapist Jimm Harrison recommends lavender essential oil for its calming, stress-reducing properties. Chamomile, whether in essential oil form or in tea, can also soothe the body and promote sleep. Valerian root is another good herbal remedy that has been valued for its calming effect for thousands of years. Melatonin, a hormone produced naturally by our bodies, is available in supplement form and can help reset your body's natural rhythm. Melatonin supplements can be helpful but should be used in the smallest effective dose possible.

KEYS TO A GOOD NIGHT'S SLEEP

Other recommended ways of regulating your internal clock include eating your meals at the same time each day, and getting up at the same time each day. Performing light exercise earlier in the day can also help your body wind down later on. In order to prepare your body for sleep and to let go of the day's worries, you need to relax and reduce stress. Try a warm bath and a cup of hot milk (milk contains tryptophan, an amino acid used by the body to make serotonin—turkey also contains tryptophan, although a turkey sandwich may not be all that appetizing right before bedtime). Hopefully, some of these tips will help you get the rejuvenating good night's sleep you deserve.

❖ ❖ ❖

From a foundation of conventional treatments, we now turn to complementary and alternative treatments. Some are exciting and controversial, some have been around for a long time, and others are just being developed, but many of these approaches can provide you with new ways to manage your illness, gain optimum energy, and find enjoyment in your life. The search for your own special treatment program may be a bit of a rocky road, but don't be discouraged. Along the way, you'll meet new people and try new things; some therapies will work for you, some won't, but by the end we hope you'll have found not just an effective treatment program, but also a positive way to look at life with FM and CFS.

Chapter 8

Chiropractic, Osteopathy, and Bodywork

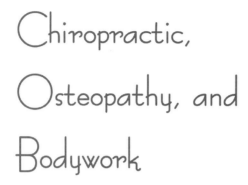

Illness is the doctor to whom we pay most heed. To kindness, to knowledge, we make promises only. Pain we obey.

— Marcel Proust

AN ESSENTIAL PART of living well with FM and CFS is giving your body the opportunity to move in a way that puts less stress on the musculoskeletal system. There are many ways to accomplish this, either through hands-on manipulation or through movement therapy classes that teach you how to move your body in a healthy, natural way.

Chiropractic, osteopathy, and bodywork (such as massage, reflexology, and Feldenkrais) can be beneficial for just about everyone, but especially for people with FM and CFS.

You may feel a little cautious about some of these therapies because of the hands-on manipulation of your muscles and bones. As FM and CFS patients, we tend to think, "Gosh, my muscles already hurt so much, without having someone pressing down on them." However, when tailored to the soft tissues of an FM or CFS patient, chiropractic, osteopathy, and bodywork can be wonderful healing techniques and an important part of your pain-management program.

Sharon W. from Seattle started getting massage treatments a number of years ago, and they felt so good she kept them up. She says, "I discovered

111

it wasn't a luxury; it was something I needed to do on a regular basis to feel better."

Erin P., also from Seattle, participated in Feldenkrais classes and says, "I went in because of my knees and came out with almost a whole new body. It was amazing."

All the therapies featured in this chapter retrain your brain to move your body in the way it was meant to move—leading to proper alignment, increased blood flow, less pain, and a greater sense of well-being. As somatics educator Eduardo Barrera says, "Life is infinitely easier if the body goes along with ease."

✤ Chiropractic Technique

BY DR. MICK TIEGS, D.C.

Dr. Tiegs is a chiropractor with a family practice in Seattle, Washington. He attended Western States Chiropractic College in Portland, Oregon, where he earned his degree in 1995 as a doctor of chiropractic. He earned his B.S. in pre-medical studies from Boise State University in 1991.

Many people don't realize that chiropractors are doctors. Just as a medical doctor attends four years of medical school, chiropractors attend a four-year chiropractic college. The programs are quite similar during the first two years, with the majority of studies covering basic sciences, microbiology, cell biology, biochemistry, and anatomy and physiology. The last two years of graduate school are where medical and chiropractic schools differ. In chiropractic college, students are trained to help the body heal through spinal adjustment, nutrition, exercise, physical therapy, and soft tissue therapy. The medical approach is to treat the symptom or problem using medication or surgery.

In the United States, chiropractors are recognized as primary-care physicians. We diagnose a full range of conditions and then either treat the patient or refer them for the appropriate course of care. Chiropractors excel in conditions known as neuromusculoskeletal (NMS) disorders. These NMS conditions affect the nervous system, muscular system, and skeletal system. FM and CFS are two conditions of this type that chiropractors have very good success in treating.

The primary focus of a chiropractor is to detect and correct spinal subluxations—a vertebra or group of vertebrae that are out of alignment and/or lack normal movement, thus interfering with proper nervous system function. If the spine is misaligned or there is restricted movement, the

nerves and muscles will be adversely affected, creating pain and dysfunction. Your nervous system provides constant communication between your brain and the rest of your body. Pressure or tension in the nervous system interrupts the normal communication between the brain and body. Chronic pain patterns seen in FM and CFS patients can be due to pressure on the nervous system.

Before treating any patient, a thorough examination allows the chiropractor to find areas of vertebral subluxation and also allows the patient to become aware of the area of dysfunction. A thorough examination involves a postural evaluation, palpation (gently moving the spine and muscles), chiropractic tests, and orthopedic tests, all of which aid in determining the areas of vertebral subluxation. X rays are often utilized to determine structural misalignments and to rule out other possible underlying problems or pathologies.

A typical chiropractic examination is very hands-on—the chiropractor needs to test the range of motion of the vertebrae and spine to determine which areas are moving freely and which areas feel bound or restricted, and the muscles need to be assessed to determine where there is abnormal tension or spasms. With FM and CFS patients, the examination will vary based on how much pressure can be asserted, especially when using palpation. Since the muscles and tissues are hypersensitive, a relative measure of sensitivity must be taken into account.

A chiropractor's primary treatment method is the spinal adjustment. The most common type of adjustment is hands-on. The chiropractor applies appropriate force (ranging from very gentle to firm) with his or her hands to an area of the spine that is out of alignment, thus returning the spine to a more normal position and improving function. When the vertebrae are returned to normal alignment and motion is restored, pressure is taken off the nervous system, and the body begins to heal properly. An adjustment can also be delivered through the use of a number of adjusting instruments. The goal of all adjustments is to improve the function of the spine and nervous system.

There are many different chiropractic techniques. The biggest concern for some people is whether the adjustment will hurt, but a chiropractic adjustment is rarely painful. The response I usually get from people who were concerned is, "That wasn't bad," or even, "That felt great." Be sure to let your chiropractor know what your concerns are; a good chiropractor will utilize adjustment techniques that you will be comfortable with and that will also achieve positive results. Good communication will help alleviate other concerns you might have.

113

I have taken care of a number of FM and CFS patients over the years. Most patients have already been diagnosed with FM or CFS when they come to my office, and they are usually very well informed. Chiropractic is unique in the way it helps people with chronic pain. In a state of chronic pain, the same signals are continually sent from the body to the brain and then from the brain back to the body. Over time, these pain signals become predominant. Chiropractic adjustments interrupt the chronic pain loop. By interrupting the irregular pain and dysfunction mode, new input is introduced into the joints and nervous system.

Some FM patients require very light force or the use of an adjusting instrument, while others require more pressure. I tend to limit soft tissue work with FM and CFS patients prior to their adjustments, as sometimes the muscles will react, making an adjustment more difficult. Conditions such as FM and CFS challenge the body's healing process, making it even more important for patients to play an active role in managing their health. With all patients, I make it a point to discuss the body as a whole. By focusing on the nervous system, chiropractic can help our bodies heal, especially in combination with healthy eating, careful exercise, and a positive outlook. ❈ ❈ ❈

❖ Getting Relief with Osteopathy

BY DR. CATHY LINDSAY, D.O.

Dr. Lindsay is a doctor of osteopathy in private practice in Seattle. She has been practicing since 1988. Dr. Lindsay helps patients with FM and CFS return to functionality and attain a greater level of health.

Osteopaths find restrictions and misalignments anywhere in the body, and then provide bodywork to help realign them. Osteopathy works on a structural level, but it also works because the body is a whole organism—everything is interrelated, and the body has an inherent healing mechanism that works best when all parts of it are moving freely.

Osteopathic medical training includes all aspects of a medical education, with a focus on the musculoskeletal system and diagnosing and treating with our hands, and with an emphasis on viewing the body, mind, and spirit as a whole. When that philosophy is incorporated, the patient's own healing potential is utilized as an essential part of the treatment process.

Osteopathy assists patients with chronic pain in two major ways. People who are diagnosed with chronic pain often have conditions that can be

addressed and resolved by an osteopath. Assessing and treating chronic pain using the patient's self-healing mechanism (which osteopaths call the Cranial Concept) can be very effective in decreasing pain, improving vitality, and enhancing a general sense of well-being.

Thorough diagnostic evaluation is completed before any osteopathic treatment is started. We begin with a full medical history, an injury history, and a birth history. We also do a thorough assessment of the patient's current symptoms and a review of the body's systems, just to see what other things are going on. Then we do what's called an "osteopathic structural evaluation," as well as a brief neurological evaluation. These evaluations assess the relationship between structure and function in the body. We look for areas of misalignment as well as functional restriction and freedom of motion—we look at how your body actually moves when it's taken through its full range of motion. Then, using these structural and functional assessments, we address the relationship between the body's soft and bony tissues. If we find dysfunction that can be improved with osteopathic treatment, we begin treatment on the first visit.

Osteopathic treatment is difficult to describe until you've actually experienced it for yourself. Usually it's quite gentle; I use a subtle approach. Many of the treatments are gentle movements of the body, and we use the body's responses to direct us in the therapy, telling us where to move the patient in order to free up restrictions or unwind twists in the connective tissue and to restore alignment. For some people, treatment is so gentle that they think I haven't done anything. But after they leave, they find that they feel better or have experienced noticeable, positive changes.

When I perform an osteopathic treatment, I apply gentle pressure to the tailbone or to the head of the patient to unblock any restrictions I find. I may also use this type of treatment on other areas of the body.

Osteopathy is different than other healing methods that try to directly break up restrictions in the body. It can be more effective than other approaches because it is so gentle. We do have some direct approaches, and spinal manipulation is one of them. Osteopathy doesn't tend to irritate the tissues as much as other therapies, and in people with FM, the tissues tend to be easily irritated. However, there is no specific approach for any particular condition—all patients are treated as unique individuals. Sometimes osteopathy helps people with conditions such as FM and CFS, and sometimes it does not. It depends on the individual and what may have contributed to their condition. ❈·❈·❈

✤ Massage Therapy

BY NOREEN FLACK

Noreen Flack is a licensed massage practitioner, specializing in many different massage techniques and therapies. She graduated from the Brian Utting School of Massage in 1993, and she is a member of the American Massage Therapy Association. Noreen lives with her family in Seattle.

Massage can provide many benefits for people with FM and CFS—it's just incredible. If you have had a bad experience with massage therapy, I encourage you to go to someone who has experience in treating FM and CFS. Massage can be very beneficial when done correctly, but it can also be very painful if you go to the wrong person. If you can find a massage therapist who is experienced in working with your illness, I think you'll feel much better.

I usually listen to a new patient's story first. With an FM or CFS patient, many times there's a huge emotional component that I also try to address, because they have been suffering not only physical pain but also emotional pain. They're often frustrated; they've seen very few results by the time they come to me, so they're discouraged and even depressed. I can empathize with their plight, because in addition to their symptoms, they are experiencing the stress response (a reaction by the sympathetic nervous system to the pain and the stressful situation that they're in). Their muscles are constricted, their breathing is usually shallow, and they are very "bound up" in their bodies. There are a lot of holding patterns; there's a lot of guarding.

In order to start working with patients, the massage therapist needs to create a safe place; the goal is to enable patients to feel calmer, to have the sense that someone is trying to help them and has empathy for them. I try to make a connection with patients on an emotional level without doing any actual counseling. Many of my patients also see mental-health counselors and are trying to deal with their emotional issues.

Providing a safe environment is vital, especially in the first few sessions, so that the patient can decide whether they like you and if they like being touched by you. Chances are that they're going to relax more and they're going to have a better healing response in a safe and comfortable environment than if they feel uncomfortable and the practitioner is just digging away into their tense, rigid muscles. I like to keep the massage room on the warm side, so the patient can relax easily. The lighting is low, there's a bit of

116

aromatherapy in the air, and the music is soft. This enables the patient to feel comfortable and to relax their mind as well as their body.

The first session is critical in assessing the person and getting a feeling for where they are with their illness. If a person has been recently diagnosed with FM or CFS, I am very cautious and conservative in their treatment. Often, people who have just been diagnosed with FM are feeling pain in certain areas of their body, and they want me to really dig deeply into those painful areas. But addressing those specific points can actually cause a much more severe flare-up the next day, so I have to explain to them how massage affects their body—the manipulation may feel good during the session, but the areas that have been worked on may be so painful the next day that you've actually done a lot more harm than good. That is why it is important to treat people with FM or CFS very lightly in the beginning.

It's really interesting to work with people with FM and CFS. It's also challenging, because there is no set groundwork, and your skills have to be very diverse to be able to help everyone. Even with the same FM or CFS patient, you wouldn't necessarily do the same treatment every time, whereas someone with a muscle strain or sprain would usually be treated the same way every time you see them.

A lot of what I do is just to give clients the opportunity to get grounded for themselves and go inward—their own healing response will actually address the points that they've been complaining about. When one gets into a cycle of resistance, it's so much harder to get anywhere; it's like bumping heads rather than going with the flow.

Massage is good, but one shouldn't expect to be cured by massage. In conjunction with other therapies, it can be very beneficial and allow you to make more rapid progress, because it helps to stimulate healing within the individual. It can get you on the road to recovery a lot faster and also help you feel better on a day-to-day basis. ❖❖❖

❖ Trigger Point Therapy

BY JOANNA FORWELL, N.D.

Dr. Forwell is a naturopathic physician who brings 13 years of clinical experience to a diverse and well-rounded practice. She has a special interest in addressing acute and chronic pain and injury. Originally from Canada, she fell in love with the Pacific Northwest when she came to study at Bastyr University and now calls Seattle home. In her spare time, she plays soccer, dances tango, and rides her motorcycle.

MYOTHERAPY

The pain from taut, knotted muscle fibers can be excruciating. There are a great many ways to release trigger points—the most popular is "myotherapy," applying manual pressure with the thumb or forefinger. Myotherapy can release the pain and muscle spasms of a trigger point. The myotherapist sustains the pressure until the tissues relax and become softer, and eventually the pain subsides. Myotherapy re-educates the muscles to prevent spasms from returning. Myotherapy is a technique that the patient can easily learn to do by themselves.

MYOFASCIAL TRIGGER POINT INJECTIONS (MFTPI)

In the case of FM and CFS, sometimes the pain is so pronounced and the tissue so sensitive that manually pressing on points causes the patient to feel worse rather than better.

An alternative to manual release is injection into the muscle trigger point using a fine needle. A small amount of solution is introduced into the area. The injected fluid dilutes nerve-sensitizing substances released by the body. My preferred solution is comprised primarily of a local anesthetic (preservative free), with a little magnesium and vitamin B_{12} added. The local anesthetic acts to increase circulation in the area, thereby improving oxygen and nutrient delivery and enhancing the removal of metabolic waste products. Additionally, and perhaps most importantly, the temporary numbing effect of the anesthetic effectively allows the pain signaling mechanism in that portion of the muscle to "go to sleep" for about 20 minutes. The effect is similar to rebooting a computer. The pain cycle is temporarily interrupted and the system has a chance to normalize itself when it resumes functioning.

MESOTHERAPY

Mesotherapy is a unique style of injection using pharmacologic and natural preparations. The technique was developed in France and has been used extensively in Europe for the treatment of pain conditions. Specialized techniques used in mesotherapy involve various superficial injections using small, short needles, which are relatively painless. The premise is that solutions injected just under the skin remain in the area longer than a deeper injection because they are slower to be cleared by the circulation. It has been found that the injected solutions continue to penetrate the deeper tissues. Mesotherapy, therefore, appears to be a novel technique to administer medicines, an approach in which the skin acts as a natural time-release

system. The French have developed successful protocols for FM and CFS patients which are comprised of a combination of vitamins, local anesthetic, and substances to improve blood flow and relieve pain.

INTRAVENOUS MICRONUTRIENT THERAPY (IVMT)

Administering nutrients by IV is a popular modality among naturopathic doctors for the treatment of acute illness, chronic disease, and pain syndromes. IVMT has the ability to achieve blood concentrations of trace nutrients that far exceed what is possible when taking them orally. There is a standard nutrient IV protocol commonly used called a "Myers' cocktail," which contains several B vitamins, vitamin C, calcium, and magnesium.

When treating pain, much of the benefit of the Myers' cocktail is believed to be derived from the magnesium content. Magnesium is known to provide an analgesic effect for a number of conditions. In addition, magnesium plays a role in modulating brain neurotransmitters like serotonin, important in mood and sleep disorders. In fact, magnesium has been found to be low in the cells of FM patients, suggesting a problem in magnesium regulation. In order to adequately replenish the cells with magnesium, it may be necessary to attain high levels in the blood, which is not possible when taking magnesium orally.

In addition to magnesium, injected vitamin B_{12} has been used experimentally to treat CFS. It has been suggested that oral or sublingual (under the tongue) administration does not achieve the effects seen with injectable B_{12}. The other B vitamins are important in optimizing the nervous system and managing stress. Vitamin C is well known for its tissue repair and immune regulating properties, to name only a few of the potential benefits.

In my practice, as part of a comprehensive and individualized program, I may utilize any or all of these injection techniques for treating my patients, depending on their needs. The effectiveness of incorporating injection therapies in the treatment of FM and CFS has been significant, as patient outcomes are much improved. ❖❖❖

Another popular treatment is dry-needling for the relief of trigger points, a technique in which thin needles are inserted directly into the trigger point, stimulating the muscle. Dry-needling is a modality similar to acupuncture. Saline, lidocaine, or Botox may sometimes be injected. Botox is a chemical neuromuscular relaxant used most often in the smoothing out of wrinkles; surprisingly, it's effective for pain control, too.

119

❖ Reflexology

BY KANDI BURKE

Kandi Burke is a licensed massage therapist and reflexologist who has been practicing reflexology since 1988. She cofounded the Washington Reflexology Association and testified about reflexology at President Clinton's White House Commission on Complementary Healing. Kandi lives with her family in Duval, Washington.

Reflexology is a healing science, based on the theory that all of the body's organs, glands, muscles, bones, and tissues can be located and palpated (touched) in the microcosms of the ears, hands, and feet. It is practiced in all the world's cultures as a viable and effective aid to one's health and well-being. Very specific thumb and finger techniques are applied to reflex points on the ears, hands, and feet. Calluses or sensitivities in any point alert a practitioner to a condition that is acute or chronic. Calluses and tenderness will vanish as affected organs or body parts return to homeostasis.

Reflexology is regarded as a science because its results are measurable: Research indicates that blood pressure drops, pain is interrupted, the body is helped to relax, and overall physical energy is revitalized. Science is also based on results that are consistent, and reflexology has been found to consistently create a relaxed state, enabling the patient to breathe more deeply; it also improves circulation.

My own experience with reflexology began when I crushed the 5th lumbar disc in my back after a fall. As a result, I developed acute bouts of sciatic pain down both legs. The pain was so intense, I couldn't bend over to trim my toenails and had to get a pedicure as a result. When the pedicurist saw my pain, he began reflexing my foot as soon as I was seated. To my shock and surprise, I had an immediate cessation of pain. I pestered him with a ton of questions about what he was doing. He told me that it was a technique called reflexology, which he had learned from books. He recommended two: *Better Health with Reflexology* by Dwight Byers and *Hand Reflexology: Key to Perfect Health* by Mildred Carter [see Bibliography]. I bought these two books on my way home and began to tend to myself as the books directed. The results became apparent immediately: My pain decreased and my brain fog lifted; I was able to fall asleep and had a better sleep experience. Even though I was very much a beginner, the results were often dramatic. I began to tell everybody I knew about what was taking place within my body, my mind, and my spirit. So many people kept asking me to "check their feet," that I eventually left my job and began a massage and reflexology business in 1988.

I encourage folks to learn reflexology to benefit their own health. I love reflexology because it makes me slow down my life and focus on how I am feeling. It is easy to learn and I use it for tuning myself up each day. Daily spot treatments can create lymphatic drainage, improve blood flow, relax the nervous system, and make breathing easier. Just increasing oxygen flow in the body is a tremendous help to health. As all these energy systems begin to move into balance, and pain vanishes.

LOVE YOUR FEET

The foot is a unique structure in the body. No other body part is asked not only to support all that we are, but also to carry us forward in life. So many folks feel that since the feet are "down there," distant from our brain, they aren't that big a deal! Yet when our feet are manifesting pain, can any of us overlook them? No. Things actually come to a screeching halt until a way is found to get rid of that pain! I think we should be bowing to our feet each day in thanks for all they do for us. ❖ ❖ ❖

❖ The Feldenkrais Method

BY JANE MCCLENNEY

Jane McClenney is a certified Feldenkrais practitioner. She has practices in both Redmond and Ellensburg, Washington. Jane lives with her family, dog, and horses in Ellensburg. She works with both people and horses.

Moshé Feldenkrais began developing his method of movement in the late 1940s. With a Ph.D. in physics and mechanical engineering, he worked with Fredric Joliot-Curie in nuclear research. He was also the first European to earn a black belt in judo and was largely responsible for bringing judo to Western culture. After suffering a crippling knee injury playing soccer, Feldenkrais went to physicians to see what could be done for his knees. Surgeons gave him a 50/50 chance of ever walking again, due to damaged cartilage.

But Feldenkrais was determined. He studied anatomy, physiology, and human development; with his knowledge of judo (which means "movement" in Japanese) and mechanical engineering, he began to teach himself to walk again—without pain or re-injury. He then began exploring how to teach others what he had learned.

121

I have been a practitioner of the Feldenkrais Method for ten years. I love assisting people to learn in an enjoyable way—teaching them to move in ways that are pleasurable and relatively pain free. And the bonus for me, of course, is being able to take care of my own injuries or movement patterns.

Much of my background has been in the corporate and art world, two very different disciplines. For many years, I also volunteered with a therapeutic horseback program for disabled children and adults. I began to notice that movement on horseback "woke up" the most comatose of brains and I began researching how this might occur. One day, one of our 14-year-old boys who had extreme cerebral palsy came "walking" into the barn. No wheelchair! We had always helped this boy onto his horse from his wheelchair. His walk resembled that of the TV character Lurch, but he definitely walked without assistance. His mother explained that he had been taking lessons from a Feldenkrais practitioner. I had no idea what Feldenkrais was, so I found a practitioner who was teaching classes. Before long, I enrolled in a training program so I could learn this work. I left the corporate world behind, and now my "art" (aside from photography) is my ability to enable people to learn to move more reliably.

WEEKLY CLASSES

Classes are a great form of maintenance for FM and CFS patients. The Feldenkrais Method is a gentle, relaxing way to perform specific movements of the body, while engaging the brain. Both body and brain work together, making movement easier and more comfortable. There is no strain or powerful effort required. Students only make movements that are within their comfort range. When the muscles and the brain are given better information, and are "invited" to work, both can make a better choice, for a better response. After a class, students feel much lighter, more comfortable, and move with greater ease. And they often become more curious about how their body moves and works.

During an Awareness Through Movement class, students lie on mats, sit in chairs, or stand and walk. Students are verbally led through a series of specific movements that help the student find for themselves *how* they move. This requires inner listening and "awareness." Through the lesson they experience other ways in which they *might* move, plus a sense of safety about making the movements; they are provided an environment for learning. As they notice these changes, movement often becomes more pleasurable, even in the first lesson.

INDIVIDUAL THERAPY

In an individual session, or Functional Integration, the practitioner works one-on-one with an individual for about an hour, guiding them through movement with slow, gentle touch. These movements send new information directly to the neuromuscular system, helping the student develop more efficient movement with less effort. This session is custom-tailored to the specific needs of the student.

Some students come to weekly one-hour classes and use the classes to maintain their condition. Others come for individual appointments once a month or more, depending on the severity of the condition. A common timeline for students to experience how effective the Feldenkrais Method can be is about one to two months. There is a learning curve, during which students find that their habitual thinking begins to change and they adopt new possibilities of movement. Then they begin to see real results.

FM students find their pain lessens and their ability to breathe improves. They report that sleep is frequently better. Movement becomes easier, and they learn movements they can do themselves at home or the office, which allows them to continue their progress. By inviting the muscles to make small, gentle movements, muscles are not as restricted and begin to respond in a more normal fashion. CFS students find similar relief because the movements are slower and not as strenuous as exercise, yet they enable students to have better control of their movement on demand. Of course, there are ups and downs with both illnesses, so there are times where the condition worsens, and students lose ground. Often, however, they can get back to where they were more quickly with Feldenkrais.

One of the best ways to learn the Feldenkrais Method for oneself is to take Awareness Through Movement classes from a practitioner. Students initially learn from interactions with the practitioner and with class members. The practitioner watches each student's movements in class and facilitates their learning. If no classes are available near you, there are many audio recordings available, as well as books with Awareness Through Movement lessons [see the Resources section]. Individual sessions are another great way to learn, since most practitioners will suggest movements one can practice at home, and students experience the results more quickly.

In the past several years, the scientific community has teamed with Feldenkrais practitioners to combine research attempts and share data. This is exciting, because many of the hypotheses of Moshé Feldenkrais are now being proven accurate by the scientific community.

The Feldenkrais Method does not work for everyone. People who are firmly entrenched in the Western medicine philosophy that a pill or a quick fix is what they want do not do well with Feldenkrais. On the other hand, those who are proactive about their health and are interested in furthering their own responsibility toward their health usually respond well.

✤ Hanna Somatics

BY EDUARDO BARRERA

Eduardo Barrera is a somatic educator in the tradition of Thomas Hanna and a nationally certified resistance training specialist. Diagnosed with FM several years ago, Eduardo credits Hanna somatics for the fact that he is now completely symptom-free. He operates the GravityWerks clinic in Freeland, Washington, and describes himself as both a student and teacher of Hanna somatics.

Hanna somatics is defined as the body experienced from within. The work is hands-on and is accompanied by movement patterns and guided exercises. Somatics allows a person to unwind and reeducate their nervous system.

My clients regain control over their voluntary movements. They are able to move pain-free, with ease and comfort, less stiffness, and less awkwardness. They have overall freer movements, enabling them to enjoy life's activities, whether they include simply sitting and lying comfortably or more advanced physical pursuits, such as gardening and walking.

Using a hands-on approach allows me to feel where the client is stuck or stiff, or can no longer sense how to move with comfort. It also clues the client's brain into how to undo these mechanisms of "stuckness, stiffness, and chronic holding."

My life has improved significantly through this approach, as I am my own student of somatics. My skiing has improved, without training specifically for it. Each year, my ability on the soccer field also improves. In the senior division in which I now play, others seem to stand still as I run by easily. My ability to walk with ease and comfort allows me to hike and bike effortlessly. It's such a joy to move that I cannot remember moving this well as a younger person. The FM no longer limits me physically since I practice somatic movements daily. There are times when my energy level is low, yet I live comfortably within myself. I'm more able to remain awake, sleep wonderfully, and be well in my body most of the time. When I incur an injury,

124

I'm able to recover quite readily, although for a brief time there may be a reminder of my past experience with FM, but that relinquishes rapidly. I feel that I've completely overcome FM. My life is infinitely better than it has ever been, and I know that my work with somatics will continue to support this positive change.

Before I got well, I would think, "Each day I will improve my ill-being." After some time, when I had regained my health, I realized I could change that thought to, "Each day I will improve my well-being." Now, when I'm temporarily under the weather, I continue to think that thought, and I'm renewed again.

Find a Hanna somatics educator or become one yourself! Find movement programs that benefit you. Get outside. Hang out with friends or social groups. Make your health a priority. So many people think they are supporting their health but they live otherwise. Work and pursue activities that you truly enjoy. Your lifestyle can be one of bliss if you so choose it.

FM changed my life. It pointed me in the direction I now enjoy: teaching others how to regain control within their body and mind, and serving as an example of such an accomplishment. It is work, it is a commitment, and the payoff is the day-to-day miracle—witnessing your former self (the FM or CFS self) now enjoying another, more joyous side of your life.

Meditation has all sorts of wonderful benefits, and the somatic practice is a moving meditation—another path to my wellness. Both practices make up the foundation of my daily health plan, in addition to a balanced program of nutrition. My day usually begins with an hour of meditation, followed by some somatic movement. The great benefit is I'm now able to handle stress more effectively at all levels.

I love teaching people how this can be achieved so easily through Hanna somatics. I love all the smiles and looks of satisfaction, bewilderment, and joy amidst the transformation. Now I'm blessed to share with others what I've learned through my own self-care. ❧❧❧

❧ ❧ ❧

The healing forms discussed in this chapter enable you to move more freely, with less pain and stiffness. Once you have achieved a greater range of motion and are more attuned to your body, it's time to think about adding regular exercise into your life.

Chapter 9

Exercise

Whatever your mind can conceive and believe, it can achieve.

— Napoleon Hue

FOR A PERSON WITH FM or CFS, exercise isn't an option, it's a necessity. Exercise can reduce the debilitating symptoms of FM and CFS, giving you more energy, strength, and stamina. Exercise also increases the production of endorphins, the body's natural painkillers.

For Tom O., exercise is an essential part of the day, "In the morning I stretch, do push-ups, leg lifts, and other exercises," he says. "I just lie on the floor and roll over, back and forth, moving every little thing I can think of."

❧ Get Moving (Gently)!

Just 15 minutes of low-impact exercise a day can improve your mobility and health. To avoid flare-ups, start slowly, exercising a few minutes every other day, and work your way up to longer exercise sessions. We want your experience with exercise to be a positive one, so don't overdo it! We recommend checking with your primary-care provider before beginning any new exercise program.

Exercise can be problematic for people with CFS, people who simply don't have the energy to spare. Dennis H. says, "I used to play a lot of basketball, slow-pitch softball in the spring and summer, tennis, coed volleyball, water-skiing, and jogging. I didn't have other hobbies; I just did the sport of the season. I enjoyed getting a lot of exercise. I'm not able to do all those activities now. I have no energy, and my body is all stiff muscles and joints. I go out walking in the evenings when I've had a temporary remission of my symptoms; those are my best times. Then I can break into a jog without my muscles and joints hurting."

Dennis has some wise words that are important to remember before beginning to exercise again: "Don't compare what you can currently do to what you used to do, or else you'll just drive yourself crazy." We couldn't have said it better ourselves.

In this chapter we'll give you some ideas to help you get moving. Dr. Kim Bennett has some essential advice for easing your body into motion; FM patient Gerry L. inspires us with her story. But first, Dr. Robyn DeSautel encourages us all to "Get out and move those muscles!"

❖ Exercise for People Living with FM or CFS

BY DR. ROBYN R. DESAUTEL, D.C.

Dr. DeSautel is a chiropractor with a private practice in Seattle. Her practice emphasizes creating overall balance and improving energy flow to the body through chiropractic adjustments. She also specializes in exercise as a way to return her patients to health.

Exercise is key in dealing with FM or CFS—with the right exercises a patient can actually get their life back!

Motion is life. Lack of motion and resting too often create deterioration and poor blood flow to the muscles, organs, and tissues. Without movement, the muscles of a patient with FM or CFS can literally become immobile. It is important to keep the tissues soft and pliable through movement, or they will harden and become even more painful and stiff.

The right exercises decrease pain and depression, increase mobility, increase blood flow, increase flexibility, and improve self-esteem and outlook on life.

I highly recommend any exercise that is nonjarring and also enjoyable. Some great exercises are walking, cycling, swimming, using exercise machines (such as ski, stair, or elliptical), Pilates, yoga, and low-impact dancing. Exercise should be performed in increments over the course of the day, so that it totals at least an hour.

The patient who does more of the right kinds of exercise will experience a huge decrease in pain compared to the patient who is immobile most of the time. Simple stretching exercises, performed so they do not cause pain, also have many symptom-relieving benefits for the FM or CFS patient.

I recommend that patients avoid weight training. Normal muscle tissue responds to weight training and stress by quickly repairing any muscle fibers that were broken down or torn. This response leads to increased muscle strength and size. But an FM or CFS patient responds (and repairs) much more slowly, due to a lack of blood and oxygen flow to the tissues. Often the micro trauma in their muscle fibers takes so long to repair that the tissues become hard, rigid, and very painful to the touch. A patient who experiences this will be discouraged from forming an exercise habit. And, in order to be life changing, exercise must become a daily habit.

In my practice, I have added a series of specialized and individualized exercises that can permanently change the muscles and ligaments supporting the postural balance of the body. The exercises include cervical traction (which increases lumbar disc circulation), diaphragm strengthening, spinal curve stretches with fulcrums, and the use of isometric weights for postural correction. When patients adhere to their exercise routine, the amount of change we can achieve in reducing chronic pain is remarkable.

My patients who regularly exercise are much more pain free and happy than those who do very little. They are often able to stop taking medication and spend less time and money in my office. ❖ ❖ ❖

❖ FM- and CFS-Friendly Exercises

There are plenty of exercise options that are ideal for FM and CFS patients. As Robyn mentioned, walking, swimming, and cycling are just some of the activities that can give your cardiovascular system a workout while still being gentle to your muscles and bones. Of course, it is possible to push yourself to extremes in all these sports (we're not suggesting Lance Armstrong–type feats).

A simple walk can clear your head and benefit your body. For example, Susie S. told us she resolved to get up and go, no matter how she felt: "When I was really sick I made myself take a shower and get dressed. I would go outside and watch the birds or walk around the backyard and look at the flowers. Now I can walk around the neighborhood and ride a bike a short way. Being outdoors really helps."

Walking is an all-around excellent exercise. Even if you are only able to walk half a mile or just around the perimeter of your house, it's a great way to begin exercising. Try to do it every day, and gently increase the distance. Beginning a walking program is more than just healthy for your muscles and cardiovascular system—it is a way to relax your body and calm your mind. Mindful walking is different than walking during the day at your job

or running errands. Walking for exercise can become a special time just for you (and maybe a dog or two who would love to come with you). Don't just walk around a track at your YMCA, walk around your neighborhood, and enjoy the added benefit of meeting your neighbors and their pets. Varying your routes will keep your walking regimen new and interesting.

Karin L. has taken to wearing a pedometer to track her activity level from day to day. "My goal is to increase my activity by 100 steps a day, every week," she says. "Ultimately, I'd love to be able to do a little jogging but for now I'm happy to be doing what I can to increase my activity."

CYCLING

Cycling gets you outside and into the fresh air. It's particularly great for your leg muscles and provides good all-round conditioning. But be cautious, cycling gives you such a rush of freedom that you may get carried away and suddenly realize you are quite far from home. Remember to take your return trip into consideration. This goes back to our earlier tip about managing your energy bank. Be sure to leave some energy in your bank for the trip home!

SWIMMING

David A., an FM patient from Seattle, tries to swim everyday. "I started out swimming ten minutes or so, and now I'm up to about 45 minutes," he says. "I actually feel completely healthy the moment I get out of the pool, but after about an hour, of course, a lot of my symptoms return. But over the long-term, swimming really improves my circulation. I've tried other exercises, but swimming is the only one that doesn't cause significant pain the next day or a few days afterward."

If you don't swim, consider water aerobics in a warm pool. It's a great way to get used to being in the water. You can also find swim classes that address any fears you may have about swimming.

WATER AEROBICS

Have you ever tried aerobic exercise in the water? It's a pleasant experience that makes movement much easier on your muscles by reducing gravity. In many areas, water aerobics classes sponsored by the Arthritis Foundation are provided in an accessible pool. The water must be at least 89 degrees, with only a slight difference between the temperature of the air and the water. These classes are set up for rheumatoid arthritis patients but are open to anyone. Check with your local YMCA for classes—you don't even have to be a swimmer to enjoy them. Sherril J. says, "Water aerobics have been

129

invaluable in getting me moving again after major flares. In between times it makes me feel even better, as if I've just oiled all my moving parts."

IT'S A STRETCH!

Stretching works wonderfully for FM and CFS patients. It's a great form of gentle exercise, easily incorporated into your daily wellness routine, and it's an effective way to cool down after your walk or swim.

Gentle stretching relaxes your muscles and actually stretches them out, lessening the sensation of tightness. Stretching also helps your circulation and increases your flexibility. It's good to stretch before and after your workout. It will lessen your chance of injury, and it feels great, too. When stretching, it is important to move slowly and be aware of how your body responds.

✤ A Patient's Story: Gerry L.

> Gerry L. lives in Lemont, Illinois. Despite having FM, she has become an award-winning runner. You can read more of Gerry's story in her informative pamphlet *So You've Been Diagnosed with Fibromyalgia*. To request a copy, e-mail Gerry at tamingfibro@comcast.net.

Through years of research and trial and error, I have learned how to manage the challenges that severe FM presents. It's been a long journey with many setbacks. It meant finding that center or balance, that time of surrender and acceptance (not giving in or giving up, but surrendering). This has given me the strength to find my path to a healthier, happier life.

Surrendering helped to set me free so I didn't need to ask the question, "Why did this happen to me?" This difficult journey transformed me from a frustrated, pain-debilitated woman, forced to quit a satisfying nursing career, to a seasoned survivor—and incredibly, a runner with a mantle of trophies. Combining alternative therapies with Western medicine, I learned to deal with repressed anger, pain, new physical limitations, the skepticism of family and friends, and the medical community's lack of knowledge.

Some years ago I could hardly get out of bed and was barely functioning. I knew only pain, fatigue, and nonrestorative sleep, which perpetuated the cycle of unproductive, depressing days.

Today I run 5K races, lift weights, and do other exercises. I enjoy my family and friends again, and I feel at peace with my body. The FM is still there, and some days are better than others, but I have my life back.

I remember vividly what it was like to be disbelieved and judged by doctors because I couldn't exercise, yet they were unable to get me to a point where I could begin and not fail. It has been very encouraging to have found supportive doctors, who look at me and tell me I am "amazing" and "an inspiration" because they understand the pain and the continuing daily struggle I experience. We wonder together how I am doing what I do. And they encourage me to stay the course in spite of the pain and difficulties encountered because we have all seen the difference it has made in my life. I cry when I run. But I am also free when I run—there is no FM for a time. I smile too, especially when I see the finish line.

Most doctors will tell you to exercise, but they do not provide any advice on how to go about it. This is a scenario designed to fail, since typically you'll begin with enthusiasm, thinking you're making progress, and then you'll experience a severe flare-up that keeps you out of commission for weeks or months.

I was in no condition to just start running. I began with physical therapy in warm water. I was then gradually taught stretches and other types of exercises. I evaluated the outcome of each one and eliminated or modified those that caused physical difficulty.

When I started walking it was for two minutes at a time. Increasing my endurance took years of hard work and tenacity, since exercise can induce painful flares. But after a while I began to see a difference in my range of motion and pain level. I began to learn what my body could do. Under guidance I became fitter, and in spite of muscle soreness, I realized that I was doing better. I was beginning to feel whole and I gained a sense of freedom.

Sometimes after a run or a workout, I needed to take medication to head off a flare-up and shorten my recovery time, so I could continue with exercise and become stronger. But gradually, I started to glimpse the person I used to be and the new one I was becoming. I still take pain medication as needed, but my dependence on it has diminished greatly.

Warm-water classes were and still are an important part of my exercise training. You become the water and are protected by the healing balm of the warm water. My favorite class is a combination of yoga and tai chi in the water. I need to go inward to obtain the healing necessary to continue my running, and warm-water exercise helps me take care of my inner self.

One very inspiring book for me was John Bingham's *The Courage to Start: A Guide to Running for Your Life* [see Bibliography]. Bingham reminds us that runners come in all shapes and sizes. As a former couch-

potato-turned-marathoner, his motto is, "The miracle isn't that I had the courage to finish; the miracle is that I had the courage to start."

What form of exercise you choose matters little: warm water therapy, walking, tai chi. What is important is to incorporate regular exercise into your daily living. The results may be gradual but they'll be amazing. ❖ ❖ ❖

❖ Ease into Motion

BY DR. KIM BENNETT, P.T., PH.D.

Dr. Bennett, who wrote the section on physical therapy in this book, is a big proponent of exercise. She is involved in training people to be able to teach the Arthritis Foundation's exercise courses.

Initially, people with FM or CFS should use their fatigue or their pain as a limit, because sometimes they won't know for 24 hours if what they're doing is too much. If you start an exercise program, start with one or two exercises on the first day, do them for only a minute or two (but no more), and see how you feel 24 hours later. If you're okay, then you might consider adding one more exercise.

As a physical therapist, this is the area in which I experience the greatest challenge with my patients, especially if they have worked out in the past. When one has a chronic condition, it's important to reframe your attitude toward exercise. Instead of patting yourself on the back because you've just run two miles, you have to pat yourself on the back because you've held back and only exercised at the level you are able to. Having the discipline necessary to progress slowly means increasing a few minutes a session no matter how good (or how bad) you might be feeling.

It takes people with FM or CFS longer to work into an exercise program that is really helpful. Once you have established an exercise routine, consider the advice of a physician I know who tells her patients, "On a good day, don't do more than you usually can, and on a bad day, don't do less than you usually can either!"

I truly believe that exercise can put you in a different state of mind; it increases endorphins and gets you away from the world of stress and worry.

❖ ❖ ❖

We agree, Kim! Find an exercise you love to do and lose yourself in the fun of it. Depression, pain, anxiety, and fatigue can all be powerfully affected by a regular, healthy exercise routine. If you haven't tried exercise as a part of your healing program, talk to your doctor first. Make sure you exercise safely and be sure to begin slowly—your body will thank you for it.

The exercises in this chapter are meant to get you thinking about moving in ways that benefit your overall health. Walking, swimming, cycling, and warm-water aerobics are all activities you can have fun doing. Find an exercise you enjoy and, as Kim Bennett says, "Do it mindfully," meaning, concentrate on the exercise and nothing else.

Chapter 10

Eastern Medicine and Healing Arts

I have learned never to underestimate the capacity of the human mind and body to regenerate—even when prospects seem most wretched. The life force may be the least understood force on this Earth.

— Dr. Norman Cousins

TRADITIONAL EASTERN MEDICINE is an ancient system of treatment, thought, and practice. Its many disciplines include traditional Chinese medicine (acupuncture, Chinese herbal remedies, and tai chi), and Indian Ayurveda (herbal therapy, cleansing, yoga, and meditation). These disciplines—and other Eastern practices—share the philosophy that the human body is an interconnected organism, which should be treated holistically and spiritually.

✤ Connecting with Life Force

Practitioners of Eastern medicine believe that the body contains an energy, or "life force." In Chinese medicine this energy is called "chi" or "qi," in Japanese medicine it is "ki," and in Ayurveda it is "prana." This energy can become unbalanced, stuck, or deficient in a number of ways. When this happens, physical conditions may develop, which we refer to as "illness" or "disease."

Tai chi and qigong instructor Kim Ivy explains, "All organic life has chi. Chi is defined as 'vital life energy,' and all health and disease is a matter of chi, or life energy and balance. Strong health and vitality are signs of abundant and flowing chi; weaker health and health concerns signal chi blocks and depletion."

There are five major categories of chi:

1. Organ chi, the chi that energizes each of our organs

2. Acupuncture meridian chi, which is the energy that circulates throughout the meridian pathways of the body

3. Nutritive chi, which you derive from food

4. Protective chi, also known as "superficial" chi, which defends the body against infection and other types of illness and regulates body temperature

5. Ancestral chi, which is the chi you are born with, given to you by your parents

From an Eastern-medicine perspective, FM and CFS are the result of stagnant or blocked chi. As Kim Ivy tells us, "Many of the FM tender points correspond directly to significant points along the chi lines (the acupuncture meridians). The tender points are areas of possible energy stagnation that reflect or create imbalances such as tension, fatigue, and pain. Those with CFS often suffer internal organ weakness and this, in Chinese medicine, is seen at least partially through the lens of a chi imbalance." The Eastern medicine philosophy also includes the movement and meditation practices of yoga, tai chi, and qigong. At the end of this chapter, Vijay Elarth tells us about the many benefits of yoga, which originated in India more than 2,600 years ago. Vijay also recommends some cleansing poses to try at home. And Kim Ivy shows us how tai chi and qigong can heal both body and soul.

The medicines and healing arts in this chapter have the power to significantly impact the pain and fatigue of FM and CFS. All share the same life-affirming philosophy that the path to wellness lies within ourselves.

❖ Acupuncture

BY ANGELA HUGHES, M.AC LAC

Angela Hughes received her initial training in acupuncture and traditional Chinese medicine in 1989 from the London School of Acupuncture. Additionally, she holds a masters degree in acupuncture and herbal medicine from the Northwest Institute of Acupuncture and Oriental Medicine in

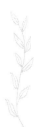

Seattle. Angela is an adjunct clinical faculty member at Bastyr University and specializes in the treatment of chronic pain and disease, especially in the elderly. She currently has a private practice at the Healing Arts Partnership and at Bastyr's practitioner care clinic.

Traditional Chinese medicine is a system of healing that is based on the theory that there are energy channels that run all over the body under the surface of the skin. These channels, or "meridians," bring vital substances to every part of the human body, including the cells, organs, skin, bones, and joints. As well as bringing blood, fluid, and a type of electrical energy, or "chi," to each part of the body to keep its systems functioning, the channels also provide "homeostasis," a correct balance of fluids, temperature, and hormones to keep the body functioning properly.

There are 14 major vessels on the body, and these branch into smaller channels, forming a complete network that brings nourishment to various areas of our physical landscape. Thousands of years ago, the Chinese discovered that there are specific points along the meridians where chi energy is concentrated. They also found that the body's homeostasis and health could be influenced by placing pressure on these points, a theory that led to the development of acupressure and acupuncture therapy. In acupuncture, the practitioner inserts specialized needles as fine as a strand of hair into the surface of the skin at these sites. The goal of treatment is to create changes in the flow of chi and "vital substances" (circulation of blood, lymph, and other body fluids) in the affected meridians.

Each of the 14 major vessels either originates or ends in a major organ system. As long as the flow of chi and vital substances is unrestricted or unobstructed, the organs associated with each meridian will be well nourished and perform their function properly.

According to Chinese medicine, the maintenance of good health and balance in the body is based on two simple concepts:

1. In order for the body to function properly, there must be sufficient chi and vital substances in circulation.

2. The flow of chi and vital substances to the organs must be unobstructed.

Disease happens, therefore, when there is deficiency or obstruction:

1. Deficiency occurs when there are not enough chi and vital substances in the body.

This can happen for a variety of reasons, including poor diet, poor absorption and assimilation, an imbalance in the input/output of energy, or long-term illness, which can deplete the body's vitality.

If there is a deficiency of chi and vital substances, it is more difficult for the body's systems to create new energy and to repair and rebalance itself.

Symptoms of deficiency in a meridian are often experienced as weakness, numbness, or coldness along the meridian itself, and malfunctioning of the organ system with which the meridian is connected.

2. Obstruction occurs when one or more of the vessels are obstructed.

Here the mechanism can be compared to throwing a log into a stream. If the flow of chi is obstructed, there will be a backlog in one area and a deficit downstream, beyond the obstruction. The longer the meridian is obstructed, the greater the backlog and the deficit it causes. Obstruction can occur due to varying factors, including stress and tension (which causes the meridians to constrict and block the flow of chi) and physical trauma (which creates swelling and bruising that obstructs the flow of chi).

Symptoms of obstruction in a meridian are often experienced as pain, heaviness, or heat along the meridian itself, and malfunctioning of the organ system with which the meridian is connected.

DIAGNOSIS

The principle aim of diagnosis according to traditional Chinese medicine is to determine which meridians are deficient or blocked and why. Due to the interconnectedness of the meridian system, symptoms of deficiency or obstruction such as numbness or pain in a meridian may have their origin in a completely different part of the body. It would be an easy option to just target the area in which the pain or numbness is manifesting. However, treatment is far more effective and long lasting when the root of the problem is fully understood and addressed.

Diagnosis is an important aspect of all acupuncture treatment. Depending on the severity and chronic nature of the problem, it may take some time for the acupuncturist to find the real root cause(s) of the patient's condition. For this reason, an initial diagnostic session with an

acupuncturist may take an hour or more and the diagnosis is reevaluated on an ongoing basis in all later treatment sessions.

Once the imbalances have been identified, treatment is aimed at restoring the flow of chi and vital substances in the affected meridians and organs. Chi is rebalanced by stimulating points known to affect the relevant sites. Chinese herbal therapy is often used in conjunction with acupuncture. Treatment may also include massage, heat therapy, and recommendations on diet or exercise.

ACUPUNCTURE FOR FM AND CFS

In terms of traditional Chinese medicine, there are three different diagnoses for FM and CFS.

Each diagnosis includes aspects of deficiency and obstruction:

1. Trapped heat

    This refers specifically to the imbalances that occur when a viral or bacterial infection invades the body and is not fully resolved. This can occur when the patient's defenses are compromised due to stress or lack of rest. If the pathogen is not expelled, this in turn can further weaken the body's defense system. In this case, the result is often a type of trapped heat (inflammation) that becomes aggravated whenever the patient becomes run-down or experiences a lot of stress. Pain in this case is often of a burning nature. Other accompanying symptoms include fever (especially at night), frequent sore throats, mouth sores, a burning sensation on the skin, insomnia, restlessness, fatigue, and irritability. Treatment is aimed at cooling the body by using points that specifically clear heat and restoring the flow of chi and vital substances in the affected meridians.

2. Dampness or dampness mixing with heat

    Traditional Chinese medicine uses metaphors from nature to describe physical symptoms. In FM and CFS, conditions referred to as dampness are reflected in an accumulation of fluid, such as mucus discharge, swelling, or edema that blocks the meridians and organs. This can be the result of an imbalance in the body's digestive or kidney system. It can also be due to a diet too rich in sweets and in foods that cause the body to retain fluid and produce phlegm. In this symptom pattern, pain is often accompanied by a sensation of heaviness, numbness, and swelling. Other symptoms

can include swollen glands, nausea, poor appetite, loose stools, heavy headaches, weight gain, lethargy, inability to stay awake, or depression. If the damp condition mixes with heat trapped in the body, then the pain will be of a heavy nature but will also be burning. In addition to these symptoms, there may also be signs of toxicity: oily hair and skin with frequent skin eruptions, pungent bodily discharges, irritability, and severe insomnia.

3. Deficiency of chi and vital substances

In these cases there is a history of gradual decline in the body's vital energy. This could be a result of a long illness, a trauma involving a major loss of blood, a chronically poor diet, burning the candle at both ends, or a habit of too much exercise of a depleting nature. The meridians and organs of the body become malnourished and are unable to function properly, causing a further decline in health and an inability of the body to sustain good circulation and keep the substances moving in the meridians, causing obstruction.

The nature of the pain experienced in these cases is dull, and it becomes worse with any activity. Other accompanying symptoms can include poor circulation, pale complexion, a tendency to feel cold or to numbness, palpitations, fatigue, breathlessness, dizziness, or poor balance.

In summary, if a patient who has been diagnosed with FM or CFS experiences any of the symptoms mentioned above, acupuncture treatments can be very helpful in alleviating these symptoms. ❖❖❖

❖ Chinese Herbal Medicine

Traditional Chinese medicine has long used herbs and tonics as the center of its healing modality. Chinese herbal medicine dates back to the third century B.C., when ginseng roots were discovered in Chinese forests and found to be powerful remedies to treat illness and to increase sexual vigor. In ancient times, ginseng was reserved only for the emperor. Thankfully, it's available to all of us now.

Chinese herbal medicine and dietary supplements support the body's natural defenses, boosting the immune system and reducing infections, while gently strengthening the body. This is a complete system of medicine. Based on the philosophy of yin and yang, the goal is to restore balance and harmony to the body, to allow the natural flow of chi. The focus is on

correcting internal imbalances that are the root cause of the illness, rather than concentrating only on symptoms.

Although it is an ancient system of treatment, Chinese herbal medicine is still a vital, continually developing modality. In China today, it is used in the treatment of a broad range of health conditions; for example, to relieve pain, improve digestion, and fight cancer.

On a visit to China, you will see herbs being carefully weighed at traditional Chinese medicine dispensaries. Remedies are available in both traditional and modern formulas. Traditionally, dried herbs are boiled to make a tea or broth. Now they are also available as freeze-dried powders or tinctures.

Some examples of Chinese remedies that address the imbalances of FM and CFS include:

- *Croton crassifolius*, or Geisel, a Chinese shrub used to regulate vital energy to alleviate pain
- Maitake mushrooms, which enhance the activity of the immune system
- Dong quai *(Angelica sinensis)*, which improves hormone balance in women
- Ginger, used to relieves aches and pains
- Astragalus, which enhances immune activity and restores energy
- Ginseng, used to increases energy and stamina

Chinese herbal remedies produce results more slowly than their Western pharmaceutical counterparts but do not involve the toxicity associated with some medications. Although pharmacologically active, herbal medicine has fewer side effects than Western pharmaceutical medicine. It is interesting to note that herbal remedies cannot be recreated artificially—for example, we know the chemical compounds of ginseng, but if we put them together in a laboratory, using the exact formula, we could not reproduce true ginseng. These combinations are found only in nature's pharmacopoeia.

If you are interested in adding Chinese herbal medicine to your treatment program, we recommend consulting a professional Chinese herbalist and getting a prescription. Chinese herbal remedies are a delicate balance of precise formulae. Just as in Western medicine, it is important to consider what you are putting into your body, the affect it will have, and the way it will interact with other medications you are taking.

✤ A Patient's Story: Ellen J.

Ellen J. is working on her master's degree in counseling psychology at
Antioch University in Seattle. At 45, she is living with FM, CFS, and multiple chemical sensitivities. She has found that Eastern medicine and healing arts are the only healing forms that have consistently helped her to live
life to the fullest. She lives in Seattle, surrounded by mountains and flowering plants, all of which she finds healing to body and soul.

In 1992, I moved myself and all my possessions west, from Champaign, Illinois, to Seattle. I came to attend Bastyr University, the world-renowned
college of natural healing. My intention was to become a doctor of naturopathy, but I ended up becoming my own patient.

I was in tremendous pain and couldn't sit in class long enough to take
notes. My hands were seizing up, my muscles were spasming from head to
toe, my jaw trembled, and I had headaches and diarrhea. I saw several doctors, who had no idea what was wrong. At that point, the dean of the school
recommended that I see a rheumatologist, and in no time at all, he diagnosed me with FM.

As my illness progressed, I found that alternative healing arts, particularly Eastern medicine, were the modalities with which I had the most
success, both when treating myself and when advising others. (For years,
I have always been the person that friends call when they have a health
question.)

I have been receiving acupuncture treatments every other week for the
last ten years. I have been treated by acupuncturists from two different traditions—Chinese and Japanese. The difference is in the type of needle used
and how deeply the needles are placed. Both have been very effective treatments for decreasing pain, for recovering from acute illnesses like sinus infections and the flu, and for improving my digestion. They have also helped
me cope with depression and express my anger. I notice that whenever I
take a break from this treatment, I have less stamina and get infections
much more often.

I have practiced yoga for the past three years with so much success that
I was discharged from physical therapy because I was doing so well with
my yoga classes and home yoga program. I practice ananda yoga, a form
of hatha yoga that involves traditional physical postures. I have also been
trained in kriya yoga, which is a meditation technique that was brought by
Paramhansa Yogananda from India to the United States. I meditate once or
twice a day for 30–60 minutes.

141

I take Chinese herbs and use principles of Chinese nutrition in my daily cooking. My acupuncturist has given me lists of foods that help to build and nourish chi and blood. Before trying Chinese nutrition, I was primarily a vegetarian. I now add a portion of fish or chicken to my meals once a week. I also eat many more root vegetables (sweet potato and parsnips) and work on balancing different flavors (sour, bitter, sweet, pungent, and salty). I make sure that the whole foods I eat are prepared in a way that best supports my particular needs. I use ginger, turmeric, and coriander in my cooking, particularly in squash and bean dishes, and in soups. These herbs are known to aid digestion, and when I digest my food well, I notice that I experience less pain and swelling in my joints and connective tissues. I eat steamed vegetables and brown rice when I need to detoxify due to exposure to allergens and chemical toxins. I try to focus on using food to heal my body, rather than just eating on the run as a way to fuel my body between activities, as I did before I got sick.

I learned several years ago that I will probably be in pain for the rest of my life due to osteoarthritis and a bone spur in my hip. But I can choose how I will respond to that pain. My choice is not to suffer. Since I made this determination, there has been a radical shift in my whole being, a paradigm shift in which my pain and fatigue, while still very much present, have shifted into the background instead of being the whole picture. My life itself has become the foreground, and the colors, textures, and tastes are sharper and brighter now. ❋❋❋

❖ Ayurveda

BY WENDY BODIN, B.S., CKP, CHP

Wendy Bodin is a certified herbalist trained in traditional herbal systems of the world. She was trained in Ayurveda by Karta Purkh Singh Khalsa and Kumu Dini Shoba. Wendy's Luminary Health Institute is located in Albuquerque, New Mexico. You can find her website at www.luminary health.com.

Ayurveda is the natural healing system of India. It is built upon a strong foundation of thousands of years of research and devotion. Today it is a comprehensive and affordable system of health and healing that is based on spirituality, yoga, meditation, the healing properties of plants and minerals, lifestyle, and environmental factors. It offers healing for the physical body as well as mental, emotional, and spiritual healing.

Ayurveda is believed to be the oldest existing healing system in the world. Originating in India, it spread throughout Asia and beyond, influencing all other major healing systems. Healers from around the world have journeyed to India to learn from Ayurvedic teachers, as well as to share their healing knowledge.

Ayurveda suggests that the root of all disease is caused by separation from our spiritual source. If we allow ourselves to disconnect from that source, we first lose touch with the mind and then the body falls ill. When this flow of divine or innate universal intelligence is blocked, due to fear or other imbalances, disease will manifest. In India, this energy source is called prana, "the breath of life." A complete cutting off of this flow will cause the body to die.

The basic premise of Ayurveda suggests that if we look at the structure of the universe of which we are a part, then we will know how to heal ourselves.

The first Ayurvedic teachers, the rishis, described the structure of the universe in components. The first three are

1. Purusha: Existence. It is the consciousness, sentience, and spirit of being. It creates desire.

2. Prakriti: The creativity that produces the manifestation of desire or will; it is the motivating force that takes action. It creates and is productive.

3. Mahat is the combined force of purusha and prakriti. It is the cosmic intelligence within each of us, which allows us to manifest according to what we create. The choice is ours.

THE GUNAS

The three gunas are basic qualities that exist throughout nature, as well as in all people—sattwa, rajas, and tamas. They also describe the life cycle of birth (sattwa), life or maintenance (rajas), and death or dissolution (tamas).

Sattwa is defined as the manifestation of subjective consciousness, or spirituality and purity. It is the pure state of mind that is reflected in a healthy body, mind, and spirit. A person who is sattwic is calm, considerate, alert, and kind. They remain balanced and grounded in times of stress or in the presence of discordant energies. This is the desired state of being to which we can all aspire and ultimately attain.

Rajas is controlled by the flow of energy. A person who values rajas energy seeks power, authority, prestige, and control. Too much rajasic energy

143

creates an unbalanced state of indecisiveness, irritability, unreliability, hyperactivity, or anxiety. People in whom rajasic energy predominates find it difficult to sit still and tend to lose focus on priorities.

Tamas is defined as potential energy. People who live under the influence of tamas energy are not fully realizing their potential or following their true path. Too much tamas energy will manifest as living in a state of fear, compromise, servitude, having unmet needs, depression, self-destructiveness, addictions, or degenerative diseases. The minds of tamasic people tend to become dull and lethargic.

Ayurveda maintains that rajas (overactive energy) and tamas (underactive energy) are the spiritual and psychological causes of disease. Since we are all multidimensional, throughout our lives we accumulate characteristics of the three energies that we must balance. For example, a person who is both tamasic and rajasic can seek balance by exercising to reduce tamasic influence. They may also practice meditation to encourage Sattwic energy into their lives.

THE DOSHAS

Along with these three gunas, there are three constitutional types or doshas that correspond to physical attributes. Individual physiology will fall into one predominant category, with some influences of the other categories.

Vata: Formed by air, or ether, people in whom vata qualities predominate tend to be wiry, thin, and highly active.

Pitta: Formed by fire and an aspect of water, people high in pitta energy are characterized as muscular, athletic, of medium stature, and may have fiery temperaments.

Kapha: Formed from water and earth, people who manifest kapha energy are large, big boned, and generously proportioned.

Each of us was born with an inherent constitution reflecting one of the three doshas that will remain with us for life. We have the ability to improve the balance of our physical and mental constitution with herbs and other therapies.

Since Ayurveda includes food and herbal therapies, the principles of the gunas and the doshas apply to the foods we eat as well. They are gifts of nature and the universe, so they also follow the same laws, providing parallel healing qualities to help us restore our health and balance.

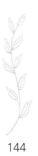

An easy way to begin is to eat foods and herbs that are sattwic in nature, foods that promote calm and tranquility. However, we still need to take into account our own constitutional type in order to make the best choices. For example, oats are very soothing—they have sattwic characteristics and can be quite beneficial. However, since oats are starchy, they are not the best choice for people with kapha constitutions, who have a tendency to weight gain.

The body, mind, and spirit seek balance and reflect imbalance in the form of disease. We have the choice to respond by allowing natural healing into our lives. In Ayurveda, health is believed to be the natural state of being, as it is in harmony with nature and the universe. Disease is believed to be an unnatural state of being, caused when the ego separates the individual from nature and the universal source.

The goal of Ayurveda is to live in harmony with the universe and its divine intelligence. Since our bodies are made up from the same elements of the universe, if we follow the laws of the universe, we can return to a natural state of health and live a long and contented life. ❖❖❖

❖ Yoga

BY VIJAY ELARTH

Vijay Elarth is a registered yoga teacher and founder of the Karuna Integral Yoga Center in Seattle. He holds "Fibromyoga" classes for FM and CFS patients. Vijay has practiced yoga since 1979. He became certified to teach Integral Yoga in 1984, and in 1985 he became certified to teach advanced classes. Vijay has received national accreditation from the Yoga Alliance, at the highest category of proficiency.

Yoga is an Eastern exercise and movement therapy designed to restore harmony, flexibility, and function to the body. The ancient philosophy teaches that the body should be healthful and that the mind should be peaceful. I didn't begin yoga until I was in my mid-forties. It made me feel so good that I wanted to do more with my body than just sit around and watch television. Many people tend to think that yoga is only stretching, but yoga practice also strengthens and nourishes the internal organs and other systems of the body. I also like the benefits of the deep relaxation that occur when the body is quiet; then the energies of the body flow into the immune system, and this also helps keep the body vital.

Four Cleansing Yoga Poses

Janusirshasana

Cleansing poses are among the most beneficial for people with FM or CFS. Janusirshasana, often translated as the "head-to-knee pose," is one of the best of these postures. For this pose, sit on the floor with the right leg straight and the left knee bent, pressing the sole of the left foot against the inside of the right leg wherever comfortable. Then fold your body from the hips over the right thigh. As you lower your body and your abdomen comes closer to the thigh, the liver is squeezed and the kidneys are stretched. Beginners should hold this pose for perhaps fifteen seconds, and then repeat it. Those more experienced in the pose will be able to hold it for up to one minute. After folding over the right thigh, re-verse the legs and lower your body over the left thigh.

There is one caution about this posture, however. If you have low back pain, do not attempt this pose without the guidance of an experienced teacher.

People with lower-back problems will increase the tension in their back mus-cles during the forward bend unless they move into the pose correctly and very slowly. To avoid creating too much tension in this area, inhale deeply to extend the spine upward before folding over either thigh. Then, holding the breath and the extension, fold until the body reaches its limit of comfort, and then exhale. At this point, the head can be relaxed so that it drifts toward the knee. Sometimes after this pose, people say they have a slightly bitter but not unpleasant taste in their mouths. I believe that this is the result of moderate compression and stimu-lation of the liver. After this pose, I usually offer a sip of water.

Uddhiyana Bandha

This posture, which benefits digestion, is also known as the "the stomach lift." Stand with the feet about shoulder width apart, then exhale completely and lean forward. The knees are slightly bent. Place the hands on the knees, then raise your head. Lift the abdomen in and up, hold it until you feel you need to inhale, then release the abdomen and stand, and inhale gently. It is beneficial to repeat

---

YOGA FOR PEOPLE WITH FIBROMYALGIA

My interest in FM and CFS began when a student told me that she had FM and felt 90 percent pain free as a result of my class. This gave me the idea to design a class especially for people with FM and CFS. In this class, we assume that there is pain; our goal is to stretch and move without in-creasing the pain.

this three times, and to do so while the stomach is empty of food. Caution: This cleansing practice may increase the flow of blood during menstruation; it is best to avoid it at that time. This practice is said to help prevent or cure digestive problems, especially constipation.

Arddha Salabasana

Much pain is caused by poor posture. An important pose for strengthening the spinal erector muscles is *arddha salabasana,* the "half-locust pose." Lie on the abdomen with the legs straight and together. Place the hands, palm up, under the thighs or hips. Then stretch the right leg and lift it slightly into the air. The knees should be kept straight. The right foot can be held in any comfortable position. Beginners can hold this pose for perhaps fifteen seconds, rest for a moment, then repeat. As the body strengthens, the pose can be held for up to one minute. Repeat the pose, raising the left leg. During the pose, as during most poses, avoid the temptation to hold your breath. Simply breathe naturally.

Deergha Swasam

I believe breathing practices are of great benefit to those with FM or CFS because they help to release toxins and impurities from the body. The basic breathing practice is *deergha swasam,* the "three-part breath." This can be done while sitting in a chair with the spine straight but not stiff.

+ First, take control of the breath and then exhale deeply from the abdomen.
+ Now let the inhalation begin in the abdomen, flow through the lower chest, and then rise into the upper chest.
+ When the inhalation reaches the upper chest, the collarbones may slightly rise.
+ Then begin exhaling from the collarbones, and let the exhalation extend deep into the abdomen.

This is one breath. In the beginning, continue the practice for a few minutes, gradually lengthening the time up to five minutes.

I try to keep the "Fibromyoga" class very small. Each client's needs are different. Several have visibly physical problems; others do not. One cannot do twists; another has hip and knee problems that inhibit movement. All realize that their bodies are their own teachers; they are empowered to do what is beneficial and to ignore what is not. A yoga teacher once told me that when she walks into a class and all the students are doing the same thing at the same time, she knows she is in the presence of a poor teacher,

147

one who has not empowered the students to be their own teachers. Despite my individualized approach, there is structure in my classes.

A GENTLE CLASS

Students enter my studio through a Japanese-style garden that contains pools and running water. The studio is carpeted and there are many blankets and pillows. There is a fireplace, and on cold mornings I build a fire and heat stones for people to hold in their hands. Students are encouraged to enter the room, lie down, and relax. They can also warm their bodies with the stones, if desired. At that point, we each check in, expressing how we feel and reporting whether or not there have been any major developments in our bodies since the last class.

At the beginning of the class we sometimes chant "Om," simply to pay homage to the ancient tradition of yoga. We do eye movements and breathing practices, and I teach abdominal cleansing practices that are designed to cleanse the digestive system. We then do the Sun Salutation as a warm-up practice. The core of the class is made up of backward-bending poses, standing poses, twisting poses, and forward-bending poses. I teach postures that involve very gentle movements, and after we move for a short while, we rest in what is called a restorative pose. The resting poses, in which the body does little or no work, allow the body to be renewed. This approach, when combined with gentle stretching and deep relaxation, also strengthens the immune system. The class ends with a deep relaxation exercise. Sometimes I play soft music in the background; in warm weather the windows are open and we can hear natural sounds, such as running water.

FINDING A YOGA TEACHER

A good yoga teacher should have several qualities. First, they should be certified. They should be a student of some other teacher, preferably of a different tradition of yoga than the one they teach. (There are many traditions of yoga; some are very gentle, which is what I teach, and others are very strenuous. The yoga teacher should have experience with all these traditions.) The yoga teacher should have basic knowledge of the structures of the body and how the systems of the body work. They should be able to name the primary muscles. If you ask a teacher where the biceps are, and he or she says, "In the legs," go elsewhere. They should also be able to name the major bones of the skeleton.

I teach "integral yoga," a gentle form of practice in which the majority of the postures are performed in a sitting position or while lying down, with many periods of rest. If you have FM or CFS, you may need to avoid other more vigorous styles of yoga. For example, Iyengar yoga is quite strenuous, with many standing poses. "Bikram yoga" is also strenuous and is performed in a very hot room. Power yoga requires extra strength and stamina because it involves a continuous series of poses that flow from one to the other, without resting.

Yoga is beneficial because we become completely absorbed by what is happening in the body. We can, for a moment, forget the past and the future; the mind settles into the present wherein there might be joy and peace. We may even for a time forget the pains of the body. This engages our awareness on a spiritual level, while on a physical level, it simply feels good to move without causing pain. ❖❖❖

❖ Tai Chi and Qigong

BY KIM IVY

Kim Ivy is a certified tai chi and qigong instructor. She has worked with FM and CFS students for over ten years. Kim is the founder of Embrace The Moon Taijiquan and Qigong in Seattle. Kim's work has been published nationally and internationally, and it was featured (with coauthor Susan Schmidt, M.D.) in *Back Pain,* by Andrew J. Haig, M.D., and Miles Colwell, M.D. Kim's website is www.embracethemoon.com

Tai chi and qigong are movement and meditation practices that originated in China, and they are practiced by millions of people in China and millions more all over the world. Qigong, the study of vital force, or "qi" (the Chinese spelling of chi), is considered to be among the first practices ancient man created for health and spiritual development. At this time, it is believed there are more than 10,000 different forms of qigong, some dating back over two thousand years, and some developed in modern times by qigong experts. Qigong is often categorized into five major groups: medical, martial, Buddhist, Taoist, and Confusion. As a therapeutic practice, it is a fundamental branch of traditional Chinese medicine and, along with acupuncture, massage, and herbs, is used prescriptively for many health-related issues, such as lowering stress and blood pressure, boosting the endocrine and immune system, and strengthening the cardiovascular system.

149

Tai chi ch'uan (grand ultimate boxing) traces its roots back to the early 1600s. Tai chi was cultivated predominately by several main families as an art of self-defense, but modern tai chi is most commonly thought of as a form of mindful exercise. It is considered a type of qigong and its benefits are similar to those of qigong. Additional benefits of tai chi include balance and overall movement control, especially in the lower limbs.

Tai chi and qigong routines vary widely, yet all are characterized by relaxation, coordinated diaphragmatic breathing, fluid movement, and a calm mental state. The pace of the exercises ranges from still and meditative to active and quite vigorous. Generally speaking, tai chi and qigong forms move continuously and for the most part slowly, through a sequence of complementary movements. The routines have a rhythm within which they develop from stillness into movement, each movement flowing smoothly into the next, and then finally ending by returning to stillness. The whole body and mind are thoroughly engaged. In contrast to other traditional exercises that emphasize the physical body by building or stretching muscles, tai chi and qigong are designed fundamentally to first build and balance chi.

Qigong and tai chi are exercise forms that offer good news for those with FM and CFS. Relaxation, mental focus, and enhanced breathing are integral to these exercise arts. Through this practice, chi stagnation and blockages are released, enhancing blood flow, tissue repair, and organ function. Because the fundamental operating principle of tai chi and qigong is relaxation, these practices also result in enhanced ability to influence one's own autonomic, sympathetic, and parasympathetic nervous systems more efficiently. This translates into the ability to shift out of the stress response more easily.

As with the highly tuned athlete, a tai chi and qigong practitioner enjoys many health benefits. Research in China and a growing number of Western studies show that meditative exercise can lower blood pressure, increase cardiac fitness, strengthen the immune and musculoskeletal systems, provide better coordination and balance, and increase one's overall sense of well-being.

Unlike other more vigorous athletic endeavors, the tai chi and qigong student achieves these results without the possible harmful effects caused by overtaxing the physical body. Tai chi and qigong, when practiced correctly, will not cause muscle tears, spasms, or depletion of electrolytes. And because none of the movements involve a strong muscular contraction (like weightlifting) they do not produce an excess of adrenaline to be pumped through the body. This is especially important for those who have health concerns such as FM or CFS whose bodies have difficulty processing adrenaline.

A SUCCESS STORY

In the mid 1990s a physician at a local hospital contracted me to develop a program using tai chi and qigong for his chronic-pain patients. The movement and exercise system I created was designed to give patients some pain relief and enable them to function without requiring such frequent treatment at the pain clinic. Most of the people who joined this program had debilitating pain and health conditions, including FM and CFS. Together, we learned to integrate tai chi and qigong principles and movement for chronic pain and fatigue syndromes.

Candace S., one of the participants in the program, was a woman in her early 50s, an athlete and landscaper. She had been thin, muscular, and vital her whole life. About two years prior to joining the program, she came down with the flu and never recovered. When Candace joined the eight-week program she was 50 pounds overweight and all but bedridden. Having confounded the medical system for some time, Candace had been recently diagnosed with CFS.

When Candace first began taking my classes she was unable to stand for more than two minutes without having her heart rate exceed 200 beats per minute. During the course of the eight weeks, Candace followed the movements as well as she could, although she rested every two minutes. During the rest time, Candace would watch very intently, imprinting the simple arm, waist, and leg patterns into her brain. When watching became too fatiguing, she would close her eyes and follow the voice instructions. Candace became skilled at visualizing the movements and would practice them mentally at home. Within four weeks of practice, we watched Candace begin to stand and practice the movements with the group for at least half of the class time.

Candace continued to develop her tai chi and qigong skills in this way and over the next four years came to practice for hours several days a week. She became a top student, expanding her studies with other teachers to become a competent assistant instructor. It was not that Candace's CFS had been obliterated, nor did she only rely on her qigong and tai chi practices to improve her health, but they were instrumental in helping her symptoms to recede and in increasing her quality of life dramatically.

Perhaps the greatest gift tai chi and qigong practice have to offer a student with FM or CFS is that of awareness. Because there is so much

emphasis on conscious alertness during the slow continuous movements of a practice, a student learns to become more sensitive to all his or her movements—not just in practice, but in daily life, too. Training teaches a student to become self-reflective and make changes in their form as needed for greater balance and fluidity. This is a skill that can easily be applied to life in general. FM and CFS students can learn to become aware of general movement patterns that cause pain and then change them. A student may also learn to identify thought patterns that lead to stressful movement and change them.

FINDING A TAI CHI OR QIGONG TEACHER

It is important to find a good teacher and the right instructional environment when embarking on a tai chi or qigong practice. Although these are ancient practices, they are relatively new on the landscape of exercise in general, and even newer when considered as a type of therapy. It may take a little research to find the right fit. Specifically, I have observed that tai chi is a little more useful for people who have severe FM because it involves more movement and less standing. For people who have CFS, qigong tends to be more useful because less movement is required and it can be quite easily modified into sitting and lying positions. However, it is always best to allow yourself a chance to explore what works for you.

For people with FM or CFS, we do not advise learning from a video or DVD. The forms look simple, but the structural and energetic alignment is specific. It is difficult for anyone to self-correct, and if the forms are done incorrectly, they can cause a flare-up, spasm, or injury.

FINDING THE RIGHT TEACHER

1. *Look for the teacher's heart and style rather than a certification.* It is great if you can find a certified teacher but certification programs are rare. Find a teacher who is flexible and willing to listen to your needs and limits. The teacher must also be willing to explore modifications of the form for your comfort.

2. *Work with a teacher who has themselves been practicing for several years.* Your teacher should have an excellent sense of both energy and physical alignment, and a well-developed compassionate teaching style borne of working with many people.

3. *Find an instructional environment that works for you.* Classes should be noncompetitive, friendly, and fun—you should want to

come to class. If necessary, remind your teacher that fragrances such as perfume and incense need to be left out of the training environment. There should always be a comfortable chair for you to sit and rest, if necessary.

BEING A GREAT STUDENT:

1. *Be proactive in your learning.* Ask if the form can be done sitting down. Ask if you can rest between exercises. If your teacher is good, they will say yes!

2. *Go at it slowly.* Tai chi and qigong are subtle, but they can still be overdone. Stay conscious, stay aware, and stop sooner than you think you need to. A little goes a long way.

3. *Be patient.* The benefits of tai chi and qigong are cumulative and take time. These are practices that are approached differently than the way we commonly view movement and exercise. Focus on the process. Allow the practice to become a path for you, rather than a goal.

Tai chi and qigong are wonderful for restoring balance, for lessening pain, and most importantly for returning a sense of joy about living in one's body. I have noticed that tai chi and qigong can provide real health benefits for the FM and CFS patient. However, they are superior when practiced in combination with other modalities such as acupuncture, physical therapy, nutritional counseling, and emotional coaching. No matter which approach you choose, the key point of these practices is to proceed slowly and mindfully, always seeking relaxation. Modify them liberally for your own comfort, and communicate directly with your teacher. Tai chi and qigong, like life, actually work best when we learn to relax and allow our natural fluidity to emerge. ❖ ❖ ❖

❖ ❖ ❖

In this chapter we have described how to support the "life force" or "chi" with various practices of Eastern medicine. In our next chapter, we look at the ancient art of energetic healing, which taps this life force through another approach. From an energetic healing perspective, our bodies, thoughts, and emotions are pure energy. Learning to harness this energy for ourselves is not only possible for each of us, but is also an inevitable part of the medicine of the future.

Chapter 11

Energetic Healing

Intuition is part of healing.

— Sharon Franquemont
From *You Already Know What to Do*

LIFE FORCE ENERGY, whether called "prana," "mana" "chi," or "ki," or is known worldwide as the Universal Energy that is tapped into by healers. In this chapter we talk about ways to affect your life force energy for the betterment of your health.

Energetic healing is the ancient art of raising your life force energy in a way that can alleviate pain, quiet the mind, and open the spirit. Perhaps more than any other branch of complementary healing, energetic healing demonstrates the powerful connection between mind and body. Patients we interviewed about their participation in energetic healing reported less pain overall, a feeling of lightness and centeredness after a healing session, and most all reported the need for less pain medication over time. There are many doorways through which to access healing energy, including Reiki, Quantum-Touch™, and energy psychology. Most are practiced by an energy therapist (metaphysician), a Reiki master, or a registered counselor and are either applied directly to a client or conveyed through distance healing. Some energy therapies are quite simple to learn and lend themselves well to self-healing. These include visualization, meditation, and progressive relaxation. In every person lies the ability to learn to heal themselves and to help another to heal.

You have the choice of finding an energetic healing practitioner and working together to raise your energy, or learning to use this form of healing yourself. There are many methods of healing available: color healing, chakra clearing, pendulum work, and crystal and stone healing, to name just a few. These types of healing open the chakras for the betterment of health by improving energy flow and relieving pain, both mental and physical. The energy therapist does not heal you; he or she simply helps you to harness your own natural healing abilities.

In this chapter you will meet energy practitioners and therapists who show us that some of the best healing can be done within ourselves. We begin with Reiki, one of the earliest forms of energetic healing.

✤ Reiki

BY MAUREEN BRENNAN

Maureen Brennan is a Reiki master/teacher, who has been practicing Reiki since 1992. Her psychic ability assists in her healing practice. Maureen has three children and lives with her family in Seattle.

Reiki is part of the oldest form of healing in the world—the laying on of hands. Reiki practitioners channel universal (rei) life force energy (ki) through the palms of their hands. The hands are placed on or slightly above the fully clothed body of the client. The hands are held in a particular position for about two to three minutes and then moved. The Reiki practitioner is intuitively guided to what each area of the body needs and the length of time needed. Commonly, the client experiences a warm sensation and sometimes waves of energy. Clients may experience a decrease in pain. When there is inflammation, that area may feel cooler following a treatment.

The client is encouraged to relax, let go, and receive the healing Reiki energy. Reiki is gentle, loving, and peaceful, yet very powerful because healing occurs on all levels—physical, mental, emotional, and spiritual. Reiki improves the immune system, relieves energy blocks, soothes pain, allows for deeper relaxation, relieves depression and backaches, and can do much more than that. Reiki masters are humble, openhearted, open-minded, and in the moment. The ego has no place here. The Reiki master's only intention is to be a pure vehicle of healing.

During the initial phase of a session, touch is applied to the front of the client's body. The session then continues with light warm touch to the back of the head, the shoulders, back, torso, the backs of the knees, backs of the ankles, and the bottoms of the feet. By the end of the session, the client is

usually very relaxed. As a general practice I thank the client, the client's spiritual guides, and my guides. On the level of physiology, as relaxation deepens the body usually shifts into the rest and repair mode (of the parasympathetic nervous system). In this mode, it is beneficial to drink plenty of water to promote the release of toxins, and to stay relaxed for the rest of the day, avoiding any strenuous activity. The healing will continue for the next three days or so. It is important to be aware of any changes that occur in the body, mind, emotions, or spirit. Honor the healing process by being gentle with yourself. Ultimately, this approach involves cradling another human being in loving, divine spiritual energy.

A man came to me about a year and a half ago with symptoms resembling mononucleosis, although the doctors were not sure exactly what his problem was. I didn't focus on mono, since I was not familiar with the symptoms. Intuitively, I knew he had a sore throat. When my hands came to the throat position, I was guided to ask him if I could place my hands gently on his throat. I usually place my hands slightly below the throat area so that the client doesn't feel uncomfortable, but it was clear to me that direct contact was necessary. He agreed, and I was guided to keep my hands on his throat for more than ten minutes, which is much longer than usual. I explained this to him and he responded that his throat was really sore.

I explained to him that the throat chakra is the energy center for expressing one's truth. There it was—the crux of the matter! He went on to describe a life issue he was struggling with—he was learning healing techniques and felt guided to continue on his new path as a healer. His wife was threatened by this, as it went against her religious beliefs. My client was at a crossroads. If he followed his intuition to be a healer it could mean the end of his marriage. If he didn't become a healer, could he live with himself? We talked at length about his challenge and how his body was giving him clues about how to heal himself and unblock his energy. After a short period of time, his sore throat faded. I have spoken with him several times since then. After careful consideration, he has decided to divorce his wife so that they may each be set free to follow their own path. He is a loving, happy person who has dedicated himself to helping others heal.

In another incident closer to home, recently I received a frantic phone call from my daughter Jen in New York, who was recovering from a car accident. She was in so much back pain that all she could do was cry. I spoke soothing words to help her relax as I mentally sent healing Reiki energy. I reminded her to let go and allow herself to receive healing. She listened,

breathed, and relaxed slowly as I spoke. Within a few minutes, the pain had subsided and she stopped crying. She was able to remain relaxed. I encouraged her to breathe and relax on her own. She has had Reiki I training so I reminded her to continue self-healing practices daily. Due to the nature of her injuries, her healing process is slow yet steady. Clearly there are many situations in which it is vital to seek medical care, but it is always important to engage the immune response and the body's other healing systems.

To learn Reiki, one needs to find a master teacher. It is important to meet first to see if you feel a connection with the teacher. I encourage students to trust their intuition in this matter. Reiki is passed on from the master teacher to the student during an "attunement," the culmination of everything the student has learned. Attunement to Reiki is a physical, mental, and spiritual passing of knowledge, symbols, and energy. Reiki is usually taught at three levels, the third attunement being the master level. In certain branches of Reiki, further classes and attunements may be offered.

When I work with clients, friends, or family, I work with total trust. I move forward in my approach knowing that Reiki energy always guides me to the highest intention for all. Within that framework of trust I am able to let go and allow healing to occur through me like wind through a hollow reed. It is this approach of balancing technique with intention and intuition that I teach my students.

There have been many advances in Western medicine, although treatment often focuses on effect rather than cause. Now we are learning to balance East and West. We are coming to realize that our essence is wholeness itself. There can be no separation between body, mind, emotion, and spirit. People of all religions and spiritual paths are supported in the process of Reiki, as are those with no particular path. Touch is acknowledged in all cultures as a source of healing.

How wonderful it is for us to have access to both Eastern and Western medicine. Let's take good care of ourselves, pay attention to the body's own wisdom, and seek out care that honors and supports our wholeness. Choose wisely; a true healer, whether doctor or alternative practitioner, is focused on the intention to heal, listens to the wisdom in your body, and supports your own innate ability to heal yourself on all levels. The general public is becoming more aware of this. As we each heal ourselves, returning to wholeness, we heal all of humanity and planet earth. Within ourselves lie the answers to our own questions. ❖❖❖

❧ Quantum-Touch™: "The Issues Are in Your Tissues"

BY CINDY ROTHWELL

Cindy Rothwell is an ordained minister and has 18 years of experience as an intuitive counselor. For more information about scheduling healing sessions or attending a workshop with Cindy, you may access her website at www.cindyrothwell.com.

Quantum-Touch™ is a powerful hands-on healing technique that is easy to learn. It encourages the innate wisdom of the body to heal itself through breathing and body awareness techniques that help people learn to focus and amplify their life force energy. The effects can seem miraculous, such as bones moving effortlessly into alignment, pain vanishing, and chronic ailments disappearing.

The practitioner surrounds the area of pain or illness with their hands, enabling the focused energy to course through the client. This is called "running energy." At the same time, the practitioner begins a pattern of breathing and visualization. The patient may feel heat or a tingling sensation. The pain or other symptoms usually begin to move to another part of the body and, eventually, out of the body. Clients sometimes experience instant relief of their symptoms.

I first learned Quantum-Touch™ by reading *Quantum-Touch: Your Power To Heal* by Richard Gordon [see Bibliography]. This book explains all of the techniques that are taught in workshops worldwide. I then had the opportunity to receive a hip alignment from the author himself. By gently placing his hands on my hips and "running energy," my hips moved into perfect alignment. I felt the effects of that three-minute healing for days and decided to take the workshop. I have been practicing Quantum-Touch™ for five years now and continue to be amazed by the healing I witness in others and myself. I feel I have an energetic first aid kit that is available to me at all times!

I have assisted many people with chronic back pain, often providing profound relief in short periods of time. I have also assisted numerous people and animals in pain through long-distance Quantum-Touch™ healing. Sometimes long-distance healing is more effective than a hands-on approach, especially if the recipient is defensive or skeptical. Last Christmas, I assisted my mother-in-law, who was having trouble breathing and did not feel well. After a forty minute Quantum-Touch™ session she felt much

more energetic and wanted to get up and make Christmas dinner. Seeing such an amazing shift in her health was the most precious gift of the day.

You have the power to heal within you; it's built in. Everyone does. Life force energy sustains all life. Quantum-Touch™ amplifies life force energy, assisting your body to be healthy and in balance. From DNA to bones, all cells and systems respond effortlessly to a highly charged energy field and focus intention, applied through Quantum-Touch™. ❖❖❖

Reiki and Quantum-Touch™ are available to anyone who is ready to open their heart to new experiences. The best part about becoming a Reiki or Quantum-Touch™ practitioner is not only being able to help yourself, but also being able to give treatments to your loved ones too.

❖ Kinesiology

BY WENDY BODIN

Wendy Bodin is a certified Kinesionics practitioner and a certified wellness kinesiologist. In her practice she offers comprehensive therapies utilizing kinesiology testing, nutritional and orthomolecular therapy, herbal therapies, intuitive energy healing, neuro-linguistic programming, Emotional Freedom Technique (EFT), flower essence therapy, and guided Buddhist spiritual healing. Wendy's website is www.luminaryhealth.com.

Applied kinesiology is a diagnostic technique developed in the 1960s by chiropractors. The concept has led to a mushrooming of techniques that have arisen from their initial work. I use a method of kinesiology testing called Kinesionics, which references over a thousand different acupressure and acupuncture points, (called evaluation points) to identify imbalances in the body.

Kinesiologists test muscle responses to receive information from the individual's internal body wisdom. Kinesiology allows the receiver to experience the knowing of his or her own body wisdom. It is a way of reaching the subconscious mind and the issues that have been hidden from the conscious mind. By experiencing kinesiology testing, the patient can feel and recognize the responses to the testing. This gives the patient the unique experience of actualizing and participating in their own healing process. This is an empowering experience for the patient, because it gives them a unique understanding of what they can to do to heal themselves.

I practice three methods of kinesiology:

1. *Nutritional kinesiology*: which addresses optimal dietary, nutritional, and herbal therapies

2. *Specialized kinesiology*: which addresses appropriate therapies for mental, emotional, and spiritual issues

3. *Structural kinesiology*: which focuses on physical issues or problems within the physical body

When I work with a client, we first sit down and discuss their current situation, when the symptoms began, and what happened at that time or just prior to the development of the symptoms. We also discuss and determine the patient's short- and long-term goals for a health and recovery plan. Then I proceed with kinesiology testing to gain information from the physical, mental, emotional, and spiritual bodies of the individual. We identify which issues need to be addressed first and then begin planning a health program for the client. Each individual's care and plan will be different, depending on their unique situations. We don't make assumptions prior to testing because many similar symptoms can be caused by unsuspected factors. I always get signals from an individual's body that help me decide what the best therapies will be for each stage of healing.

There are several acupressure/acupuncture evaluation points for candida yeast, mold, and fungal infections, as well as for other types of parasitic infections.

I then test remedies against these evaluation points. The remedies that "test in" with a strong muscle response are those most likely to be effective in assisting the body to heal this issue. It is important to go beyond this by identifying a balanced formula in conjunction with the indicated remedy. This way, the body will have the ability to release the toxins safely without side effects and promote healing at the same time.

I look for food allergies by testing uncontaminated, isolated samples of suspected allergenic foods in the person's energetic field. This can be done using specific evaluation points or using standard nutritional testing points. It is important to consider what other ingredients may be contained in a food that is suspicious. For example, a person may be reacting to the pesticides on a peach rather than reacting to the peach itself. We can also test for combinations of foods that may aggravate the condition. Sometimes a person may find that they are not actually allergic to bread, but instead they are reacting to the yeast in the bread. I have found that yeast and mold in-

fections can be causal factors in many chronic illnesses, including FM and CFS. Once we get the body cleansed and on track again, most of the allergic reactions will disappear or minimize over time.

Each person is different, but the more I work with these issues, the more I see patterns evolve that are relatively easy to treat. My practice is designed to accommodate these issues, as they have become such an integral part of my work.

For people who come to me with symptoms of FM or CFS, the most common complaint I hear is a nagging malaise and discomfort that nothing seems to help. When I test people and work with them, we find the apparent underlying cause of their problems and then work on removing it. Among these clients, symptoms reflect a range of many different issues. The key is getting better, and working with the cause of the problem.

❖ Energy Psychology: Thought Field Therapy

BY MARTI MACEWAN, M.A., LMHC

Marti MacEwan is a licensed mental-health practitioner. Thought Field Therapy, woven into the traditional therapy process, is her primary approach. She lives with her husband and two daughters in Seattle. Her website is www.energytherapist.com.

Energy psychology is an emerging field, and there are a growing number of practitioners throughout the United States and the world. The catalyst for this new field was Thought Field Therapy, Dr. Roger Callahan's creative joining of kinesiology and acupuncture. Callahan has combined these existing disciplines and applied them in a new and unique way that can bring relief from emotional pain.

I have been in private practice as a therapist for more than 20 years. During most of that time I used traditional talk therapy approaches to address eating disorders, depression, anxiety, and trauma recovery. In 1996, I came across what was then a new technique, Thought Field Therapy.

The premise is that emotional issues take the form of disruptions in the subtle energies of the body, in the same energy meridian system that acupuncture accesses and balances. Callahan's theory suggests that by clearing the energy system of these disruptions, emotional issues can also be cleared. This was a fascinating idea to me, and one that I saw borne out in practice. I began observing exceptional "cures" of long standing emotional distress.

161

When Dr. Roger Callahan discovered Thought Field Therapy in 1980, he was already a well-established and seasoned clinical psychologist specializing in, among other things, the treatment of phobias. Callahan was searching for a faster, pain-free, medication-free, and more effective approach for his clients to be relieved of their symptoms. Among the theories he was exploring were applied kinesiology, acupuncture, and acupressure.

CASE HISTORY

His experience in one particular case was instrumental in the development of Thought Field Therapy. He was treating a woman named Mary, who was overwhelmed by fear and panic whenever she encountered any type of water. She had intensely fearful reactions to puddles, baths, showers, and even rain! Dr. Callahan was treating her at his home, where he had a swimming pool, in hopes of gradually getting her accustomed to the water using cognitive-behavioral therapy and desensitization techniques. It was a slow and emotionally painful process for Mary.

One day, during a treatment session, Mary mentioned that when she looked at the water she felt sick to her stomach. Dr. Callahan knew that the end point for the stomach meridian (in acupuncture) was just under the eyes. He asked Mary to tap firmly under both eyes (applying an acupressure technique to the stomach meridian). To the total amazement of both Mary and Dr. Callahan, her reaction to the water rapidly disappeared. Within minutes, Mary's fear of water was totally gone, and it has not returned to this day, more than 20 years later!

Mary's experience turned out to be just the starting point. Dr. Callahan dedicated himself to finding out why this had happened, how to recreate this healing with others, and how to apply it to other types of emotional and psychological distress.

Dr. Callahan spent the next two decades developing his therapeutic technique and presenting his methods to other mental-health professionals. He has created a very effective system for treating many forms of emotional distress (and often their physical symptoms as well). These techniques have proven themselves to be effective and are now available to all.

Other professionals who learned these techniques from Dr. Callahan, including myself, have continued working on the expansion and variation of their application. Therapists all over the world are successfully using energy clearing techniques in various forms to relieve trauma-associated stress, anxiety, addiction, depression, and other mental health conditions. Thought Field Therapy is also increasingly used to treat physical conditions that are affected by, and affect, the energy systems. ❖ ❖ ❖

❖ A Patient's Story: Stephanie E.

Stephanie E. is a psychotherapist and also a FM patient. She uses energy psychology and energy medicine in her practice in Bellevue, Washington.

I was initially diagnosed with FM by a physician, using the tender-point criteria. I had never heard of fibromyalgia until a client described her symptoms to me and I realized that that was what I had: exhaustion, fever, swollen glands, muscle aches, and other flu-like symptoms, and frequent migraine headaches. I also had irritable bowel syndrome. In terms of my intellect, I felt as if I were living in a mental tunnel, and I was no longer my normal quick-witted self. I tried many traditional medical treatments. Doctors treated me with various kinds of antidepressants, which didn't help and caused even more problems, including headaches and sleep disturbance. Pain medications weren't good for me, either. I tried massage and acupuncture, which weren't the answer. Now I know that the acupuncture didn't work because my energies were so scrambled, "homolaterally," as we say in energy medicine, and this needed to be corrected first. Eventually, I combined several energy techniques and developed my own method to correct my energy scrambles. I used that approach regularly, and it began to help.

The emotional issues of a chronic illness are massive. There is discouragement, shame, and grief, as well as a whole bouillabaisse of emotional trauma and travail. Clearing up the emotional aspects of having the illness using Thought Field Therapy was a large part of what helped me recover.

I used Donna Eden's daily energy routine to keep my energies running in the right direction. I started wearing a watch and setting the alarm on the hour. I did my energy corrections as often as I could on the hour for a good four or five months. I also kept strengthening my energy system using Thought Field Therapy to clear any stressful experience, whether physical, emotional, or psychological, whenever it appeared.

I see over and over again in my practice that fundamental energy imbalances lie at the heart of FM. There are energy corrections that help tremendously in strengthening our energies overall and contribute to our recovery from chronic illness.

Intention to heal plays a big role. Don't buy into negative beliefs about the possibility of healing. I had always heard that you couldn't recover from FM, but I just would not believe that this was a permanent illness. I continued to look for ways to heal that would work for me.

Be open to a combination of remedies, including nutritional, psychological, and energetic therapies. Different remedies may be useful for you

163

at different times. In my own case, my work with essential oils was very valuable at one stage, and a nutritional approach helped most at another stage.

The results don't necessarily show up immediately. Often there is a cumulative effect. It's helpful to remember that results happen little by little. If you slip away from working with yourself, don't be self-critical; just come back to it. Know that the recovery process will sometimes be two steps forward and three steps back. Even though some symptoms might persist, it doesn't mean there isn't progress. It took me a good four years of actively working on myself to truly heal. Stay with it.

Resist the temptation to make your illness the central focus of your life. Be committed to getting better, and then as you do get better, let it recede in importance in your life.

Regard FM as a teacher and learn what it is there to teach you. For me, it was to be in sync with myself. This has enabled me to come into my own by becoming attuned to subtle energies, learning to use my gifts, and not letting circumstances control me. ❖❖❖

❖ Meditation

Since breath is life, the basis of all energetic healing, including meditation, is breath work. In Chapter 10, we learned a three-part breathing practiced in yoga. One form of meditation requires us to simply notice our breath. The ageless act of breathing in and out, while relaxing the body, is a basic meditational tool for the beginner, as well as for those who meditate daily.

MINDFUL MEDITATION

Try this easy meditation. Relax in a quiet room, sitting in your favorite chair, with your arms and legs uncrossed to allow the movement of energy. Close your eyes and exhale. Push out all of your breath. Then, as you slowly breathe in, notice the rhythm of your breath. The expansion of your lungs as you inhale, also raises your abdomen, filling your belly with air. Exhale and feel the tension leave your body. Do this several times. You are now ready to quiet your mind. As thoughts come, let them pass; don't get hung up on creating the perfect void of nothingness. If you have a song in your head, a grocery list, a problem you're mulling over, you aren't the only one. It's human nature—don't worry that you seem incapable of clearing your mind for meditation. Be patient and just try your best to simply notice the thoughts that come into your mind; then let them comfortably pass as you breathe in and out, in and out.

You may wish to try concentrating on a word that holds special meaning for you; for example, the name of your child or of a pet may work. Visualize the face of the individual you are naming. Meditation is an intensely personal act and no one does it in the same way.

PROGRESSIVE RELAXATION

Another approach to meditation is to begin with gradual relaxation of the body—this often seems to do the trick and helps people get to the point at which real relaxation begins.

* As you breathe slowly in and out, imagine that you are going to progressively tighten and then relax the muscles in your body from head to toe.

* First feel the skin gently tighten on the top of your head and around your skull. Keep the muscles a little tense for a slow count of five, and then slowly let go. Breathe out for five seconds.

* Proceed to your shoulders. Hunch your shoulders and tighten your upper back, holding the tightness until once again you let go, feeling the relaxation. Remind yourself to breathe from your diaphragm slowly, in and out.

* Now move your attention to your upper body and arms. Brace yourself for tightening of the muscles and hold them tight for a count of five seconds.

* Your middle section is next. Proceed to your belly, and hold for a full count of five seconds. Release now and feel the tension being carried away by your breath.

* Now tighten your buttocks and thighs firmly for five seconds. Notice that these big muscles need a bit more tightening. Hold for two more seconds and let go blissfully, breathing out to a count of five.

* Your lower legs and feet are last—tighten your calves and then the small muscles in your feet. There are a lot of muscles in your feet, so hold them gently, and then let your breath go.

* Now you are ready for extended meditation.

One good approach to meditation is to make an audio recording of the above instructions that you can play for yourself when you are practicing meditation. Use a calm, well-modulated voice, and speak clearly. Set it up so it's all ready to go when you are. Keep some eye shades and a blanket by

165

your chair so you can easily meditate for fifteen minutes every day, which is a good way to start.

✤ Visualization

You don't have to be a psychic or a student of the metaphysical to be able to find the pain in your body and use your mind to change it. (We know this from the discipline of biofeedback and the extensive research conducted in the field of psychoneuroimmunology—the effects of the mind on the nervous system and the immune response.)

To get a feeling for visualization, try this simple exercise. All you need is a quiet room and time to close your eyes. The aim is to distract yourself from your pain—to break the pain cycle, allowing your muscles to relax and the pain to lessen.

There are five steps to accessing your pain: identify it, isolate it, examine it, change it, and let it go. Sit in a chair rather than lying down if possible, because you want to be awake throughout the following visualization:

- ✤ Focus on the pain you want to change.
- ✤ Isolate it from any other bodily sensation. Direct your attention to that exact spot.
- ✤ Turn it over in your mind—what color do you imagine your pain is?
- ✤ What size is it? What is its shape? Picture your pain as an object in your mind.
- ✤ Begin by lightening its color. If the nugget of pain is a dark color, picture it gradually lightening.
- ✤ Examine it for size. Is it smaller?
- ✤ Now picture the pain becoming a lighter color and becoming even smaller.
- ✤ Continue examining and changing the pain picture until you have reached sparkling white light; then allow yourself to rest in this beautiful light, knowing that the pain has lessened.

As with meditation, using an audio recording can help enormously with visualization. When pain overtakes us, listening to a recorded visualization can help distract us from the discomfort or agony long enough for healing to occur. (See the Resources section for some suggestions of audio and video visualization self-help tapes.)

166

Each person experiences visualization differently; Char M. uses visualization while doing her stretching routine: "I see my muscles as a waterfall and imagine that I am floating on clouds." Linda Martinson describes the power of visualization in the poem "Migraine," excerpted from her anthology *Poetry of Pain.*

MIGRAINE

I awake to pain.
My head is heavy,
encased in cement;
I cannot move.
My eyes open;
molten agony flows
through spread-eagled limbs
to innocent feet.
Still life on a bed;
frozen in place.
Except for my mind,
my tripping, ticking mind
that says *Enough!*
Refuse to be involved,
for to dwell on pain
is to feel it twice over,
with madness not far behind.
I must steal pain's energy
and think it gone:
From my pores I will birth flowers,
Tiny seeds of pain
will bud and bloom
with the grace
of time lapse photography.
Blossoms will fall from my skin
wherever I hurt,
soothing me and comforting me
with soft color and
gentle scent.
My head is pillowed in flowers
fallen away in sweet abundance.
Each throb produces more.

167

My feet are massaged
By velvet petals.
I am covered with flowers,
mounded with flowers.
I am adrift in a sea of flowers.

© Linda Martinson 1997

❖ ❖ ❖

You can decide if you want to receive energy healing from a practitioner or if you want to learn to use these techniques yourself. In our next chapter, we'll look at nutrition and the use of herbal remedies, many of which have been around since ancient times.

Chapter 12

Nutrition, Naturopathy, Homeopathy, and Aromatherapy

Let your food be your medicine, and your medicine be your food.

— Hippocrates

THE OATH THAT today's physicians take before receiving their license to practice originates with the father of modern medicine, Hippocrates. In Hippocrates' day all medicine was "natural," meaning it was derived from nature. Today's natural health-care providers are still strongly grounded in the theories and ethics of that time. They know that the role of nutrition and natural health care is central to physical and spiritual healing.

The use of natural remedies requires patience and participation to be effective. Your body needs time to absorb the nutrients and to activate your own inner healing mechanisms. While the remedies in this chapter are natural, they may still have a volatile effect when the wrong dosage is used and may not combine well with prescription medication. You will have to consider how each vitamin, herb, or supplement affects your body and how each remedy you take interacts with the others. Don't forget, it is essential to have one practitioner on your healing team who is aware of everything you are taking, including all your medications and natural health-care products. At the back of this book, in Appendix A, you'll find a reference table of vitamins, herbs, and supplements found effective by many of our respondents and recommended by practitioners.

In this chapter, Dr. Jenefer Scripps Huntoon and Dr. Maryann Ivons provide an overview of naturopathic medicine and homeopathy. Diana Pepper talks about her healing practice, which includes herbal remedies and flower essences. We begin, however, with nutrition, something that should be an important part of every FM and CFS patient's treatment program. In the following pages, you'll discover that what you eat can have a surprising effect on how your feel.

✤ Eating for Optimum Health

BY JOLEEN KELLEHER, R.N.

Joleen Kelleher is director of the Light Institute for Health in Olga, Washington. This nonprofit organization teaches people how to make sustainable changes in health habits that will allow them to live life in harmony.

Nutrition is of utmost importance for anyone dealing with a chronic illness. Ideally, we view your food as a living substance, a reflection of nature's energy, which can help supply the necessary nutrients for your body and your inner balance. Then your food becomes a reflection of how you nourish yourself physically and spiritually.

Our society has distracted us from this balance, through advertising and fast food restaurants. This has created a false belief that food is something other than nourishment, that we should eat primarily as a social activity or for pleasure. Often we may be acting on incomplete information. Consider the problem of lactose intolerance, for example. Enzyme supplements are available that contain lactase, to support the digestion of dairy products. For some people, these products make it possible to continue to eat dairy foods despite lactose intolerance. However, many people are intolerant not only of milk sugar (lactose) but also of milk protein (casein). In this case, taking these supplements only masks the body's discomfort at having to process dairy foods. This illustrates how complex food is and that we may be unaware of the powerful effects of food on our health or mood. When we feel miserable and overstuffed after a meal, that is the body telling us it is out of balance. We then know that what we have eaten is not something the body can easily assimilate.

Awareness is critically important: awareness of the food we're taking in, of how that food is being digested by the body, and of how our system feels after eating a particular food. Our bodies use food in two ways: for fuel and as raw material for repair. When someone has a condition such as FM or CFS, their symptoms are an indication that the body is very low on energy (in terms of their internal life force).

I find that most normal "healthy" people have real energy problems (research shows that the average American reports energy at about 60 percent of optimum). This means that most of us also don't have enough energy to digest our food. Digesting the typical American diet requires about 60 percent of the body's internal energy. That means that if you're only operating at 60 percent of your normal energy and you have a typical American meal (which tends to be overcooked, overprocessed, and contains a lot of sugar and red meat), it's going to take all of your energy just to digest your food.

One way that people with a chronic illness can heal is by improving their diet and increasing their internal energy. A bad diet will not help to repair and heal the body. And the energy used for digesting an unhelpful diet detracts from the energy the body needs for healing. One of the goals, then, is to prevent healing energy from being used up in the process of digestion.

I recommend two steps you can take to improve this problem. One is fasting. Fasting frees up energy in your body and can help detoxify your system. That's one of the reasons people feel "lighter" after a fast. They're feeling more energy because energy has been freed and the body has been detoxified. The other solution is to simplify your diet, so that you're eating closer to nature and eating less processed food.

THE BENEFITS OF FASTING

Fasting can be an important approach in healing chronic illness. Many people are afraid of fasting because they think of it as deprivation process. Done intelligently and with moderation, it is a way of resting the body while healing takes place.

However, many people who fast inappropriately immediately resume eating the way they did before. When a fast is broken, the body is vulnerable and hungry for new nutrition. Like dirty footprints on a clean carpet, the harmful effects of poor nutrition are immediately apparent after a fast. If a person takes in healthy food after the fast, however, it is quickly absorbed and metabolized, creating a higher level of health than that which existed before the fast. Following a fast, it is beneficial to eat foods that contain naturally occurring enzymes. Doing so helps to bring energy into your system and aids in digestion. Plants convert solar energy into matter

171

through the process of photosynthesis. The closer we eat to this natural process, the easier it is for our digestion, and the more we bring in the basics we need.

For a beginner, a fast should last for only one day, unless it's done under the guidance of a physician. A "healing fast" can last from three to five days. One problem with this type of fast is that it can cause "a healing crisis," a period when the body detoxifies, causing symptoms such as achiness, headaches, or fatigue. It may feel as if symptoms have been exacerbated. Although that is a normal reaction, many people become concerned the first time this happens because they believe they are getting worse. As long as the symptoms are not serious, the solution is to just hang in there until the crisis is alleviated.

In a simple juice fast, always use fresh juice, made either in a blender, a juicer, or from fruit squeezed by hand. Drink juice throughout the day, as well as water, and do some simple walking. Moving becomes very important, as it not only flushes out your system but also helps your lymphatic system. Read, meditate, relax, and listen to music; do this for twenty-four hours, and as you're coming out of the fast, add lightly steamed vegetables or fresh soup. The next day, you can add rice or other grains to the fresh veggies and fruit.

When the body detoxifies itself, it releases energy that was used to hold or process toxins. Once those toxins are eliminated during fasting, that internal energy is freed, and to some extent your internal life force is also freed. Fasting can bring the benefits of nutrition to bear on your emotional, mental, and spiritual life.

WORKING WITH A NUTRITIONIST

If you're seeking a nutritionist, look for someone who understands about life force, someone who knows that food is more than just calories. By doing some reading, you will be able to ask educated questions to gain a sense of whether the nutritionist is in harmony with your own philosophy. There are a number of books that address the issue of eating for health. One is *Healing with Whole Foods*, by Paul Pitchford; another is *Conscious Eating*, by Gabriel Cousens (see Bibliography).

You will also want to consider the nutritionist's philosophy on spiritual nutrition. Most nutritionists stay at the purely scientific level, teaching that the body needs so many carbohydrates, so many proteins, a certain amount of vitamin C to heal, etc. This information is all helpful, up to a point. But when dealing with a body that contains a great many toxins and

a weakened life force, there are additional factors to consider, beyond simple nutrition. Someone who is experiencing tremendous fatigue doesn't feel like running a mile. Why? Because they have very little life force. Yet many nutritionists don't think in terms of life force—they don't realize that food has a certain life force of its own. A fresh apple is alive, but applesauce that has been cooked to mush does not have any life force. It has calories and sugar, but it has no life force. What people with chronic illness need is food that has life force.

MAKING THE CHANGE

Where you decide to begin making changes is an individual choice, based on your own awareness. Some readers may have already made the shift to a more natural, wholesome diet. But such a change may not even be in the consciousness of others. You, as an individual, ultimately make changes based on your own priorities.

Our judgment of ourselves often prevents us from making the move to a healthier diet. You know you should have an apple, but you really want to eat some chocolate. Go ahead and eat that candy; eat with deep awareness and joy. Then take that awareness to the next level, which is to notice how you feel afterward. Ask yourself, "Is that how I want to feel?" And sometimes you'll decide that it doesn't matter. At other times, you will find that you don't want to feel that way. Peace comes from learning how to bring joy and awareness into your life. If you have joy and awareness, you don't have judgment.

COOKING WITH LOVE

Have you ever heard the saying that it takes a special person to cook with heart? This means that person has a deep love and awareness about nourishment. If we bring awareness to our food preparation, we infuse that food with our love and joy. The food tastes different, and it has a different quality to it. I encourage everyone to practice this—prepare a simple dish with mindfulness. See what you notice about it as you prepare it; think of it with deep awareness as a gift of nature you've chosen to nourish your body.

THE BASIC RULES OF EATING

+ Try to keep your meals on a regular schedule, but if you don't feel hungry at mealtime, then fast until the next meal.

+ Eat slowly, because your mouth is the juicer for your body, and it begins the digestion process.

- Eat only about four or five different kinds of food at one meal, because complexity makes digestion difficult.

- Eat until you're only half or three-quarters full. That should make you feel as if you've not really eaten. If you don't feel too full after eating, you've eaten the right meal.

- Maintain a peaceful attitude during meals, because if you infuse your meal with energy, your body experiences it on a higher level.

- Try to fast once a week or once every couple of weeks.

- Eat at least one raw salad a day, and try to shift from heavily cooked foods to lightly steamed or sautéed foods.

- Always remember that you're eating to live, not living to eat.

✤ You Are What You Drink

Your body is 95 percent water. Your brain, when properly hydrated, is 80 percent water. Yet few of us drink enough water. We need to drink water regularly, not just when we feel thirsty. When the body becomes rehydrated, natural thirst will return.

Doctors and nutritionists recommend six to eight 8 oz. glasses of water per day. Unfortunately, soda, tea, and coffee don't count, because the caffeine in these drinks actually dehydrates the body by forcing the kidneys to expel water. Dehydration also produces free radicals—unstable atoms that speed up the aging process and increase our risk of degenerative diseases, such as cancer.

Begin to watch your body for signs of dehydration. One obvious sign of dehydration is wrinkles, particularly on the hands and face. If you're well hydrated, your skin will appear smooth and you will radiate overall health.

Here's a simple analogy. When a houseplant doesn't get enough water, its leaves begin to droop. Left unwatered, its leaves wither and dry up. Sure, it perks right up again when you give it some water, but this continued cycle of drought and rehydration is not good for the plant—the process compromises its overall health. Your body reacts the same way. So next time you skip your daily eight glasses of water, think of yourself as a withered Peace Lily!

Practically every system in your body requires water in order to function optimally—from your cells, nerves, muscles, and lungs to your lymphatic system. Water allows your cells to produce energy and increases your metabolism. In fact, properly hydrating your nerves and muscles may help to alleviate some of the symptoms of FM and CFS.

Drinking more water is something you can easily do to make a big difference to the way you feel. Try leaving a pitcher of water on the kitchen counter; every time you walk past the pitcher you'll be reminded that you need to drink more water (room temperature water is easier to slug down). Buy a water bottle and take it with you everywhere, remembering to fill it up a few times each day. If you have difficulty drinking your eight glasses, try chugging down half a glass, as if you had just run a mile. It beats sipping ice water any day and is far better for your digestion. Your stomach can immediately put room temperature water to use, while ice water must come up to body temperature before being utilized in digestion.

❖ A Patient's Story: Erin P.

Erin P. is a 41-year-old acupuncturist. A healthy diet has made a dramatic difference to the way she manages her FM. Erin lives with her partner in Seattle, Washington.

I was just 26 when I was diagnosed with FM. My life was in such a great place when I first began having difficulties. What I miss most are my high energy, physical strength, and mental acuity. None have been fully restored to pre-FM levels, and each of these factors has a tremendous impact on how one's life is lived. On an emotional level, I feel that my life was better before. On the other hand, I've had to learn to take better care of myself, which must be a positive. It's forced me to mature in ways I might not have otherwise, or perhaps wouldn't have done as soon. FM has also opened the door to alternative medicine, where I finally began experiencing some relief. My entire life has changed as a result, for the better. But I still miss being a highly active adrenaline junky.

In my process of healing, the most life-changing event happened when my boyfriend and I took part in a three-week detoxification program at the Optimum Health Institute in San Diego. The cornerstone of the program is an all-raw-foods, vegan diet. I know it sounds kind of boring, but I have been doing it at home and it's great. I have a lot of sprouts and no animal products of any kind. Wheat-grass juice is a big part of it, too. Other parts of the program include colon cleansing, since the colon is phenomenally important in all bodily functions. If you have a lot of gunk built up in your intestines—which most of us do, due to our lifestyles—it permeates your

175

whole body and clogs up everything. They taught us how to do a specific type of daily lymphatic exercises—the lymphatic system is another waste disposal system in the body that can clog up. It's very easy to do and consists of leg lifts, stretches, and walking. It's very low impact, and it gets your lymphatic system moving. They also taught us ways to cultivate a positive mental attitude.

Many people go for one week, just to do a simple cleanse. By the time most people get through the first week, they feel a lot better. I felt terrible at first. I experienced all my FM symptoms three times worse than usual during that first week. It wasn't easy. But my body was going through the detoxification process. All that stuff was coming out of my core and bubbling to the surface, and I was re-experiencing it both mentally and physically while it was being eliminated from my body.

By the middle of the second week, I started feeling much better. I ran up the same stairs that I had had a hard time walking down just two days before. I slept a lot better. My face started to look different. My boyfriend and I would both look in the mirror and go, "Oh, my God!" There was light emanating from my face. I felt a lot lighter and more unclogged. I felt clean inside, and it was easier to move and easier to think, because things weren't gunking up my system. It was really surprising.

The complete program runs for three weeks, and I'm really glad I was able to stay for the third week. It tied things together. You go to classes the whole time you're there, and you learn about how your body works and how the foods you eat affect your body. Not only are you doing the cleansing process, you're also learning about why it's good for you, which really helps.

I was amazed by the difference in my health after completing the program. I didn't have any expectations initially, but I found that I was able to sleep better than I ever have in my life.

However, despite feeling so much improved, I eventually fell back into my habitual workaholic ways (working and going to school, both full-time). Lifestyle habits eroded, and once again I began to have difficulties, primarily with sleep and fatigue. Early in 2004 I came down with a raging case of mononucleosis, which almost forced me to go the ER because I had severe airway constriction. Shortly after, I was also diagnosed with a hypothyroid condition. Now, after a number of false starts, I'm just starting to get back on my feet.

I'm still so immensely grateful for my experience at the Optimum Health Institute, and I hope I can put the lessons I learned there to good use. My goal is to feel whole again and to live a full life. But at present, my rewards in life are having a relatively normal day—talking to friends or visiting with them, doing yard work, cooking dinner, laughing, taking a walk, doing errands, and washing the dishes. I've never been so happy to wash a sink full of dishes before! I expect to widen my circle of rewarding activities as things continue to improve, but it's kind of nice just to enjoy these simple activities so much.

Diet is fundamentally important. This point cannot be stressed too much. Nutrition, nutrition, nutrition. There's tons of information out there about this all-important topic. I join the entire health profession in shouting this from the rooftops.

* Avoid white edible substances (processed foods such as white sugar, flour, white rice, etc.) Why? Each of these substances is highly processed and depletes your body of nutrients.

* Avoid coffee. It's a diuretic. It dries you out. The caffeinated type drains your adrenal glands. And caffeinated or not, it does a number on your kidneys. Try green tea instead. If you need a lift, there are so many other, healthier alternatives.

* Avoid dairy and flour products. Dairy products can produce mucus and phlegm. A mucous environment in your gastrointestinal tract is a playground for yeast overgrowth, such as candida, and for parasites. Flour products that contain yeast, such as bread and pizza, cause big food cravings. Flour products that are sweet bounce blood sugar around. Too many sweets can cause extreme emotional highs and lows and irritability, as well as brain fog, confusion, and difficulty with concentration.

* Avoid highly processed and packaged foods. Most lack useful nutritional value and are typically loaded with sugar, sodium, and chemicals.

* Consider acquiring a good produce juicer and make it one of your new best friends.

* Enjoy plenty of whole foods: grains, beans and legumes, and fruits and vegetables.

* Make sure you get enough protein from sources like soy, nuts, protein powder, fish, chicken, and lean meat. Insufficient protein can lead to a number of problems, including low blood sugar, impaired immunity, and thyroid problems.

* Eat organic foods if and whenever you can.

177

❖ Eat regular and balanced meals.

❖ Take it slowly. Changing your diet can be challenging. It's not the things you do once in a while that are most important; it's what you do every day (habitually) that has the greatest impact on your health. ❖❖❖

❖ Naturopathy

BY DR. JENEFER SCRIPPS HUNTOON, N.D.

Dr. Scripps Huntoon graduated from the National College of Naturopathic Medicine in 1975. She has practiced at the Naturopathic Clinic in Seattle for the last 30 years. Dr. Huntoon specializes in the treatment of FM and CFS, digestive conditions, autoimmune disorders, and musculoskeletal imbalances. She lives with her family in Seattle.

Naturopathic physicians are trained as general practitioners to treat a variety of conditions. The naturopathic approach involves a range of nontoxic methods to strengthen the immune system. Treatments include botanical medicine, nutritional and vitamin therapy, spinal manipulation, and overall preventive care.

Originally, all doctors were naturopathic physicians. Hippocrates laid down two basic laws of medical practice: "Let your food be your medicine, and your medicine be your food" and, "In treating, do nothing that will harm your patient."

In accordance with "Let your food be your medicine," naturopathic doctors prescribe nutritional programs and herbal remedies using botanicals derived from plants. In accordance with "Do nothing that will harm your patient," naturopathic doctors also use the latest diagnostic procedures (those which do no harm to their patients).

A natural foods diet is important for everyone. A patient may take all the right remedies, but working with diet is also essential to improve their health. In general, I recommend eating natural, whole foods instead of white flour and processed foods. In other words, if you are going to eat rice, select brown rice over white rice, and if you eat bread, eat sprouted wheat or sprouted multigrain bread instead of white bread. The better a patient complies with a nutritious diet, the quicker the results.

Most people need to dramatically reduce the amount of sugar in their diet. This is a challenge because sugar is so addictive. There are naturopathic remedies to help reduce the craving for sweets. Sugar depletes the body because it offers no nutritive value. It lowers immune function and contributes to the growth of candida yeast and harmful bacteria. Candida occurs in the body normally, but if it is fed, it takes over, depleting the immune system and contributing to musculoskeletal pain—worsening the symptoms of FM and CFS.

Most people don't realize the sugar in fruit juice is almost as bad as table sugar for feeding yeast. People need to limit fruit to perhaps two servings a day and to load up on vegetables.

Both pharmaceutical and herbal treatments can be used to kill candida yeast, but these remedies by themselves don't necessarily solve the problem. They kill the yeast, but the yeast may come back even stronger if the patient doesn't also change his of her diet. Diet is extremely crucial in treating candida, but there are also a number of herbs, botanicals, and enzymes that will help get the yeast under control.

TREATING FM AND CFS PATIENTS

I recognize that each person is biochemically unique. Extensive testing is used to evaluate each individual's body chemistry. This testing includes a comprehensive physical exam and blood and urine analysis.

Frequently, I am able to reduce the underlying causes of FM and CFS by using high potency plant enzymes. FM and CFS are often a result of toxicity, inflammation, and/or infection, and I have found enzymes to be clinically beneficial in these conditions. Enzymes can be used to digest yeast, viruses, bacteria, or parasites. Plant enzymes are found in all raw fruits and vegetables. Ideally, we should be eating diets that are 70 percent raw foods. Since this is difficult for most people to do, we recommend that patients take capsules containing plant enzymes with meals.

I use the plant enzymes in two ways. First, enzymes are necessary for the digestion of all foods. Poor digestion of food results in toxins. When leaky gut syndrome occurs, digestive toxins are released into the bloodstream and can lodge in joints and muscles, causing inflammation. In the long-term, inflammation can result in pain. Toxins can also affect organs and glands, causing inefficient metabolism.

Second, these enzymes can be used to accomplish therapeutic goals, such as reducing inflammation, removing toxins, and dramatically reducing infection and parasites. I use a high protease formula, which digests foreign proteins, including, bacteria, candida yeast, fungus, viruses, and parasites. We also use an enzyme that is high in amylase to improve digestion of carbohydrates and improve joint flexibility.

179

Plant enzymes are a safe, nontoxic approach to these problems. Most patients see some improvement of their symptoms within two to three weeks of treatment. However, it can take from three months to a year to achieve complete recovery. The response to treatment varies, based on the cause of the problem and the duration of the symptoms. We have numerous patients who were originally diagnosed with FM or CFS who are now living healthy, productive lives as a result of these therapies.

SUCCESS STORIES

Amy, a 30-year-old CFS patient, became severely fatigued after experiencing significant stress in her life. Eventually, she had to take a leave of absence from her job. Her exam and lab tests indicated over-worked adrenals, liver congestion, hypoglycemia, and candida yeast.

Amy's energy improved within two weeks, through the use of plant digestive enzymes and enzymes to control candida and help her liver. After three months she was able to work part-time, and after six months, she was able to return to work full-time. She told us enthusiastically, "I feel even better than before I got sick."

Don, a 45-year-old FM patient, had musculoskeletal aches and pains. This greatly limited the activities he could enjoy, such as bicycling and hiking. His exam revealed that a vertebra was pressing on his spinal cord and that he was low in vitamin C complex and had candida yeast and a virus.

I provided several spinal correction treatments. This relived the pressure on his spine and gave him some immediate relief. He was also given vitamin C complex from a whole-food source. This strengthened his connective tissue, reducing pain and increasing his resistance to infection.

Don was educated about a natural foods diet and agreed to eliminate sugar. He began to notice significant improvements following two weeks of therapy. In four months, he was feeling better than he had in years and resumed his exercise program of biking and hiking. ❖❖❖

❖ Homeopathy

BY DR. MARYANN IVONS, R.N., N.P.

Dr. Ivons is a registered nurse and naturopathic physician. She has a private practice in family medicine with a homeopathic specialty. Dr. Ivons is a former nursing educator and is a member of the faculty in the naturopathic medicine program at Bastyr University in Seattle. Her professional ties include being chairperson for minor surgery for the International Naturopathic Medical Board tests. She is the author of *Homeopathy for Nurses*.

Homeopathy is a therapeutic modality developed by Dr. Samuel Hahnemann in the late 1700s. Dr. Hahnemann was frustrated with the medical practice of his day because the toxic substances used in treatment were often harmful or even fatal. He began to experiment with the available medications, giving smaller and smaller doses. Eventually, he found a point at which the decreased dosage had a therapeutic effect and virtually no side effects.

As a man of science, Dr. Hahnemann strove to explain what he observed. Research at that time was not well advanced; there was a limited understanding of anatomy and almost no knowledge of physiology or any of the basic sciences we take for granted today. In order to explain his observations, Dr. Hahnemann devoted the rest of his life to careful observation, to "prove" the remedies he had discovered and develop the science we now call homeopathy. The major premise of homeopathic treatment is that "Like Cures Like." That is to say, a substance that can cause a set of symptoms when used in material doses can cure them when used in minute homeopathic doses.

The process that makes a homeopathic medication homeopathic is called "potentization." Any substance can be potentized. The process involves dilution and "secussion" (shaking) of the chosen material. The dilutions can be either a one in ten (x potency) or one in one hundred (c potency). The number of times that the dilution/secussion process is repeated determines the potency of the remedy. The most common potencies used today are 12c, 30c, 200c, and 1M (1000c).

To understand how homeopathic treatment differs from allopathic treatment, it is important to consider the concept of "vital force." The vital force is that property which animates, or gives life to, every organism. The effects of vital force can be seen on all aspects of the person—mental, emotional, and physical.

According to homeopathic theory, when the vital force is imbalanced it attempts to rebalance by expressing symptoms of increasing severity. Genetic problems within the body can cause imbalance—for example, sickle cell anemia. Each individual has certain areas in the body that are vulnerable or weaker, and if the vital force becomes imbalanced the symptoms are

181

usually expressed in the weakest areas. Poor eating habits, lack of exercise, and lifestyle choices such as smoking or alcohol consumption may all contribute to an imbalance in the vital force. And, in our society, one of the most important and ubiquitous problems we face that causes imbalance is stress.

Every person's vital force is unique, and each person will exhibit symptoms in a unique pattern when their vital force is imbalanced. A homeopath finds the unique pattern of imbalance for each patient. The pattern is matched with a remedy that will reestablish the balance, and therefore reestablish health.

In allopathic medicine, the mind and the emotions are treated separately from the physical symptoms of the body. Focusing only on physiology can impede treatment when trying to heal a person with physical symptoms that have an emotional origin. This is particularly important in a diagnosis like FM, which can be triggered by posttraumatic stress.

Stress imbalances the vital force, and the vital force, in order to correct the balance, elicits physical symptoms that can manifest as pain. Physiologically, we now know that stress increases inflammation, which can eventually result in pain symptoms. When a physician cannot find a physical cause for pain, it is labeled "psychosomatic."

While homeopathy can be extremely effective in the treatment of FM and CFS, if not done by a qualified professional with experience, it may cause more trouble than it cures. Ineffective home care means that the patient is not receiving treatment. Since we really don't understand how homeopathy actually works, giving repeated doses of medications without good indication may well cause harm. In conditions such as Lyme disease, which mimics FM, delay in treatment can have disastrous consequences.

❖ ❖ ❖

Ellen J. has used homeopathic remedies as part of her treatment plan for more than fifteen years. "I started by reading books and trying various low-dose remedies. I regularly use the remedy *Arnica montana* for sore muscles and to prevent bruising after I bump into things. Before and after dental treatment and any surgical procedure, I use *Hypericium perfoliatum* to prevent and treat nerve pain and injury. I have also used *Rhus toxicodendron* to relieve joint pain related to arthritis. I highly recommend beginning with a good basic book on homeopathy to learn low-dose homeopathy first-aid."

❖ Aromatherapy (Essential Oil Therapy)

BY JIMM HARRISON

Jimm Harrison is a certified aromatherapist, licensed cosmetologist, and cofounder of Spirit of Beauty Nutritional Skin Care. Jimm has been conducting workshops and certification courses in essential oil therapy for accredited massage, spa therapy, cosmetology, and medical institutions across the country since 1993.

The therapeutic use of essential oils, known as aromatherapy, is a powerful and diverse healing modality. Essential oils are volatile fatty-acid extracts derived from plants and composed of organic chemicals. Like all plant medicines, essential oils have a natural harmony with the human body. Essential oils contain pharmacologically active compounds, giving them unique and sometimes surprising healing results.

I have developed many formulas for clients diagnosed with FM or CFS. I formulate a "full spectrum" essential-oil blend that contains anti-inflammatory and soothing oils, as well as those intended to address nervous tension, immune function, and cell regeneration, in order to support and balance the whole body. Emotions are also addressed through the olfactory and limbic response to essential oils.

A full-spectrum philosophy is very effective when treating inflammation as both a symptom and a cause of other symptoms such as muscle aches, joint pain, or headache. Similarly, in a full-spectrum formula, the possible causes of the inflammation, such as stress, nervous tension, immune response, infection of parasitic microorganisms, or environmental stress, may be addressed and relieved.

ESSENTIAL OILS WITH A FULL-SPECTRUM COMPOSITION

There are certain oils that contain a chemical structure resulting in a diverse set of properties that may include at once, stress relief, anti-inflammatory and antimicrobial activity. These oils are excellent additions to a full-spectrum formula and can be used to address many symptoms or conditions simultaneously, but they may also be used alone.

Lavender (*Lanvandula angustifolia*): Lavender is an all-purpose essential oil with beneficial tonic effects. Lavender's main components are linalool and linalyl acetate. These are the compounds that provide lavender with its sedative, stress reducing, and anti-spasmodic properties.

Rose *(Rosa damascena):* Rose is an extremely complex oil. Like lavender, it has wide-ranging benefits for use in holistic health. True rose essential oil is quite expensive, though this does not make rose a cost-prohibitive oil since it is used effectively in small amounts.

Geranium *(Pelargonium asperum):* Geranium is considered an "adaptogen," an oil that adjusts to the conditions or requirements of the body. This, along with geranium's wide-spectrum antibacterial, antifungal, and antiviral activity, makes it a unique and favorable addition to any formula. Geranium is also highly recommended for women, especially when hormonal imbalance is an issue.

STRESS REDUCTION AND SOOTHING ACTIVITY OF ESTER COMPOUNDS

The essential oils that are most calming and balancing to the nervous system and emotions are those containing ester compounds. Lavender is the most popular ester-containing oil. Each of the following essential oils has therapeutic benefits derived from its ester content.

Roman Chamomile *(Anthemis nobilis):* This is very soothing and relaxing to the nervous system. It is an effective treatment for muscle tension and also works as an antispasmodic.

Neroli *(Citrus auranthium):* Neroli is derived from the orange blossom. It has a floral citrus fragrance, which adds to its therapeutic benefits and emotionally uplifting quality. Neroli is tremendously advantageous for conditions of anxiety.

ESSENTIAL OILS TO REDUCE INFLAMMATION

There are quite a few choices when selecting essential oils for inflammatory conditions. The sesquiterpene content is generally recognized as supplying this property to the oil.

Everlasting *(Helichrysum italicum):* This is an ideal oil for inflammatory conditions, due to its sesquiterpene hydrocarbon content. Everlasting also provides soothing and nervous tension relief from an ester compound. It has wound healing properties and is an absolute must for use in skin care.

German Chamomile *(Matricaria recutita):* The blue color of this oil is due to the chamazulene sesquiterpene compound that has powerful anti-inflammatory properties. ❖❖❖

If you're interested in essential oils, we recommend that you consult a professional aromatherapist. As Jimm explained, essential oils are pharmacologically active, and as with any medication, care must be taken in their use. Be aware that essential oils will be labeled with details concerning their correct usage and any relevant cautionary information.

✤ Herbal Remedies and Flower Essences

BY DIANA PEPPER

Diana Pepper is an interfaith minister and Reiki master. She has worked with a number of FM patients to help them with stress and hypersensitivity, primarily using flower essences and sometimes using energy balancing and clearing. Diana lives with her family at Tree Frog Farm, Lummi Island, Washington. She and her partner John Robinson have a website, www.treefrogfarm.com.

I have always had a closeness with nature, but I didn't really begin a working relationship with it until 1998. That was when I read *The Findhorn Garden* by the Findhorn Garden Community and *Behaving As If the God in all Life Mattered* by Machaelle Small Wright [see Bibliography]. I was again reconnected to the consciousness of everything, including plants.

When we moved to Tree Frog Farm, I fell in love with our land. I'd walk around, letting the plants draw me to them and talk to me, so I could practice listening. I learned to do land energy clearings, to plant and tend gardens, and to care for the woods in cooperation with nature. It was there that I began making my own flower essences.

In my experience, people who have FM or CFS are by nature sensitive people. Many are locked into the stress response—"fight or flight"—and the result is often a hypersensitivity to just about everything. The first essences that I use in these cases encourage a reduction in hypersensitivity and the sense of trauma from the body-mind-spirit continuum. Flower essences I commonly use in these situations are pennyroyal, lady's mantle, comfrey, bleeding heart, and moon shadow rose. Sometimes I also use mock orange, self-heal, and purple passion rose.

Pennyroyal: Calms the sympathetic nervous system. Spiritually, it provides strength to stand firmly in your center, then to relax as the perceived danger dissolves. (This addresses mostly a kidney system/adrenal gland survival issue.)

Lady's Mantle: Brings deep spiritual peace to your whole body and being, by balancing the sympathetic nervous system. (This addresses mostly shock to the emotional heart that activates the sympathetic nervous system.)

Comfrey: Aids in the healing of wounds so deep and traumatic that they affect your soul's journey.

Bleeding Heart: Supports compassion for yourself during challenging or stressful situations. Aids the process of shifting from wanting to change another person or situation to realizing you can only change yourself and your reactions to situations.

Moon Shadow Rose: Encourages us to stop chasing shadows of our past and open up to the lessons that can be gleaned from them.

Mock Orange: Draws out emotional residue and clears your cells.

Self-Heal: Promotes the state of balance from which whole body/being integration flows, by balancing the chakras along the spine.

Purple Passion Rose: Aids in releasing interwoven karmic patterns.

Primarily, my clients take the flower essences orally, one drop in the mouth or in a glass of water. I sometimes put a drop of pennyroyal, comfrey, or self-heal flower essence on my fingers and place it on the tender points at the base of a client's skull. Lady's mantle and bleeding heart are helpful on upper chest points and those on the front of the neck.

Anyone can use flower essences for self-care. However, people who have FM or CFS often can only take one drop a day, or sometimes one every other day, initially using no more than three essences at a time. If you are lying down, the flower essence can be applied from the dropper directly onto points on your torso or arms. Or you can apply the essence to your finger first, and then lightly touch the tender point. Care needs to be taken so the dropper doesn't touch the skin or anything else. If that happens, just rinse the dropper with warm water before returning it to the bottle.

My philosophy is that all of us are sparks of the creative life force, going through experiences in order to learn more about ourselves. Often we forget who we are. Learning experiences can be traumatic and become locked in our bodies, creating physical symptoms. I encourage my clients to remember who they are and to release old energetic holdings layer by layer, in order to learn and continue to grow on their spiritual journey. ❖❖❖

❖ ❖ ❖

We hope the practitioners and patients who have contributed to this chapter have shown you that natural remedies provide a gentle way to treat your FM and CFS, and are invaluable if your body is oversensitive to pharmaceuticals. Remember that a healthy diet is one of the best weapons we have against illness and should be an essential part of your treatment program. And don't forget those eight glasses of water a day! When you are living with FM or CFS, it's important to keep your body, mind, and soul healthy. Our next chapter looks at the mental health and spiritual equation.

Chapter 13

Mind, Emotions, and Spirit

The greater part of our happiness or misery depends on our disposition and not on our circumstances. We carry the seeds of the one or the other about with us in our minds wherever we go.

— First Lady Martha Washington

WHEN WE LIVE WITH FM and CFS, we often find ourselves on a roller-coaster ride of emotions: anger, guilt, fear, grief—our minds struggle desperately to understand and cope with what our bodies are experiencing. As we lose touch with our bodies, we also often lose touch with our spiritual side, and we may question beliefs we once held strongly.

It is not hard to see how profoundly FM and CFS can affect one's mental well-being. When our functioning is impaired and our daily lives are constrained due to FM or CFS, it is natural that we grieve that loss. Grief is not just triggered by the death of a loved one—it can occur in response to the loss of anything that is special and important to us. As FM and CFS patients, we must grieve the loss of our former selves.

Our respondents graciously shared their most private emotions with us, in the hope that it would help others with FM and CFS. You may recognize a little of yourself in some of these comments:

"I feel anger and fear when I think about what would happen to me if my husband were to die or be disabled. In addition to missing him, I worry about how I would function without him there, doing what he does. Who would I turn to? Who would get me to appointments? Where would I live? I get angry at the dependence, the pain, the confusion." — Hannah D., Hanlontown, Iowa

"I get scared that no one will ever want me. I get scared that even if I have a family I won't be able to take care of them. I worry about getting so sick that I won't be able to work. Since my fears aren't the same as those of my friends, sometimes it gets very lonely."
— Kim A., Las Vegas

"I was a totally different person. I could multitask with the best of them. Now I can't even do one thing at a time well. I was able to play with my grandkids. I was active, skating, skiing, hiking, etc. Now I can hardly get out of bed most days. I am just a shell of the person I used to be." — Carla B., Jacksonville, Florida

"Guilt is my most difficult emotion to deal with; I usually push it away until I end up feeling better or until I get into a 'rage.' Just like the guilt, sadness, shame, or even happiness—each emotion serves its purpose at its time. And every day brings a new mix of all these emotions." — Chandy W., Shelbyville, Tennessee

In her groundbreaking book *On Death and Dying*, Elizabeth Kübler-Ross concluded that there are five stages of grief: denial, anger, bargaining, depression, and acceptance. We too, must go through these stages as we grieve the loss of our pre-FM and -CFS lives. It is a continual process, with each day bringing new challenges and losses. In the following section, grief counselor Dr. David Redick talks about his approach to helping chronically ill patients confront their grief.

❖ The Language of Loss

BY DR. DAVID REDICK

Dr. Redick is a doctor of energetic healing. He is also a Reiki master, Quantum-Touch™ practitioner, Thought Field Therapist, and an ordained minister. Before establishing his private practice, he served for many years as a volunteer grief counselor and support group leader for an AIDS group. His practice is located in Seattle, Washington.

The first skill I learned as a grief counselor is that a person needs to talk about their loss in order to begin the process of healing. At first it can be difficult to talk when you feel like crying or are scared to reveal such intimate feelings. I create a safe environment in my support group so that each individual is able to talk through their fears and pain.

Similarly, when someone is angry, they need a safe place to express that anger. I tell my support group members that it is okay to be angry, as long as the anger is not directed at anyone else in the group. It may take time for the anger to be expressed—often this is the first time there has been someone there to listen. This is a very important part of the healing process and cannot be overlooked.

I also think that touch is important. I do not want to invade someone's space, but a hug or a touch on the arm or hand is healing. Group members share their wounds and hearts, and I believe in acknowledging that. Listening and touch, done with respect, may bring out emotions that talking cannot.

Grief is something most of us experience at some time in our lives. In our support groups, we follow a set of steps, working through grief in stages, in order to resolve it as completely as possible.

First, recognize that what has happened to you has been a profound loss. Seek support so you do not have to go through your grieving process alone. Reach out to those who are willing to listen. When you have lost the opportunity for a normal life due to a chronic illness, you need to learn to grieve that loss.

Not everyone in your life can be supportive of what you are going through. Some may not be able to deal with your pain, grief, or anger. Like others with long-term illness, people with FM and CFS sometimes have difficulty with the fact that friends and family do not believe that their pain is real.

Often, people who have never dealt with chronic pain do not know what to do to help. The most important thing that family and friends can learn is that they cannot "fix you." They would love to be able to cure your illness, and when unable to do so, frustration sets in. Tell your loved ones that you understand and that you just need them to be there for you. Don't give up on them if they are unsupportive emotionally—they are still your family and your friends. It is your reaction to them, not their reaction to you, which you need to watch.

If your family or friends cannot or will not assist you, thank them and find someone who *can* help you. This may be an individual or a support group. Most of us are taught not to ask for help—we are taught to be independent. It is as if asking for help were a weakness. It is not. We need to learn whom we can safely ask for help and determine who will be there for us in our lives.

I began my own healing journey by going to counseling for alcohol abuse in 1982. I had been an alcoholic for more than 10 years. After spending days in a coma and then losing most of my possessions in a house fire, I knew I needed help.

It is tough to reach out but that is just what needs to happen. We are all individuals and no one deals with pain and loss in the same way. Nevertheless, it often helps to talk with others who are in a similar situation. Be open to new ideas and take what you need to assist you in your journey. Above all, learn who you are and stand up for yourself.

✤ Positive Thinking

There are things we can do to lighten our mental load. As FM and CFS patients, we've all experienced symptoms we might describe as a 9 or 10 on our own personal pain scale. Then, suddenly, a friend comes over, or a great television show starts, and even though our flare-up is still topping the scale, becoming distracted by something alters our perception of pain.

Distracting yourself can do wonders. Hannah D. offers an uplifting example: "I make an effort to think positively about my illness. It's allowed me to stay home for my kids during their last years in high school. I read a lot, which is something I have always loved to do but didn't have much time for. I am also focusing more on my spirituality."

She goes on to say:

> Our neighbor's wife, to whom I was very close, died of cancer last year. I was able to spend time with her as she fought to survive. I have also spent some time with her elderly husband as he goes through the grieving process. In addition, I volunteer as a "chemo-angel." I discovered this organization online. I am matched with a person going through surgery and/or chemotherapy. I send my "buddy" a card and small gift once a week. It really feels good to be able to provide encouragement to someone going through a difficult time.

Buy a little notebook that you can carry around with you. Each time you have a negative thought about yourself, or pop out a negative sentence, write it down. Most of us are surprised to find how many negative thoughts are running through our minds. Look at each negative thought in your notebook as a challenge—a chance to turn your life around, word-by-word. Then, after a week of recording negatives, switch and record positives. This can be as easy as noticing squirrels in the wisteria or a cat in a sunbeam.

THE EFFECTS OF STRESS

A recent experiment tested if plants are a barometer for stress. Scientists planted several gardens and exposed them to sound. In one, the plants were serenaded with soft music. The next garden was quietly talked to with gentle positive affirmations. The next was bombarded with loud, fast music. The final garden was left alone. It's not hard to guess which garden produced the best crop—it was the one that was given positive affirmations!

Masaru Emoto, an internationally renowned Japanese scientist, discovered that crystal patterns that form in frozen water change when thoughts, words, and feelings are directed toward them. Water that had thoughts of love directed toward it formed beautiful, complex patterns. But water that had negative thoughts directed toward it formed incomplete, ugly patterns. If your negative thoughts and emotions can have that kind of effect on the natural world around you, just imagine what they can do to you. (See Bibliography for information on Emoto's fascinating book *The Hidden Messages in Water*.)

THE VALUE OF COMPANIONSHIP

In the garden experiment, one group of plants was left all alone. They didn't die, but they didn't flourish either. Studies show that people who are married or living together, and those who keep pets, live both longer and happier lives. Don't forget how good it feels to go out with a friend for an ice cream or a movie. Staying indoors alone is detrimental to your mental and physical health. One of Mari S.'s favorite mottos is "My feet won't hurt any more at a movie than they do at home."

SELF-TALK

Do you constantly criticize yourself or your friends? Is that niggling voice inside your head chattering away about how you were treated last night or what was said at a party? This negative self-talk is just like having a recording of your negative thoughts playing in the background, thoughts that are being soaked up by your brain.

Try standing in front of the mirror for a few minutes each day and just look at your beautiful face. Guaranteed, you will be able to see beauty in your eyes and your smile. You could even go one step further in your search for your positive attributes by getting a friend to make a list of the five qualities he or she likes best about you. If you are a closet negative self-talker, this could be a revolutionary experience.

Treat yourself as kindly as you would a treasured friend. The words you say out loud or internally to yourself have a huge impact on your self-esteem and, ultimately, on your health. If you say to yourself, "I am not a fun person to be around," or "I look awful," the words are internalized and can become a self-fulfilling prophecy.

GRATITUDE AND APPRECIATION

Every night before you go to sleep, ask yourself, "What happened today that was special?" Maybe an old friend called or someone stopped by to see you. Or was it something as simple as a family member asking, "How are you today?" and really wanting to know the answer?

Write these positive thoughts down in your journal or on a little calendar by your bed. You'll be surprised to see what really makes you happy and thankful, and what is especially important to you. It might not be as big as a new job or car. It might just be your family playing a board game together or watching your dog fetch a ball. However, by counting your blessings, you will never have to wonder what's good in your life.

WORRY

If estimates are correct, and the average person has 10,000 thoughts or images coursing through their brain every day, how many of these are negative? How many are positive? Only you can control the negative images in your mind, so it's up to you to decide if you've had enough negativity in your life and to decide when it's time to let go.

Try using an affirmation. This really does work (even if you can't help thinking about that Stuart Smalley *Saturday Night Live* skit). Begin by choosing a positive, personal subject, and give it a good visual image that conveys an emotion to you. For example, if you needed to lose weight your affirmation could be, "It's important for my overall health that I make good food choices to nourish my body and bring it to its healthiest weight." When "worry" is the subject, the affirmation might go like this, "Worry is an emotion that serves no purpose in my life. I am free of worry so that I can spend my time on positive things."

Mary Beth M. from Houston shared her positive affirmation with us: "I stop what I'm doing and close my eyes and think: Today I am grateful for all

my body parts—the ones that work well and the ones that don't. I know it's a little thing, but it helps."

RELAXATION

Are you able to relax? Do you have difficulty unwinding? Do you feel guilty when you lie on the couch and do nothing? You may need to learn a few tips about relaxing and letting go of the guilt. If you are lucky enough to have a dog or cat in your life, you have witnessed true relaxation that occurs without guilt. Dogs and cats can lie down and be out in minutes, and they don't much care where they lie down either. Guilt? No dog or cat knows guilt.

Relaxation is vital to the FM and CFS patient. We must be able to relax in good conscience. So take a tip from our canine and feline companions—just lie down and rest whenever it suits you.

❖ Pet Therapy

A cold night? Simply throw on another dog or cat. Pet therapy is used in hospitals and nursing homes because it's been well documented that depressed and sick people respond well to the pure love and acceptance of pets. Mari S. has four cats, two dogs, and numerous fish. Helen W. has a big, fat orange cat and three black ones. Pets love us unconditionally, warts and all.

Hannah D. has a menagerie: "I have six cats and a dog. I don't know what I would do without them! They help me achieve some peace—even on the very bad days. I feel instantly soothed when I am with them. They seem to know when I need them the most. I feel such peace seeing them 'meditating' in a sunny spot or napping on my lap. I especially like seeing them curled up together. I often refer to them as our 'peaceful kingdom.' The cats get along well with our dog (who I swear thinks she is a cat). Their antics, as I watch them play and hunt, always bring a smile. Many times I have buried my face in my dog's fur and felt so comforted. I truly believe they are angels from God."

❖ A Patient's Story: David A.

David A. is 42 years old and lives in Seattle with his wife and children. David saw numerous physicians and tried several remedies before he was accurately diagnosed with FM. He recently found new energy and a sense of well-being after reading Dr. John Sarno's book *Mind-Body Prescription* (see Bibliography). David says, "The mind can be the hardest thing to work on, but if you're open to exploring it and you're desperate enough, I think there's a huge opportunity there."

Several years after I was diagnosed with FM, I went on a camping trip with my wife, our kids, and another family. I noticed how much better I felt when I was camping out in the woods. I didn't seem to be bothered as much by my food sensitivities, even though I was eating strange food out there. We also went hiking. I normally have trouble walking more than a couple of blocks. I have plantar fasciitis in both feet, so my feet hurt all the time and I don't really like to walk very far, but when we were out there camping, I just felt really good and I walked about three or four miles a day.

After I got back from camping, I began thinking about how strange it was that I felt so much better. I was familiar with the cycles of FM, and how sometimes I felt better and sometimes I felt worse, but the difference I noticed on the camping trip seemed quite remarkable to me. So I resolved to keep up with my exercise, since I knew I felt better exercising, and at night I'd take walks of about two or three miles. I did that probably every night or every other night for about a week.

Right around that period, somebody recommended a book to me called *Mind-Body Prescription* by Dr. John Sarno; they said it dealt with back pain, but that it might be applicable to me and my chronic pain. I started reading the book on a Friday night. I read it during the day and took walks at night and thought about what I was learning. By Sunday night it was as though a huge weight had been lifted from my shoulders, and I felt 100 percent better.

I went into work on Monday morning. At that time I was only working part-time, because I couldn't type very much without experiencing pain. My hands hurt and it was hard to type for more than 10 minutes at a time before I started to get sore wrists and elbows. But that day, I typed three or four hours and didn't have any pain at all. There was a sense of complete elimination of tension in my neck, shoulders, arms, and back.

Over two to three days, I had a kind of epiphany that, as Sarno puts it, the source of one's pain is repressed rage or infantile rage, as though your inner child is asserting itself (although I don't necessarily agree with how he describes it). This anger is like the impulse to rage at a red light for being red, because you're in a hurry to get somewhere and you wish it were green. I felt that I had been having that sort of reaction all day, every day, for some time.

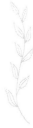

195

When I took my walks in the evening, I looked at my emotional life throughout that day in minute detail and began to see that there where many times when I carried a great deal of tension—impatience, frustration, or irritability. I also tended to have a lot of anxiety and was often driven by the need to be perfect. While reading Sarno's book, I started being able to observe all those reactions and also saw the pattern of my own thoughts. People on the outside would not have called me an uptight person or stressed-out, but I noticed that my inner emotional health was much more volatile than I had ever realized.

When you're upset or roiled emotionally in some way, having this conflict inhabit your body becomes a way for the emotion to come out through an outlet that doesn't upset the mind. It's a kind of self-defense mechanism that protects your mind from dealing with stress—but it has a negative impact on your body. Once you observe this process going on, your body no longer functions as an outlet for your emotions. Instead of processing them in your body, you can now process them in your mind. We've all seen connections between emotions and the body: butterflies in the stomach, a cold sweat, or the adrenaline spikes you feel when you're happy or giddy with love.

What I didn't understand was how my emotions were affecting me (and my body) without my even noticing it. There had been other opportunities for me to explore the mind-body connection before that point, but I wasn't open to them. Now I had gained a new awareness of the fluctuations in my health and about how they often coincided with happier times. At the same time, someone had handed me a book that stated that there is a big connection between the mind and the body. I accept this coincidence as very serendipitous.

Early on in my FM, I was in a lot of pain and I was seeing a lot of doctors. At first they said, "There's nothing wrong with you. You look great." But I didn't feel great and I didn't feel that I was getting anywhere trying to explain my pain to them. I discarded any notions that there was a psychological component to it. Basically, I felt that if somebody told me there was a connection between my attitude and my pain, then they were telling me that it was imaginary and therefore was not real pain. And I didn't really want to go there. But after five years of struggling with it, what did I have to lose?

The important thing for me was to recognize that while there may be a psychological component to it, the pain is definitely real, and it's not all in my head. And a second point was that it is also not my fault. Yes, I thought this happened to me, and yes, I may be able to dig my way out of it. But regardless of how I got there, I'm just doing the best I can like everybody else. I'm not a slacker if I can't manage it on my own.

It took a certain amount of humbleness and willingness to accept how things were. I needed to drop the barriers and not try to put up a big front. In order to move forward, I had to get over feeling defensive about the connection between mind and body.

Stress was another piece of it. I worked for a computer software company up until 1995, where I got totally burned out. After I left, I went from working 12 to 16 hours a day, not eating very well, being stressed out, and working really hard, to not working much and having free time.

Ironically, not working didn't seem to make a difference. That was one of the curious things; I felt really crappy when I was working—I was sore all over, but especially in the hands and feet, and I suffered from headaches and migraines. But then I went traveling for four months in southeast Asia and I didn't feel any better. I thought, "Hey, what's the deal here? If this is all stress, related to work, why aren't I feeling better now that I'm taking it easy?" I had acquired mental habits and attitudes that stayed with me. I was still tense and anxious, even on vacation, at least onterms of my low-level, below-the-radar reactions to the world around me. I was still a live wire. I had developed a way of interacting with the world that was high-intensity, high-energy, and full of high expectations. I felt as if I were playing a permanent video game—you get real jumpy working on a computer all day, every day, and I thrived, 70 to 80 words a minute, and I knew every keyboard shortcut to every program out there, super fast. You get programmed that way.

I tried all kinds of therapies; I had a physical therapist who worked really hard on my neck and gave me myofascial release therapy, and that helped a lot. I explored a number of different ways to change how my mind and my body were connecting, and the mental attitude was the last piece. But I don't think I could have reached that point without having changed my work environment and having a lot of treatment along the way that helped with stress reduction and reorganizing my priorities.

The other thing I have noticed is that when I wake up in the morning, if I stay in bed too long, I get really stiff and sore. It's partly because I'm lying there, thinking, and as I think, I get more tense. And as I'm lying there without moving, and feeling tense, I get more sore.

I tried acupuncture and yoga. The yoga was pretty helpful. Again, I view that as another indicator of the mind-body connection, because

although I did other forms of exercise, yoga seemed to be the most helpful. It was also the thing that calmed me down the most, got me into a state of clarity, and reduced mental activity.

Now I try to process my emotional life. I try to give myself time alone every day, and the way I do that is to take a walk at night. The first half of the walk, I look for points of tension or stress during the day that I did not address at the time—feelings or experiences that I stuffed. Whether it was an argument I had with somebody or even just an interaction that made me worried, I just acknowledge these feelings. I have a kind of internal dialogue with myself. And sometimes I'll even try to mentally solve the problem when I'm walking, "Well, okay, if you're really worried about this, go call this person tomorrow." Or, "If you're really worried about this, but, gee, since there's nothing that you can do, try to let it go." I'll spend the first half hour of my walk doing that. The second half hour, I'll just try to walk, smell the fresh air, and look at the sky. I feel my body move and experience my breathing. My goal is to connect with my body in a mindful way, without a lot of mental activity. And that seems to make the most difference, just that simple act of walking.

Although I had an almost complete cessation of my FM symptoms over that three-day camping trip, FM is still something I have to manage day by day. However, if I don't take care of myself and don't stay connected to my inward life and my emotional life, the tension comes back, and the symptoms start to come back. But the difference for me now is that now I know the source of it, and I can manage it without drugs or a lot of visits to the doctor. That's been huge—it's very empowering and a really wonderful thing. ❖❖❖

❖ Psychotherapy and Chronic Illness

BY MAUREEN SWEENY ROMAIN, M.A., LMHC

Maureen Sweeny Romain is a psychotherapist in private practice in Bellingham, Washington. Maureen specializes in counseling people with chronic illness and utilizes homeopathy and Bach flower essences in addition to psychotherapy in her work with clients. She spent nine years working with patients at the Fred Hutchinson Cancer Research Center in Seattle.

There are things you can do, psychologically, emotionally, and physically, to help your body heal. I work from the perspective that our bodies are really designed for health. Western medicine tends to focus solely on disease, and in some aspects it does an absolutely wonderful job of curing disease. But it disregards the Eastern-medicine approach, which trusts the body's wisdom and ability to heal itself. In my practice, I try to find psychological, emotional, and spiritual approaches that support physical healing, particularly when I'm working with people who have FM and CFS or complications from cancer treatment.

There are different types of psychotherapy, and a person needs to first search for a good relationship with a therapist, rather than seeking out a particular type of therapy. If a therapist pays attention in that initial session to how the person is responding, if the client has a sense of comfort or feels, "This is somebody I could develop a relationship with," this is more important than the type of technique the therapist uses or the school of thought that is followed. The capacity to really listen, and the experience of being "heard," can be powerfully healing.

Most therapists take some form of history from their clients in order to gain an understanding of the individual within the context of their lives. This is not limited to information like, "I was born in a log cabin," and it considers what the client's experiences in life have been, the significant experiences (good and bad), and the makeup of the client's family and support systems. It is important, too, to learn what the client expects to get out of the sessions. Sometimes, a client can't articulate that intent very well, but I think a therapist needs to ask this question: "How is it that you would like me to help you?" Therapy must be entered into as a collaborative effort between the client and the therapist.

I use a great many different techniques. In particular, with people who have chronic illnesses I look at the emotional and psychological baggage or unrealistic expectations they may be carrying. Just because you have an unresolved issue in your life doesn't necessarily mean that it causes your chronic illness or pain. But if your expectations are not being met and you have strong feelings about that, this can divert your body's energy. That energy is needed to help heal your body. As a result, you don't have access to all the resources that could be available to you in the healing process.

It's helpful for people to work on this factor and let go, to face and accept whatever is happening in their life. That allows them to move on, to adjust the expectations that can cause hurt, pain, sadness, or dread and to be able to focus on health.

One technique I use to address this type of issue is to ask the client to meditate on a particular word or phrase during the week, between appoint-

199

ments. Examples include "humility," "surrender," or "let go of anger and want." Clients spend time thinking about, being present with, and watching where this particular concept presents itself to them during the week. Often, the word or idea I suggest comes from the subjects we explored in session. Individuals are encouraged to apply this technique with true mindfulness, which is a Buddhist concept implying great self-awareness. Some individuals have found this to be a powerful exercise.

"Mindfulness" means having a level of awareness that allows you to use yourself as a source of information and helps you to make your way through this world. We're not often taught to operate in a mindful way, to look at our thoughts and feelings and what our bodies tell us about how we are doing. Mindfulness can be an extraordinary practice and very helpful when working with any kind of illness. This has led me to the belief that spiritual work can be an incredible healing force. I'm not talking, necessarily, about going to church, but rather about developing spiritual peace, about really connecting with a core part of ourselves that is about innate goodness and love. When we connect with that part of ourselves and live in that space (even momentarily), it puts our bodies back into balance. I believe that this is challenging work, and we are increasingly seeing the importance of it.

Western medicine tends to look only at the physical aspects of the person and to address only physical symptoms. Yet it often misses emotional aspects, mental aspects, what people think, the beliefs that they hold, the perspectives or the frame of reference through which they view the world, and how these contribute to their well-being (or ill health). In American society, too, we tend to go for the quick fix. If there's a pill for it, then we'll take it, and if one pill works, then three pills might work better and faster.

If you have a chronic illness, you are challenged not to go for the quick fix, but to work with your mind, thoughts, expectations, and spiritual life. When you are working in all four of those areas, you've reached the heart of what healing is all about. A cure may or may not come, but emotional healing has the potential to create physical health.

Some people have hesitations about going into therapy. Part of the challenge is that we live in a society that attaches a stigma to therapy. Some people believe that you're somehow weak if you talk to a therapist. However, I've always felt that it makes less sense to *not* seek some consultation when you're struggling. If we break an ankle or have acute chest pains, it isn't considered a sign of weakness to go to the doctor, but when our emotional selves are in pain, there is sometimes a social stigma on seeking help.

Today we're increasingly seeing that paying attention to one's spiritual health is a very important component of healing. In the early days of cancer treatment, researchers found that women who went to support groups experienced a better quality of life during the time they had prior to death. The support groups may not necessarily have cured their disease, but these women were able to establish friendships within the group that supported them in all aspects of their lives.

✤ Cognitive-Behavioral Therapy

Cognitive-behavioral therapy (CBT) has the potential to alleviate some of the symptoms of FM and CFS, particularly mild depression, mood swings, anxiety, and sleep problems.

In CBT, the patient plays an active role in the therapy. Working with the therapist, patients explore their reactions to troubling stimuli and identify the techniques that will help them overcome unwanted habits or behaviors.

CBT is a combination of two types of psychotherapy—behavior therapy and cognitive therapy. Behavior therapy addresses habitual emotional or physical responses that a patient may have to certain situations; for example, shopping at the grocery store makes you feel anxious, or you get into bed each night and immediately obsess over whether you'll get any sleep. Together, you and your therapist begin to weaken the connection between the situation that is troubling you and your inappropriate reaction to it.

Cognitive therapy teaches the patient about thought patterns that cause the inappropriate response. You and your therapist focus on the troubling situation and the thought processes that lead to your distorted view of that situation The patient is taught to identify the relationship between events and feelings, to maximize self-praise and avoid self-punishment.

Cognitive-behavioral therapy has a particularly good track record in curing phobias. Therapists use gradual exposure to help patients overcome their fears. For example, if the client has agoraphobia (a fear of being outside or being in crowded places), the therapist might begin by having the client spent very brief periods outside at each session, gradually increasing the time spent at each subsequent visit. Cognitive-behavioral therapy is not an instant cure, but it can be very effective over the course of a few months.

Ellen J. had learned the need for balance in her life, but going back to school tested her resolve to put her health first:

I was initially very careful to do the things that maintained my health: meditation and yoga, connecting with friends, doing my own artwork, but as I continued, I started to get a bit cocky. I fell back into the mindset of my old type-A personality and the mental dialogue that went with it, thinking, "If I can take one class and be okay, then of course, I can take two. If I can take two classes and pass them, then I can take three." And that was when the applecart got unbalanced. I started having memory problems, constant sore throats; my pain level soared back into the 7–10 range. I sought out medical attention to determine what was wrong, rather than listening to my body screaming at me to cut back and slow down. Fortunately, the CFS clinic at Harborview Medical Center in Seattle had a psychologist who specialized in cognitive-behavioral therapy. The therapist helped me examine how I think about my situation and myself. The next step was to clarify and change these messages. I turned off the "super-student" mindset. I even had to modify the "I can do anything a healthy person can do" mindset. (I *can* do anything, but slower. And it takes a little more support.) I'm now getting voice-activated software for my computer, asking for extensions on papers, and taking one class at a time.

❖ A Patient's Story: Jill M.

Jill M. was living and working near Philadelphia when she was bitten by a tick and contracted Lyme disease. A growing number of people, once infected with Lyme disease, go on to develop FM, as Jill did. She and her husband now live in Burien, Washington. Jill, now 59, discusses how psychotherapy and group therapy helped her overcome the emotional difficulties FM brought to her life.

At the time, I didn't even realize a tick had bitten me. I was living with my second husband and my daughter, who was going through a full-scale teenage rebellion. I was very ill one weekend, and could barely crawl out of bed. But it went away, so I put it down to a 48-hour bug. Six months later, I found myself getting more and more tired. My doctor ordered a blood test right away, and, sure enough, it came back positive for Lyme disease. I remember lying in bed watching a full two weeks of Wimbledon—all I could move was my head, as the ball went over the net. Thinking this was a short-term event, I even enjoyed the tennis. I thought this thing would be over in a month or so and life would go on. I took massive amounts of antibiotics and coped with the resulting yeast infection, but there was little improvement. Of all the unlucky people who get Lyme disease—which at that time was about 3,000 people in Pennsylvania and about three in Washington State—only 8 percent go on to develop FM as I did.

At that stage, denial was the order of the day. I went back to work part-time for about three months and then full-time because I could not keep up with the workload on a part-time schedule. Then I crashed with a vengeance. I used up all my sick leave and went on disability leave, which lasted six months at 80 percent pay. I finally made the decision to quit. The company would have given me a pity job, since I had more than 20 years with them and had, over the years, managed to work my way up to manager, very rare for a woman at that time. But I don't take well to pity and could not stand the thought of dealing with people who had once known me as an effective, intelligent person. I knew it was the right decision, because my stress decreased immediately and I was able to say goodbye to that part of my life. I don't think my husband had quite the same level of relief. He was hugely supportive and took care of me wonderfully, but I don't think either of us really understood that this was going to be a massive life change for both of us.

My major difficulties at this time were sleeping, widespread muscular pain, debilitating fatigue, and short-term memory loss. I took Flexeril for sleep, but I kept needing to increase the dosage to get any sleep, leaving me doped up all day. I underwent psychological testing that confirmed my short-term memory loss and knocked about 12 points off my IQ level.

My doctor prescribed Ambien, which worked well and had no side effects on the following day. I felt as if I had gotten my brain back. I started warm-water physical therapy classes, and they were wonderful. They got me back on my feet, and I started building up some muscle strength. I was feeling better.

There I was, all day with nothing to do, an ideal situation in which to return to school. (Some of us never give up!) Not just any school, but Bryn Mawr, which had started a new program for us older types. I figured I could handle a couple of courses a semester and maybe even have some fun. Fun had been sadly lacking for quite a while. My husband and I talked it over, and he promised to help with household stuff so that I could use all my available energy to study. The first semester was really hard, but it was fun. I met some neat people and managed to ace both my courses, Latin and English.

It all came apart in the second semester. My husband basically disappeared, and so did all my help and support. The company had assigned him to a new program that would be taking place in Seattle. He tried commuting for a while, flying home every other weekend, but it just about killed him, and he slept all the time when he was at home anyway, so what was the point? I learned a lot about stress; I fell apart emotionally as well as physically. I tried to keep going at school, but I found myself forgetting everything I had learned the day before. I then had to try to relearn what I had forgotten, as well as that day's quota. My brain had turned to mush. I dropped out.

By now I considered myself totally to blame for failing to get better. Why wasn't I just pulling up my socks and getting on with life? The failure to keep up intellectually was a crushing blow to me and my self-esteem.

We decided to move to Seattle. My personal style in life had always been to run away if anything was too big to deal with. I knew that I could not manage on my own and knew instinctively that I needed to run from the current situation. Life hadn't taught me yet that that the baggage always comes with you. We moved into our new house in July 1994. The process of finding the house and moving in had taken three months. Of course, I seriously overdid things, firmly sublimating any illness. By the time we actually moved in, I had developed a raging ear infection and found a local doctor to give me antibiotics. He told me to "get a life" when I kept bursting into tears.

Then I went into group therapy. There were six of us. We bared our souls, talked, and wept. I finally came to the understanding that my life had changed irrevocably. I had to learn to accept that change and to recognize and accept myself as a different person. I realized that there should be no blame and no guilt. This was easy to say and accept on a superficial level but was a whole different story to understand and accept in my soul. However, I began to settle in and feel a bit better. I had a new doctor to give me medication and a counselor who taught me cognitive-behavioral therapy and relaxation techniques. I learned to identify the things that caused me the greatest difficulties. The biggest factor turned out to be interaction with other people at a social level. These interactions plain wear me out. Since I became ill, I haven't been able to maintain any friendships with non-fibro people. It takes too much energy, and the return on the investment isn't worth the resulting fatigue.

In 1996, I developed a severe rash on my hands, lost 40 pounds, and also lost a tremendous amount of muscle strength in my legs. I had dermatomyositis—a rare autoimmune disease. In this condition, the cells in the capillaries attack one another, gradually starving the proximal muscles of oxygen, so they too die, resulting in weakness in the thigh and upper arm muscles. Luckily, I was diagnosed before any major damage had been done. (Incidentally, I had just applied for Social Security disability for my FM, and the diagnosis came through at the right time for a quick approval.)

Obviously, that was not a good year, and depression set in. My psychiatrist recommended drug therapy to counter the depression. Over the years, I had tried every depression drug on the market and reacted badly to all of them. But new ones were available, so I tried one. I had a very bad central nervous system reaction. Instead of taking me off it, my psychiatrist threw other drugs at me until I finally said, "Enough."

By this time, my brain was a sponge and my heart did not want to live anymore. It was an astonishingly seductive experience: All I had to do was go to sleep, and there would be no more pain, no more fear, no more crushing fatigue, no more anxiety attacks. Just peace, beautiful peace. Even though I ultimately decided to choose life over death, I ended up spending four days in a psychiatric unit. What an experience. They sorted me out and sent me to a different psychiatrist who specializes in mixing drug cocktails for people like me.

While my life is not exactly a bowl of cherries, I have survived. With the dermatomyositis treatment regimen, my hands are considerably better. I am back in warm-water therapy and try to go twice a week; walking laps in a warm-water pool on a regular basis strengthens my leg muscles. I am still trying, but the setbacks come as regularly as the steps struggle forward. It is often difficult to maintain an upbeat frame of mind, but I try not to lapse into thinking that it's easier to do nothing. However, life still had a few curveballs to throw at me and mine. In 2000 I was in two car accidents. In the first one, I was the passenger and I had my seat belt on (thank goodness). Nothing was broken, but somehow I had hit the windshield, because there was a lump on my head. There was bruising from the seatbelt and other bruises in the strangest of places. Bruises heal, but the soft tissue injuries, especially in my left shoulder, take their own sweet time, and I still have trouble with my shoulder.

I was back to just being able to get out of bed for five minutes, due to pain and debilitating fatigue. Gradually that improved and I managed to reclaim two of those good hours a day. Eight weeks later, to the day, I decided it was time to for me to drive again, this time into Seattle for a doctor's appointment. At the busiest part of I-5, traffic had come to a halt. I

slowed, thinking I had plenty of time to stop, when to my horror, I crashed into a pale blue van that was in front of me. Then someone rear-ended me. I thought it was completely my fault—perhaps I had tried to drive too soon, I had lost the ability to assess distances, all sorts of things. It wasn't until the police came and the officer pointed out the skid marks made by the car that had rear-ended me that I realized I had been hit in the back and pushed into the van. Again, I suffered no major injuries, but I had double whiplash and I was back to square one. My shoulder was re-injured and, although I didn't know it at the time, I had just signed myself up for two years of migraines.

Life was a nightmare. I had lost whatever impetus I had to create a successful life for myself. I was still under the care of a psychiatrist and was also in counseling with a woman whom I liked enormously. If I hadn't had that emotional outlet, I think I would have exploded. My life became extremely limited; all social contact stopped, and I even stopped answering the telephone because I didn't have the energy for a conversation. Pain, fatigue—they both intensified. I was full of anger and rage, and I just kept erupting. I started giving away things I cherished to my daughter. I never realized that all this behavior was a precursor to suicide. My poor husband, what I put him through.

I think it was about November when I had yet another outburst of rage, the one that tipped the scales. I went into the bedroom and swallowed a handful of Xanax. I just wanted everything to stop; to have no more pain, no more daily struggle, no more rage—no more feelings at all. I sat there, on the edge of the bed, contemplating whether or not I should tell my husband what I had done. He took the decision out of my hands because he came to check up on me and I told him. He dragged me to the local ER—I only went because he was so upset, and I didn't like seeing him so unhappy. So I went through the stomach pumping and swallowed the charcoal, and I don't remember anything else because I passed out. The next day I just couldn't figure out why everyone was so mad at me (except my husband, bless him). The social worker wouldn't sign the release paper until I agreed that someone else would have the responsibility for all my medications. My step-daughter, who is a nurse, agreed to take care of them and did it very compassionately, making sure that I had enough pain pills and "extras" so I wouldn't panic when I really needed them but would also not have enough to do myself any more harm.

The aftereffects of the suicide attempt? I realized it was an attempt to escape, a huge howl of pain at the universe. I underwent lots of counseling and changes to the drug cocktail—who knows what did which? But now I was educated. I recognized the precursors for what they were, and I learned the width of the path I was walking and how slippery the sides were.

Now, when I have an outburst of inappropriate anger, I stop and think—what is new? Any new drugs? What is triggering this? And I know to ask for help. After the storm, came the peace—finally. My support group provided the most incredible help in a totally unexpected way. There was one occasion when I said I was considering suing an insurance company. Almost the instant I got the words out, the group seemed to surge forward and in one voice said, "How can we help?"

This triggered in me an intense feeling of spirituality or transcendence that left me speechless. It lasted for about six months, and I can still tap into it if I need to. It brought me an enormous sense of serenity and peace. I now live one day at a time, taking into me all the goodness of the day and eliminating the negative. The group broke up soon after this and, sadly, I have never been able to tell them how much I owe them and to express the depth of my gratitude for providing such support. Perhaps this account will do that.

Now, my life is still limited to two to three hours a day. I read a lot and get a lot of pleasure from sewing and knitting, enjoying the peace of these activities and the pleasure of creativity. I get tired very easily, but I have an early warning system, because I start to sweat when I become too fatigued. I do no socializing except with my family, and, of course, I have the continuous companionship of my husband. Answering the telephone is still not possible. But even after all this time, I know if I reach out, my friends will still be there, and this brings enormous comfort. ❖❖❖

❖ Healing the Spirit

No matter your chosen spiritual path, pain and illness are universal, and healing of the spirit is attainable.

As Dharma Singh Khalsa, M.D., tells us in *The Pain Cure*, "Pain and suffering are two different things, and it is possible to experience pain without suffering." It's possible, even probable, that we will experience a life-changing moment or lesson as we go through chronic illness. We can't help but be transformed.

Ellen J.'s illness helped put her more in tune with the universe:

I try to use my condition as a way to connect with the source, rather than feeling like I've been abandoned, and my spiritual practices have really changed. I found that I could no longer go to services, so that forced me to find other ways to be spiritual, including meditation. I feel really blessed that I've had the opportunity to connect with people on a deeper level, in contrast to how I think most people in our society deal with one another. I probably wouldn't have had this opportunity had I not become ill. I've had to examine who I am and whether my life is going in the direction it should go. Even though I would not have chosen to live my life in pain, I'm finally at peace with it.

❖ Spiritual Counseling and Chronic Illness

BY CORNELIA DURYEÉ MOORE

Cornelia Duryeé Moore is a 46-year-old filmmaker and healing prayer minister living with FM. She and her husband Terry Edward Moore are raising two sons. Cornelia believes that prayer is a powerful tool in the healing of chronic illness. She doesn't take any drugs, preferring to eat a healthy diet of organic vegetables, fruits, nuts, and seeds. She sees a naturopath, a chiropractor, and a physical therapist, but her favorite therapy is horseback riding. Now she is able to work again, after years of gradual recovery. Cornelia's website, with many links on healing, is: www.CorriesLeapofFaith.siteblast.com

I have been a practicing Christian for twenty-five years. I became interested in healing prayer when I took a two-year course from a healing prayer counselor, Reverend Tilda Norberg, one of the first female ministers ordained in the USA. Her course sent me on a wonderful journey into healing. Here's one example of how healing prayer has affected me and my family. I had been sick with FM, multiple chemical sensitivities, and endometriosis for some time. Before I got married, the doctors working on my endometriosis said they did not think I would ever be able to conceive or carry a child. My healing prayer colleagues had an all-day prayer session for me—what they call "soaking prayer." Three women gathered around me as I lay just under the altar in the church. They prayed for my fertility, they sang, they sat in silence, and they laid their hands on my abdomen for hours at a time. It was one of the most glorious times of prayer I have ever experienced. Those angel women were utterly loving and generous, and I felt the spirit of God surrounding us. And my first son was born two years after I was married. It was miraculous.

Soaking prayer can be a marathon session, like the one my friends had for me, or it can mean praying day after day, week after week, being in the

presence of God and inviting God's healing spirit. And miracles always happen. The healing that takes place isn't always physical. God's agenda for healing may not be the same as mine, so I try to pray without worrying about that. God's agenda will always come to be, and it is always perfect. God effects healing in our spirits and souls, and often (but not always) in our physical bodies.

Our family experienced a terrible crisis in 1997. Within a two-week period, everything horrific that could happen did. My seventh pregnancy failed, my husband was in a terrible accident, and we were fired from our jobs in the theater we had cofounded—the theater that was our entire life. The church gathered around us in a way that was holy, strengthening, and uplifting. We didn't have to cook for a month. They brought us food, they mowed our lawn, they prayed with us and for us, and they sent us notes every day to let us know they were thinking of us. It was the most beautiful outreach of the body of Christ that I have ever experienced, and it just blessed us down to our socks. In the midst of our terrible grief and pain, the church was like a dolphin swimming alongside another dolphin that is giving birth, helping to support her as the pain fades and a new life is born. It was a perfect example of how people in the church can be family to one another.

My spiritual director gave me a prayer that has been very helpful. It's an ancient monastic prayer. You simply say "Lord Jesus Christ" as you breathe in, and "Have mercy on me" as you breathe out.

When I am in trouble, when I'm scared or upset, or wake up from a nightmare, that prayer is the first thing that comes to my mind. It's lovely to have a prayer that happens without thought. It has become my default setting, if you will. It's comforting to me, because there's great power in saying God's name.

Some people just pray by saying the word "love" or the word "peace." Anything that draws you closer to God's spirit can be used as a simple breathing prayer. It can be done daily, even hourly. It can be done in traffic, it can be done in the bathtub, it can be done anywhere. Sometimes I burn a candle and use it as a focus in my prayer. Some people hold a rock or something that reminds them of the earth. Like many women that I know, I am drawn to making altars—sacred places in my home with objects that are icons of God for me. An icon, some say, is a window to heaven. And I always need to be reminded of God's closeness, but especially when I am coping with a lot of pain, exhaustion, or brain fog.

There's a burgeoning trend within the medical community to tend to patients' spiritual well-being as well as their physical needs. I know that many nurses are learning all sorts of spiritual healing techniques, such as therapeutic touch, energy work, and soaking prayer. I've read that almost half of the nurses practicing today are open to spiritual healing. Miracles are happening every day in our hospitals and clinics, and people are becoming more comfortable with different healing styles. I hope it continues.

A very important part of my Christian practice is my raw vegan diet. I believe I have been greatly healed by eating a diet high in raw vegetables, fruits, nuts, and seeds. I eat to honor God, for better health, and for better stewardship of this fragile planet. God doesn't want me to binge on junk food; God wants me to honor the body I was given by putting clean air, water, and food into it. I really believe that you are what you eat. And I don't want to reflect the energy of a candy bar. I'd rather be like a nice organic apple.

I believe that the Creator made us as a unity, as a wholeness. The word "whole" comes from the same root as "holy," which also means "healthy," "hale," and "hearty." I think it's important to remember this, particularly when we're dealing with a challenge like a chronic illness. We are meant for more of God than we often embrace. I believe one reason I am making such good progress toward physical healing is that the Holy Spirit will not let me ignore my spiritual life. I get wonderful nudges that remind me to pray or to be mindful of God—a dream, a song, or a word from a friend, and all of a sudden I am back in communion and moving toward wholeness again.

❖ A Patient's Story: Debbie M.

Debbie M., an FM patient, transformed her life through spirituality. She now teaches both adults and children to find peace within and to overcome obstacles. You can find information about her company, Unlimited Inspiration, at www.unlimitedinspiration.com. Debbie lives with her family in Weston, Florida.

The deepest pain for me came when my mother contracted tuberculosis. I was only five at the time, but I remember her trembling as she asked, "Am I going to die?" Those five words embedded themselves in the depth of my being. For the next year and a half as she lay in bed on very high doses of medications, I became more fearful. She eventually recovered, but the emotional scars remained with me, leaving me severely dyslexic, clumsy, and physically ill.

During my days in high school and college, the darkness grew deeper. One morning I opened the newspaper to find that one of my closest friends had died in a drunk-driving accident. Once again I was shaken to the core. Over the next five years I attended five more funerals of dear friends who thought they were invincible—who thought that living life to the fullest meant drinking and drugging themselves into a stupor. I fell deeper into despair—until I met Michael, a bright light of gentle strength, wisdom, and comfort. We fell deeply in love, and he became the grounding force of hope in my life.

A year into our marriage we began a seven-year odyssey that proved to be pivotal in transforming the very essence of who I was to become. During this time period my son was born two months prematurely and later developed a severe auditory processing disorder. Another of our children was hospitalized twice with complications from a genetic disorder called Ehlers Danlos Syndrome, six immediate family members died, and I began experiencing numerous stress-related physical symptoms. Then one day I hit bottom—I felt as if someone had pulled the plug on my life force. My legs buckled and my arms trembled; pain racked my body, mind, and spirit. Every system in my body was screaming for relief. These physical symptoms led to a misdiagnosis of lupus, then of MS, and eventually to a diagnosis of FM.

On my knees I prayed, "God I can't do this anymore; show me a way out of this darkness." As I spoke those words, a wave of peace rushed over me. The next morning I was reading, as I often do, three books. Within one hour I read the same sentence in each book. *You will keep repeating the challenges in your life until the lesson is learned.* As I read these words, I was covered in goose bumps. But what could my lesson be? I went back to the books, and the next page I turned to said, *If you want peace in your life, you must create it within.* That was the key to release me from pain: I had to find ways to create peace within.

That day I was given a marvelous meditation tape. As I listened to the comforting words, I cried the most cathartic tears. It was as if the hand of God had reached through the many layers of pain and fear into the depth of my soul. I was finally letting go of embodied emotions and opening up to receive the light. I had discovered, in the midst of these challenges, my indomitable inner spirit.

Through daily prayer, journaling, Reiki, energy work, and meditation I was able to connect deeply to my source of strength. This connection allowed me to release my attachment to the pain, distress, and drama I was living. I came to realize that everything I was experiencing could help me learn and grow. Through this growth, I was able to find the blessings in the obstacles and bring light to the darkness. I learned to find peace within.

Now that I was *emotionally* strong, I began working on my physical body. Through daily exercise, stretching, increasing the nutritional quality of my diet and vitamin program, and learning to balance my life, my health quickly improved. My life began to shift from one of suffering to one of hope, health, gratitude, and reverence. This shift allowed me to help my children find peace within themselves and to become as healthy and happy as they could be.

As I emerged from the darkness, I was greeted by the most glorious light—the light of inspiring others. Although I am grateful for the opportunity to help others along their path, my most rewarding work is within my own family. I am truly blessed to have a marriage that has grown stronger and stronger. And my beautiful children are now healthy, thriving, and bringing so much joy to our family.

Although I am truly grateful for being able to transform my life, I know that without those challenging experiences I would not be at the point in my life that I am today. The words *find peace within* helped me to reach a place of reverence, gratitude, and confidence. I am now able to live a life of grace and strength. ❖ ❖ ❖

❖ ❖ ❖

Our spiritual lives are an intensely personal aspect of who we are. Spirituality means something different to every person—we hope you find a sense of spirituality that enhances your life to its fullest extent.

When you have a chronic illness, it is natural to grieve for the life you had before. But, as you have seen in this chapter, there are many rewards to be found in your new life. So what if you can't run around like a whirlwind anymore? Appreciate being able to stay home with your children, watch the wildlife in your garden, read a good book, and get to know your neighbors. In other words, "Stop and smell the roses."

We'll leave the close of this chapter to Linda M.: "On a spiritual level, I think I've become more intuitive, more caring about other people who have pain in their lives, because I can certainly relate better now. I felt like I needed to have some hope and not just focus on the dark times, so I asked myself, 'How have I changed, what have I learned?' I am so pleased to know that I have learned something from this experience. This pain, while no blessing, may yet be God's road to enlightenment."

Chapter 14

The Guaifenesin Protocol, Mirapex, Medical Marijuana, and Magnet Therapy

The brain helps start chronic pain—and the brain can help stop it.

— Dharma Singh Khalsa, M.D.

THERE ARE SOME therapies for FM and CFS that are difficult to categorize, but we would be remiss if we omitted them, because they all have the potential to be helpful in a FM or CFS treatment program.

We want you to be aware of everything that is available to you. If something piques your interest, research it more thoroughly. Look online or read a book on the subject. You'll find many interesting websites and publications in our Bibliography and Resources sections at the back of the book.

From music therapy to laughter therapy, there are many different ways to transport yourself out of pain and into feeling good.

When you are ready to take on a new method of healing, ask yourself a few questions:

1. Which aspect of my chronic illness do I want to affect (e.g., pain, fatigue, brain fog)?

2. Will I be able to afford another type of health care?

3. Does the practitioner get good results?

4. Do I feel comfortable with the practitioner?

5. How long has he or she been practicing this modality?

6. Is the practitioner convenient to my home or office?

Remember, you are the leader of your healing team, in partnership with your primary-care physician. Do not hesitate to ask practitioners any questions that are on your mind.

✤ The Guaifenesin Protocol

When we began this new edition, we sent out a questionnaire to hundreds of FM patients. When responses to our questionnaire started pouring into our inbox, one group of people stood out—they were patients on the guaifenesin protocol. Every single one of them was brimming with enthusiasm about guaifenesin therapy and begged us to include information on their treatment. Robin N. told us about her experience: "The one helpful thing my doctor told me was to go home and research my condition on the Internet. I read everything I could manage until I came across a discussion of the guaifenesin protocol. My health has improved in so many ways through guaifenesin therapy that I have less time these days for research and more time for living life." In the following contribution, R. Paul St. Amand and Claudia Craig Marek talk about this exciting new treatment.

BY R. PAUL ST. AMAND, M.D., AND CLAUDIA CRAIG MAREK

Dr. St. Amand, the physician who developed the guaifenesin protocol, has devoted a lifetime of research into the diagnosis and treatment of FM. Together with Claudia Craig Marek, he is the author of *What Your Doctor May Not Tell You About Fibromyalgia,* a groundbreaking book about FM and this protocol.

Paul and Claudia run the Fibromyalgia Treatment Center in Santa Monica, California, a nonprofit foundation that raises money for FM research, educates patients and physicians, and organizes conferences to raise awareness of FM. The Fibromyalgia Treatment Center has a network of support groups and an online group of more than 2,000 patients. Its web-

site is www.fibromyalgiatreatment.com. St. Amand and Marek have worked collaboratively on FM research for eighteen years. Both have FM.

Paul:

I have been involved in the study of FM for the past 46 years, long before it was given a name. As an endocrinologist, many patients came to me with vague complaints of fatigue, pain, anxiety, and memory problems that they assumed must be hormonal. But of course, no test ever showed that to be true.

At the time, I was doing a great deal of work with gout. There were certain similarities in symptoms, and also dissimilarities, that intrigued me. One pattern is that gout occurs mostly in men, while FM occurs mostly in women. Yet when I used gout medications on my FM patients, they got better! So I had to find out why.

It turns out that a disturbance in phosphate metabolism plays a role in both these conditions. What led me to the concept that FM can be an inherited condition involving phosphate metabolism was a patient's observation that his gout medication improved his dental tartar, because it caused the chipping away of his dental calculus. The gout medication caused an increase in kidney phosphate excretion, and I attributed the reversal of FM symptoms to that action.

I became fascinated by this improvement in patients whom no one else had been able to help—patients with a condition, which at that time, no one agreed existed. I also realized I had the condition myself, as did two of my daughters. Those were very personal reasons to find a treatment that worked. I've now been on medication for 48 years and am in better health physically and mentally than I was years ago. So I am motivated to help others because I know what it is like to be sick with FM and not be able to accomplish anything.

Guaifenesin is our current choice of medication. It is capable of this same effect. We believe that tissues that have been saturated with excess phosphate due to a renal defect are blocked from forming adequate amounts of energy (chemically known as ATP) in cells. Such cellular action occurs in most of the body compartments. When cells are deprived of sufficient energy, normal function is altered and the cells go into a metabolic hibernation. Tired cells produce tired patients. If we compare our store of energy to a checking account, that account allows only so much expenditure before going into deficit spending.

Claudia:

Guaifenesin is a treatment and not a cure. It takes time to work and the time schedule is different for each patient. Some have been ill for 2 years, some for 10 years, and some for 40 years. Response to the medication seems to be genetic; people in the same family typically need about the same dose to begin reversal. Each patient travels back through his or her own timeline to the point before they had FM. Guaifenesin only works on FM; it does not work for arthritis or other coexisting conditions, such as hypoglycemia or obesity. So one must also get healthy in other respects. It is not a miracle pill that takes your pain away in six hours or six weeks. It is part of a process. Reversal symptoms can be painful initially; in fact, the hallmark of being on the correct dose is that one has an exacerbation of symptoms.

Paul:

Because I could get nowhere with the medical establishment (who would not listen to me, a lowly doctor in private practice), I resigned myself to just helping as many patients as I could. People came from everywhere, and their families and friends came too. When Claudia came to work with me (and, as a coincidence, she also had FM), she felt we could not help enough people unless we communicated about our work and made huge efforts to get the word out.

I have developed my own system of a totally objective examination ("mapping") wherein I palpate most of the musculoskeletal system in search of swollen places. This "map" (a body-wide caricature) that I produce then serves as the basis for all future comparisons.

We probably succeed in 95 percent of the patients that we can keep under our wing and remap at appropriate intervals. Most failures occur when patients inadvertently consume products that contain salicylate-bearing ingredients (such as aspirin). Our website, www.fibromyalgiatreatment .com, has helped us communicate about the program, using both printed material and an online chat group.

Claudia:

Managing FM is no different than managing other illnesses. We focus on FM because it is ours. Anyone with a chronic illness must do some house cleaning and do what I call, "putting your health house in order." Your ability to recover from any illness, be it breast cancer, FM, or some other type of chronic condition, depends on your general health. So this advice is really generic for everyone and serves us well, even when FM has been reversed and resolved.

Get rid of stress, eat right, and exercise, however you can. Even if exercise to you only means stretching on your living room floor, it will help. If it involves starting a walking program, it will help. If maintaining a healthy diet only means cutting back on junk food or sugar, it will help. If relieving stress only entails getting organized and letting the nonessential things go, it will help. Get rid of negative people, no matter who they are, and don't watch or read depressing news stories. All of these are essential steps in accentuating what you can do and doing positive things. We laugh at self-esteem these days because it has become a catch phrase, but self-esteem, based on what you *can* do, is important. So joining a support group and helping others, doing some work to raise FM awareness, accomplishing a goal of exercising—these are not to be underestimated. It's easy to pooh-pooh things while sitting on your couch, but let me tell you, no one ever gets well sitting on their couch...*from any illness.* You can learn from groups like the Fibromyalgia Treatment Center how to get help and how to help others.

Paul:

I have restricted my practice to FM for the past eight years. My reasoning was that any endocrinologist could do the blood pressure and thyroid work —but that I had something to offer to fibromyalgia patients that no one else was doing at that time. Now we have doctors who travel here to work with us, and that's rewarding, and they are now located all over the country.

❖ A Patient's Story: Beth O.

Beth O. is a 27-year-old yoga teacher. Beth was diagnosed with FM in 2003, and she has had tremendous success using the guaifenesin protocol. She lives with her husband in Louisville, Kentucky.

Before treatment with the guaifenesin protocol, I was angry that I was sick. I lost many of my friends. I felt lonely and misunderstood. But most of all, I was terrified that I would only become worse. My pain level was an "8 out of 10" on a daily basis, and I was barely functioning.

I became desperate to treat my illness. None of the medications my doctor prescribed were working and the side affects were an annoyance. I

217

read more than 40 books on FM and CFS. I scoured the Internet. I looked for a treatment that addressed the root cause of the illness—one that was not a moneymaking scheme.

I finally read *What Your Doctor May Not Tell You About Fibromyalgia* by R. Paul St. Amand, M.D., and Claudia Craig Marek. I have some background in physiology and anatomy and everything in the book seemed like a valid and logical explanation of the entire illness. The book presents a treatment to address the cause of FM and CFS, rather than just the symptoms.

My primary-care provider treats FM with the guaifenesin protocol and is very knowledgeable about it. Due to my current treatment, my life is great! I am able to exercise and I feel physically fit. I rarely experience depression and my pain is half what it was before. Since my success with guaifenesin, I am able to do most of the things I did before my FM crash. I still don't do much heavy work and I don't stay up late, but I am very happy with my lifestyle now.

The guaifenesin protocol is the only treatment that I have read about that reverses the symptoms of FM and CFS. I haven't seen anything else as promising, and I have had great results with it. I have received great support from the Guai Group online support list and am starting a local support group for people who use guaifenesin to treat their FM and CFS.

If it were not for guaifenesin, I would not be able to fully take care of myself. I had almost reached the point of being unable to work before I began treatment and I think I eventually would not have been able to continue walking without help.

Before I became ill, I was determined to ride a bike for 100 miles at a time. I was considering multiple day biking tours. I had high goals for physical fitness and most of my goals were self-oriented. My goals now include strengthening my marriage and accepting each day as it is. I have more spiritual goals, and my faith has been greatly strengthened. Although I am interested in staying as healthy and fit as I can be, I no longer obsess about having a beautiful body or about being sexy. My goals are more modest but also more mature.

My faith, my marriage, and the beauty of life drive me. My rewards are spiritual peace and simple happiness. Enduring pain has taught me compassion and inner strength. Enduring severe depression and anxiety has taught me empathy. The gratitude that I now have brings me inner peace, and I seek to deepen that. ❖❖❖

❖ The Mirapex Protocol

BY DR. ANDREW J. HOLMAN, M.D.

Dr. Holman is a board-certified rheumatologist in private practice in Renton, Washington. He lives with his family in Seattle.

On the wall of Dr. Andrew J. Holman's office is a map of the United States. Pins of all colors dot almost every state, one for each patient who has contacted him for help. Many pins have flags on top; these signify the patients who have traveled to see Holman in person.

Dr. Holman's research into sleep and the central role it plays in FM led him to develop his own treatment protocol involving Mirapex, a drug commonly prescribed for Parkinson's disease. He theorizes that FM could be an "umbrella condition," and that by uncovering the underlying cause(s) of FM we may be able to unlock the secret to CFS, irritable bowel syndrome, carpal tunnel syndrome, and other overlapping conditions.

If you take Marines, who are incredibly fit, and torture them by depriving them of sleep, they will experience FM, even if they don't call it by that name. It doesn't matter how fit someone is, you can eventually cause fibromyalgia-like symptoms—it's just a matter of how long you deprive people of stage IV sleep, the deep sleep level at which the body heals.

In 1998 Dr. Manuel Martínez-Lavín presented some interesting data in *Arthritis and Rheumatism* on the abnormalities of the sympathetic nervous system in patients with FM. Martínez-Lavín's premise is that FM patients have an overactive stress response—excessive sympathetic activity. Think of the sympathetic nervous system as a dimmer switch that controls the fight-or-flight response. It can be turned off all the way, like when we're in a deep, peaceful sleep, or it can be completely on, like someone in a life-or-death struggle.

When the stress response is turned on almost constantly, it becomes less responsive—there's only so much capacity in the system. This constant autonomic arousal [stress response] in the brainstem prevents FM patients from achieving stage IV sleep.

THE RESTLESS LEGS SYNDROME CONNECTION

In an effort to restore stage IV sleep in FM patients, I took the first steps in developing a protocol with the drugs Ativan and Klonopin (two benzodiazepines that are used in low doses to treat restless legs syndrome in elderly people). Restless Legs Syndrome (RLS) is a condition that frequently

219

overlaps with FM. In fact, in a 1996 study, Muhammad B. Yunus, M.D., reported that RLS was more common in patients with FM than it was in normal controls (31 percent versus 2 percent).

My first thought was to prescribe these to patients who had both RLS and FM. I undertook a two-week study in which 200 patients with both RLS and FM took 2 mgs of Ativan daily. After just two weeks, most appeared to be feeling markedly better. I found there was a significant level of improvement in these patients when I prescribed a sleep medication in combination with one that affects the autonomic nervous system [which controls both the stress response and the relaxation response]. No one got better on the Ativan alone, because Ativan doesn't induce stage IV sleep (in fact, to some degree it deprives people of deep sleep). So by itself, Ativan wasn't a particularly good answer, but combined with Trazodone or a muscle relaxant, it produced clearly observable benefits to patients.

I presented this data at the American College of Rheumatology meeting in 1998, and had an opportunity to talk with many doctors who were interested in the protocol. I asked Dr. Robert Bennett, an FM expert from Oregon Health Sciences University, to give me some constructive criticism because I was less experienced and had only been practicing for five years. He thought my protocol was a little too aggressive and could produce a placebo effect; I considered that fair, because it was only a two-week study, and placebos were not included in the trial. But there was a gentleman with him who took me aside and said he liked the idea. This gentleman was Harvey Moldofsky, a doctor behind groundbreaking studies in fibromyalgia and stage IV sleep.

Moldofsky said, "Don't be surprised if you meet people who don't move at night [FM patients who do not have restless legs syndrome]." I said, "Well, I know lots of people who don't move at night. We just don't give them the Ativan." He said, "No, they don't move but they have the same brain activity on EEG testing as people who *do* have restless legs syndrome."

A pattern was becoming clear. Moldofsky's research indicated that whether FM patients had RLS or not, the majority had the same pattern of brain activity.

I had found that 60 percent of my patients didn't have any restless legs symptoms at all, so I hadn't given them the option of these medications. But with Moldofsky's encouragement, I decided to give it a try when I got back to my practice. Sure enough, every single person started to notice some benefits. They weren't cured, but I definitely saw a trend—adding the medication for restless legs syndrome enhanced the sleep response.

Although I didn't know it at the time, I was having success because I was combining a sleep agent with a brainstem agent—something to control autonomic arousal [stress response] in the brainstem.

MIRAPEX

Mirapex and Requip have turned out to be the most effective medications for restless legs syndrome that have ever been developed. But it wasn't until 2005 that Requip was FDA-approved for the treatment of RLS, and Mirapex still has not been approved (at the time of going to press) for the treatment of this syndrome.

With the availability of Mirapex, we had access to a medication that treats RLS like nothing else. Now we had to tease out the puzzle of FM, working, working, working, until we figured it out.

It took 18 months to find a neurologist willing to talk to my patients and give it a try. Dr. Christopher Lawrence in Seattle put two of my patients on Mirapex, and they did fantastically well. I slowly became comfortable with this new medicine, and we worked on the dose that suited the patients' own level of preference.

We then began a study of 200 patients. At first, the patients took about 1.5 mg of Mirapex at bedtime. Then it became quite apparent that the dose should be at least 2 mg, and probably 4.5 mg. I was able to report at the 2002 American College of Rheumatology meeting that 22 of our patients had significant improvements in all parameters.

The next step in the research was to see if we could reproduce these positive results in other doctors' offices. We had a protocol and some sophisticated evaluation tools, including a definitive rating scale of fatigue, pain, and global function We were unable to get the manufacturer of Mirapex interested, so I had to obtain samples, purchase the drug with my own money, and negotiate the study with the FDA. Initially they would not let us do a study at the higher 4.5 mg dosage level because there had been no Phase I safety data on a 4.5 mg treatment program. There is only phase I safety data on the 1.5 mg dosage three times a day, which is the highest single dosage prescribed for Parkinson's disease.

We published some data involving 200 patients in which we used up to 10.5 mg of Mirapex at bedtime; this appeared in the *Journal of Rheumatology*. We were very cautious and made it a point to increase the dosages slowly to make sure they were at safe levels. After that research was published, the FDA said it was sufficient for them to approve the study design for a larger trial. No placebo-controlled trials can be done without FDA

approval, because they not only monitor the safety of drugs on the market, they also monitor the safety of all drugs used in research. We finished the study and presented it at the 2004 American College of Rheumatology meeting. The expanded study was published in *Arthritis and Rheumatism* in August 2005 and demonstrated the highest therapeutic response of any FM study so far.

What makes our study most interesting is that it is designed differently from other studies, which are usually run by pharmaceutical companies. These companies want studies done with patients who are willing to take no other medication. This can be a problem for patients, because they have to take the risk of getting an inactive dose of the drug (the placebo) throughout the course of the study. Understandably, only a fairly small number of patients are willing to take the risk of doing without any medication at all.

In our group we decided that we would do an "add-on therapy," which was more realistic. In this approach, patients continue taking their regular medication and then take ours in addition. Patients simply had to agree not to change the dosage of anything they were taking prior to the study. In this particular trial, 57 out of 60 patients finished the study, which is an astronomically high number (and 2 of them moved away). We have never seen a study like that—these patients were very dedicated people. Approximately half were taking chronic narcotic analgesics and 30 percent were disabled. None of these patients would have participated a traditional FM study, and most pharmaceutical companies would have excluded them as "untreatable."

COMPLICATIONS OF SLEEP APNEA AND NECK PAIN

However, there were two important exclusions. Patients could not be in the study if they had untreated sleep apnea or if they had cervical pain with prolonged neck extension. One of our goals was to decrease arousal [associated with the stress response] that can fragment normal sleep. There are two arousals that we already know will limit the effect of a dopamine agonist such as Mirapex. One is the "drowning reflex" of sleep apnea, which is present in about 40 percent of people with FM. You can treat FM and sleep apnea with all the other protocols. However, if you try to treat sleep apnea patients with our protocol, it won't work very well, because the drowning reflex of sleep apnea is so powerful that it will overwhelm the effects of the Mirapex. It is important to remember that sleep apnea does not cause FM—many people have sleep apnea without the signs of FM. However, when sleep apnea is present, it interferes with this approach to the treatment of FM.

The other condition that is counter-productive to treatment with Mirapex is cervical cord compression in the neck, called myelopathy. We screened people for our study by asking if they experienced neck pain when bending their neck back, for example, in a dentist's chair or at the hair salon. We know that this is a potent autonomic arousal for people with neck issues *and* FM.

NECK CONDITIONS AND FM

About one third of the people we see for consultation have both neck issues *and* fibromyalgia. They are another special group—a subset of FM patients. It is important to treat them in a way that takes into consideration the effects of this neck condition. It is important to take care of the neck *and* the FM.

Since this study did not allow us to provide neck physical therapy, we had to exclude patients with this condition. If my patients need to be evaluated for a neck condition, we do the MRI evaluation at the beginning, before starting treatment. The radiologists at Valley Medical Center in Renton have helped us by modifying their MRI procedure, so that we can obtain flexion-extension views. We are the only facility west of Chicago that has access to information of this detail, and this is only because the radiologist will do extra views of the measurements I ask for at no charge. They actually measure the diameter of the spinal canal at each disk level. The flexion-extension MRI can be done anywhere. You do not need new technology. You just need to have a hospital and radiologists who are willing to do this imaging.

The MRI can be uncomfortable. We sedate the patients a little, and some can become somewhat claustrophobic because their fight-or-flight response is keyed up. We have developed a protocol that makes it easier for patients. It's like a biopsy; it may hurt, but it lets us know what the problem is.

We usually give everybody a chance to go the nonsurgery route, but if patients have really extreme myelopathy, we tell them kindly that they will need to consider curative surgery. Most patients are okay with this, because they see their MRI picture and they say, "Oh my God, my neck looks like link sausage." (It really does look like link sausage, but only when they look up.)

Myelopathy has predictable effects, mostly on the autonomic nervous system. As mentioned, this condition can be a potent source of autonomic arousal of the stress response. Also, if the cervical cord is compressed, this can produce referred pain over the entire body.

223

TREATMENT PROTOCOL

Basically the first stage of treatment for FM is to understand how it works —the mechanisms of autonomic arousal, how sleep plays a role, and the vital importance of sleep apnea and cervical cord compression. You can help people so much more if you know how these conditions affect the autonomic nervous system.

Mirapex is the only medication I've seen that actually cures FM. It does not produce a cure very often, and I separate "cures" from "effective treatment." Effective treatment is relatively common. A cure is unusual, but it does occur.

We have patients who have been on our protocol for a couple of years. We've tapered back the Mirapex because they're doing so well. The medication seems to reset their brainstem and help decrease the stress response. It makes some sense, because if you wind up the brainstem and then add pain, fatigue, and stress, that stress response heightens activity in the brainstem even more, and it becomes very hard to slow it down. But if patients are able to reverse that trend and become able to get restorative sleep and wake up refreshed day after day, without fatigue, after a while they really believe they're going to stay this way. Then it has a cumulative, positive, de-stressing effect, and they realize that if FM comes back, they will be able to do something about it. Patients have to watch out for sleep apnea, and they have to be careful not to injure their neck. But if they do get injured, they know that it is important to take care of their sleep at the same time that they take care of their injuries.

AN IMPORTANT WARNING

After nearly ten years of treatment with dopamine agonists, like Mirapex, and recognition of their relatively benign safety profile in patients with Parkinson's disease and restless legs syndrome, a new important concern surfaced in 2005. After rare scattered reports, a Mayo Clinic group described a possible link between compulsive behavior and these drugs in the journal *Archives of Neurology*. The group monitored their Parkinson's disease clinic for two years and found 11 patients who developed compulsive gambling, shopping, and hypersexuality while on treatment. There were no cases of compulsivity in RLS patients. It is suspected that the lower doses required for the treatment of RLS may be the reason.

However, the therapeutic dosage for FM, which is usually only administered at night rather than throughout the course of the day, is high enough to raise concern. Consequently, my office, along with David Dryland, M.D.,

in Medford, Oregon, decided to conduct an exhaustive search to determine if this problem was an issue for patients with FM or only for those treated for Parkinson's disease.

After reviewing 3,000 charts in Seattle and a database of 700 patients in Medford, twenty-five patients were identified with compulsive gambling, shopping, and even sewing/crafts habits, often leading to severe financial and social consequences. Hypersexuality was not generally noted, and other abnormal behaviors were lacking.

All twenty-five people were patients who had responded rapidly to the treatment and had been virtually FM-symptom free for many months to years. When taken off the medicine, the symptoms went away. Also of interest, their FM did not return, although a few patients noted that their high energy state faded.

As physicians, we try to alleviate suffering, and untreated FM remains a daunting challenge. We, and patients, realize that all medications can have side effects in some people. All patients are now counseled to watch for behavioral changes and to not be afraid to discuss the medication with their physicians or to discontinue taking it. Guarding against any side effect is very important, but this increased risk for developing compulsive behavior requires a thoughtful discussion upfront and the full cooperation of the patients and usually their families for monitoring.

Dopamine agonists still transform the lives of many patients with FM without side effects. It is important to not throw out the baby with the bathwater, but the issue of compulsivity needs to be an important concern when considering this approach to the treatment of FM.

CONCLUDING THOUGHTS

Most researchers in the United States, whom I know because it is a small club, believe that FM should be abandoned as a specific, unified diagnosis. They believe it is really a general disorder, which would explain why there is a variable response rate (some people get better on *this* protocol, some on *that* one.) This research has given me a different perspective. The variable response may be better explained by combinations of other separate problems, like sleep apnea or neck problems with FM.

Finally, the good thing about the Mirapex protocol is that more of our patients are doing well. We don't have all those unhappy follow-up visits any more. The protocol is three months long. In the beginning I have patients call me in a week to discuss how they're doing. If things aren't going well, we get a sleep study and wait for the results. Then I see them in eight

225

weeks, as they gradually increase the Mirapex under the protocol. I then see them for a repeat follow-up six weeks later. Either they are doing well or they are not. If they are not, we consider other treatments. Tolerating treatment for sleep apnea can still be a big problem, but now we understand why someone is not doing well. If they are well, we see them three times a year to monitor safety.

I have found that my FM patients do not have flare-ups as often and I get fewer distress calls. Generally, the only people who call me are those who have not yet completed the protocol. Before I began prescribing Mirapex and Requip, I would get calls during cold, damp weather or during the holidays, because my patients were experiencing more stress. I rarely get those calls now. My practice is completely different—it is so much easier and more satisfying. ❖❖❖

❖ Medical Marijuana

Marijuana was dropped from the U.S. pharmacopoeia in 1941. Unlike cocaine and morphine, it was not "grandfathered" in to the federal comprehensive drug act of 1970. Therefore, marijuana is not in a category that allows doctors to prescribe it for pain and nausea. But some states have legalized the use of marijuana with a doctor's prescription.

❖ A Patient's Story: Suzan B.

> Suzan B. is 47 years old. She was a White River rafting guide and auto mechanic before becoming ill with FM and CFS. Suzan is prescribed marijuana as a part of her pain-management regimen. She lives in Seattle with her cat Rabbit.

My use of medical marijuana began one day when I was in such incredible pain I couldn't move. I lay on my bed with my head propped between pillows to immobilize it because the slightest movement was intolerable. My neurological symptoms were at an all-time high, and I felt like my nervous system had been plugged into a wall socket running electricity throughout my entire body, vibrating every nerve to the key of fingernails on a chalkboard. Every muscle in my body screamed in pain. All I could do was lie in bed all day and pray.

I remember lying there just wishing I had something to help me make it through the day, to survive until tomorrow. I wanted to take a swig of whiskey, but I knew alcohol would exacerbate my symptoms, and the last thing I wanted was to make things worse. After three days of this, I remembered that I had a small film can with some marijuana in it in the bottom of a drawer somewhere. I had smoked pot in my early 20s but had decided to quit. I had kept a small container of it in my bottom drawer. Had it turned to dirt after ten years?

I expected it would help me to survive my day, but what I did not expect were the results I got. The marijuana almost eliminated my neurological symptoms. Very few things I had tried had ever helped these symptoms. My headache greatly decreased. My general malaise lessened. And this improvement did not wear off when the pot did.

Since then I've been using marijuana to help me recover from this illness. Before I became sick with CFS and FM, I used to run two to three miles a couple of times a week. After I got sick, I could not walk a block to save my life. My brain had shut down with the illness, but I instinctively knew that part of my recovery lay in being able to get even mild exercise. I started to walk a short way down my street and back. When I had worked up to half a block away, I panicked, afraid I would be unable to get home. But soon I began short walks in the woods. Nature has always been very healing for me, but in this case it held even more for me.

Out in the woods, I was able to smoke marijuana on my walks. It was incredibly painful for me to walk, and smoking helped me be able to do it. It also helped in other ways. I have always had a high drive to achieve and push myself. While this had been helpful in my career, it got me into trouble on my walks. I often pushed myself too hard and would end up sitting down, out in the woods, thinking I would never walk again as long as I lived. This was a problem. I soon found that, with rest, a lot of water, an energy bar, and, most importantly, some marijuana, I was able to get back up and walk back to my car. This has allowed me to continue my walking in spite of my fears, pain, and severe neurological symptoms. Walking has improved my condition considerably. My FM and CFS has gotten a little better every year since I've started this exercise, while I see others around me deteriorate or stay the same. I would not be able to do it if it weren't for the marijuana.

While the marijuana is very important for my condition, I must remember that it is medicine. It is a drug. The reason I quit smoking pot in my 20s was that I saw people who smoked marijuana daily turning into couch potatoes. This is the last thing I need now. I need it to help me become more functional, not less.Each medicine has its side effects and a maximum dosage. With a lot of testing I found that if I limit my intake of marijuana to about three times a week it works best. Certain other medica-

tions also need to be taken on a schedule. For example, Motrin also works best if I limit the dosage. If I take too much too often, it stops being as potent for me.

Marijuana helps my problem with input overload. If I am in a busy place with a lot going on, I get exhausted very quickly. Marijuana helps me tune out some of the noise and commotion. Marijuana, although not a panacea and not a cure, has been a fantastic help for me. It is everything from a pain reducer and energy restorer to a stress reducer. Marijuana works for me in ways no other drug has. I hope one day that more patients have access to this important medication. ❂ ❂ ❂

❖ Magnet Therapy

Due to the industralization of our planet over the past three centuries, our exposure to the natural magnetic field has decreased. Our daily lives often revolve around the use of electricity and electronic devices, and these inventions emit alternating current that interferes with the magnetic field. We also live a large part of our lives inside buildings, which futher block the earth's magnetic field. In the following contribution, Carolyn Else talks about how magnets can be used therapeutically.

BY CAROLYN ELSE

Carolyn Else is a wellness consultant. Carolyn attended Stanford University and now lives in Tacoma, Washington. She became interested in using magnets for healing after hearing powerful testimonials from a variety of people, including some in the medical profession, about life-changing experiences after using such products. To learn more about Carolyn's wellness practice, visit www.5Pillars.com/healthyorelse.

Although the use of magnets for health purposes has greatly increased in the past ten years or so, many people are still wary of their use. It is important to note that magnet therapy is not a new idea. As early as 2500 B.C., magnetic stones were being used for healing. One must remember that we all live on a huge magnet called the earth.

There are many different approaches to using magnets therapeutically:

❖ Magnetic pads are held briefly on specific points along the acupressure meridians to increase and balance the flow of energy through the body.

* Magnetic pads can also be applied to problem areas of the body to increase energy flow and circulation and to stimulate the lymphatic system.

* There are numerous other ways to experience the benefits of magnetic therapy, including sleep systems (special mattress pads and pillows), seat cushions, and insoles.

The idea is to provide a way for people to achieve total wellness through prevention. Everything I use in my wellness practice is geared toward that end. The magnetic products give the body energy from the earth, and far-infrared products give the body energy from the sun. Both technologies work to help the body heal itself or prevent illness. Individuals who use the magnetic products report that they enjoy better sleep, more energy, and mental clarity.

No medical claims or predictions are made about the magnetic products I use because they are not medical devices. Rather, they incorporate natural technologies including the natural magnetic energy that is present in the earth's magnetic field. When one exposes one's self to that magnetic energy, the body may be better able to recover.

Since deep sleep is so important to good health, a sleep system is recommended as one of the foundations of wellness. When I introduce this technology to a person, they may feel a sense of relaxation, a decrease or cessation of discomfort, warmth, and/or increased energy. Use of a sleep system may result in deeper, less restless sleep. People using these products either sleep on a mattress pad embedded with magnets, or they place magnets in their shoes or over the affected area on their bodies (for example, with a knee injury, a knee wrap can be used with a magnet tucked inside, near the injured area).

Based on client reports, I believe that everyone to whom I've introduced this technology has benefited, because the body is so compatible with the earth's natural energy, which is present in the magnetic products.

❖ ❖ ❖

In this book, we've talked about the myriad alternative treatments for FM and CFS. Another important part of managing your illness is addressing how it affects your quality of life. What can you do if you are unable to work? How do you apply for social security benefits or a disabled parking pass? What about legal issues? Our next chapter answers these questions.

Chapter 15

Work and Legal Considerations

There will come a time when you believe everything is finished. That will be the beginning.

— Louis L'Amour

MAKING THE TRANSITION from a career to a leave of absence or even retirement is difficult on many levels. One of the most difficult aspects of living with FM or CFS is the impact your illness has on your ability to earn a living. Severe pain and fatigue often leave us unable to work at all, or only able to work a few hours each week. In a two-income family, there is a lot less money coming in and this can cause tension between partners. If you live alone, especially if you are a single parent, it can be devastating.

Robin N. had no choice but to make work her top priority in order to provide for her family. "When I became so ill, I had to put all my remaining energies into working since I am a single mother who had to keep a roof over our heads. That meant missing out on my children's activities and eliminating my social life. Life was work and rest; nothing else."

❖ You Are Not Your Job

Your number one job is to take care of yourself. In order to do that, you may have to cut back your hours or quit your job entirely. Being unable to work impacts one's self-esteem. For many of us, what we do for a living is inextricably linked to how we feel about ourselves. After you're introduced to someone, the first question you're often asked is, "What do you do?" Ellen J. says, "When I first became ill, I flinched when people asked me what I did for a living, because I used to be such a 'doer.' I defined myself by my job, by what board of directors I was on, which volunteer project I was working on. Over the last few years, I've tried to change my focus from 'what I do' to 'who I am.'"

Dennis H. agonized over the decision to give notice at his job:

When you do something eight hours a day, five days a week, for as long as I did, you take a lot of pride in doing your job well. It feels like I stepped into an alternate universe. Being sick all the time requires a tremendous adjustment in your lifestyle. Dealing with it emotionally and psychologically is quite a challenge; in fact, it's almost a catch-22 situation for me. I did a fairly good job of adjusting to what has happened, and I'm not letting myself fall into the depressive state that often happens after people lose their health and job and the activities they used to enjoy so much. I thought I stopped and smelled the flowers before I got sick, but I appreciate my health even more now.

If your ability to work is affected by FM or CFS, there are steps you can take to maintain your quality of life. In this chapter, we look at ways to help you find a balance between work and healing. We also look at what to do if you are unable to work. There are laws in place to help you, but since making sense of them all can be confusing, we hope to make that process easier for you.

✤ A Patient's Story: Lois S.

Lois S. is 52 years old. Since developing chronic myofascial pain and FM, she has experienced many challenges in her work environment, from physical discomfort to unfriendly coworkers, and a human resources department that didn't recognize her illness. Lois's goal is to find a new job where conditions will be better and she can enjoy her work. She lives in Goshen, Connecticut, with her husband.

I have worked in a factory for more than 30 years; I guess it finally took its toll. My problem started in my upper neck and back, and I ended up having to stay home from work because of it for two months. I returned to work and signed up for an inspection job, which sounded great to me since it

231

consisted of moving around and not standing in one spot for eight hours. I lucked out and got the job. I felt fantastic! I didn't hurt at all, and it showed that the secret to me being pain-free was to move.

Unfortunately, after a few years, the company decided that they didn't want auditors anymore and they dropped my job. I was so depressed that I stayed out of work for a few days just trying to get my head together. Fear went through me because I thought to myself, "Where are they going to put me?" and, "Am I going to start hurting again?"

I was put on a machine where once again I was forced to stand like a robot, and it didn't take any time at all before I started to have those old symptoms. I have been the same way ever since.

It is clear to me that my employers and coworkers don't understand chronic illness. For example, at one point I had to take sick leave for several weeks, and when I came back, you'd think I'd been on a beach somewhere, the way my coworkers reacted to my time-off.

Just recently, I was put on new machinery, and someone came by and made sarcastic comments about me. Ironically, this man happens to live with someone who has had a bad back injury and is walking with a cane. But thank God his girlfriend doesn't have to come into the factory every day and try to survive. I don't think he thought of this as he was slapping me in my face with his thoughtless comments.

I also have to deal with an unsympathetic human resources department. One woman in particular loves to question me about my absenteeism although she knows about my chronic condition. She too, supposedly, has been diagnosed with FM, and peeking around her desk one day, I spotted a heating pad! It must be so great to come to work and just sit on heat. I have tried to figure out how I could come in and duct tape a heating pad to my behind with a super-long extension cord, while running lathe machinery. If anyone has a suggestion, I would love to hear from you.

Having this condition is terrible, but there is always something positive that comes out of anything terrible. I am currently thinking of leaving this place of pain and finding another quality control job. If I can find a job that is better for my health, I might be able to put my money somewhere besides pills and doctors. Wouldn't that be great? ❖❖❖

❖ Vocational Rehabilitation

BY DON USLAN, M.A., MBA

Don Uslan is a psychotherapist, a rehabilitation counselor, and the owner of Northwest Counseling Associates, a private practice specializing in treating patients with chronic medical conditions and occupational problems. Don also cofounded the Center for Comprehensive Care, which provides rehabilitation services based on the philosophy that coordinated care will produce the best patient outcome.

Vocational rehabilitation is a term that is not generally well understood. Quite simply, vocational rehabilitation helps chronically ill people to maximize their work potential. A vocational rehabilitation treatment plan depends upon many variables: the condition that a patient has, how they manage their life requirements while fulfilling their work requirements, and what changes can be made to integrate work into their whole treatment picture. Vocational rehabilitation also includes working with clients and their attorneys to gain accommodations that will allow the patient to work part-time, take time off work, go back to work, or change their job or occupation entirely if necessary.

A rehabilitation counselor may also work directly with employers, insurers, or physicians by assisting them and providing information on other possible interventions. The counselor may also make recommendations on legal issues such as disability benefits or reasonable modifications to a job or workstation. Vocational rehabilitation involves implementing plans that keep work part of the picture and make receiving disability benefits a temporary part of the treatment plan, as opposed to a long-term goal.

Should a person diagnosed with FM or CFS continue to work? Part of the answer depends upon what point in the treatment process you are talking about. Early on, people don't yet know what is happening to them. A year down the road, they may have a better sense of where they are in their illness, once they are over the initial shock of being diagnosed with a chronic disorder. Three or four years later, when they've had good treatment and are more experienced in managing their illness, work may be more appropriate.

Most people with FM or CFS require time off work to get themselves together, to focus, rest, and recuperate. Then they may go back to work. My impression is that only about 20 percent of the people diagnosed with FM or CFS can really stay on the job full-time. Even if circumstances are ideal, most people have a hard time functioning as employees in the current work environment. Usually, modifications are necessary. Some people are able to work out of their homes, which allows a lot more flexibility. Most others, though, have employers who are cooperative and can work with them.

233

It is difficult for a person with FM or CFS to work a professional forty-hour workweek. Except for a very few situations, however, permanent disability is something I do not support. It does happen, usually when a good employer cannot be found or the patient has other responsibilities, such as young children. But with proper employment strategies, in conjunction with good providers and treatment plans, people can expect to eventually return to a reduced work schedule. However, for a return to work to be successful, it requires soul-searching, adjustment, and coping with a major lifestyle alteration.

In 1989 I developed the treatment model now known as the Proactive Living Program. This sixteen-week, group-model program is designed to integrate a variety of effective treatment approaches to save costs, allow greater communication among providers, and assist patients in gaining mastery over their medical conditions. The program provides adjustment counseling, including developing self-management strategies and skills for coping with lifestyle changes, support systems, goals, and relationships. The program also provides acupuncture, active-movement therapy, relaxation techniques, physical reactivation, and rehabilitation education (including occupational alternatives, disability issues, recovery planning, access to community resources, health education, nutrition, pain management, optimal sleep strategies, stress reduction, and pacing techniques). The program staff includes a nurse health educator, an acupuncturist, physical therapists, a medical psychotherapist and social worker, massage therapists, and medical specialty consultants.

A typical patient with FM who has gone through the program is Gwen [name changed for privacy], a 38-year-old woman who was a claims examiner for a major insurance company. Gwen, who is married and the mother of two, had been recently promoted, but her growing fatigue, difficulty with concentration, forgetfulness, and pain were adversely impacting her performance on the job. She struggled with FM for more than five years. During that time, nine physicians assessed her for a variety of medical ailments (including psychological conditions). She was diagnosed as exhibiting symptoms of multiple sclerosis, cancer, and a number of other chronic conditions. Gwen spent thousands of dollars on a wide variety of prescribed medications and alternative herb therapies. At one point, a doctor suggested that she had FM but told her there was nothing to be done about it.

Finally, Gwen saw a good rheumatologist who referred her to the Proactive Living Program. Gwen met other people with similar conditions and began to realize she was not alone. While she learned about the history of her condition and what to expect in the future, she also began to experience some relief through acupuncture, careful stretching regimens, and specialized exercises. She learned how to monitor her symptoms and keep a diary. She learned techniques to help her sleep better and gave her physician more feedback about the effects of various medications. She developed new skills in dealing with other people and their reactions to her illness. She learned the limits of her strength and energy, and how to pace her exertions.

Gwen informed her employer about her condition and gradually modified her work schedule to two and a half days per week, while supplementing her income with disability benefits. She decided to enter psychotherapy to deal with some long-standing issues that caused her internal stress and anxiety. Stress-management techniques helped her create periods of profound calm and served generally to "turn down the internal thermostat." Gwen learned how to cope with the flares and cycles of her condition. She formed close relationships with other group members and learned to rely more on them and less upon health professionals.

Gwen's family members met with the program leaders and the group members to learn how they could help her improve. Gwen began to feel increased self-confidence as she gradually gained some control over many of her symptoms. For the first time, she felt optimistic about the future. During the two or three years after she left the program, Gwen continued in a follow-up group and made gradual gains (with occasional setbacks), and she is now successfully working four days per week at her job. Her pain has decreased, her sleep is better, her concentration has improved, and she has gradually recovered her energy.

Managing FM and CFS requires a strong support system. If everything is orchestrated correctly, I believe that patients can return to work (unless some other medical, physical, or psychological issues are going on). Many people who have been diagnosed with a chronic illness are in deep despair because they feel like they have lost everything. Our message is that it doesn't have to be that way. ❖❖❖

Many of our respondents described how they reluctantly left their flourishing careers, suddenly unable to deal with a 40-hour workweek, let alone some of the punishing schedules they had been working. After a period of grief for their former selves, they began to discover joy in their new lives and many of them reinvented themselves, finding new careers that better accommodated their illness.

❖ A Patient's Story: Katrina B.

Katrina B. was diagnosed with CFS in 1986. She practiced as a psychologist for more than 20 years and taught at the college level. She also facilitated seminars and workshops for educational institutions and the private sector, lectured, and held CFS/FM seminars annually. Katrina had to cut back on many of her professional activities due to her illness and was ultimately forced to close her practice in 2001. Katrina is the author of *Chronic Fatigue Syndrome, Fibromyalgia and Other Invisible Illnesses: The Comprehensive Guide,* originally titled *Running on Empty*. She presently serves on the board of directors of the CFIDS Association of America and the CFS Association of Arizona, experiences that allow her to continue her involvement in the field and to make a contribution to the world of CFS. Katrina lives in Happy Jack, Arizona, and maintains a website at www.LivingWith Illness.com.

The loss of my practice was acute, akin to losing a valuable and irreplaceable part of myself, and although I have been able to continue to be somewhat active in the field, I continue to feel this loss strongly. However, I find that although I am no longer able to practice in my profession, life offers numerous opportunities to be of help to others. Although this statement sounds corny and self-sacrificing, I must admit that the ability to help others is an act of selfish gratification since I derive meaning and pleasure from this role.

I began to seek information about CFS following my diagnosis (two years after onset) and soon became aware of the lack of literature on the subject. Filling that void became a primary motivator to write about CFS and other chronic illnesses. Because I hoped to publish it after obtaining my degree, I wrote a document that not only met the requirements for inclusion of all the elements of a traditional dissertation but that was also publishable in a modified form for the general public. (The result was a dissertation roughly the size of the Manhattan yellow pages.) I revised the work to make it suitable for patients and began looking for a publisher, a daunting task.

I received enough rejection slips to wallpaper a medium-sized room. In retrospect I am able to appreciate how risky it was then for a publisher to publish a book about a questionable illness. However, Kiran Rana, publisher at Hunter House, was sufficiently farsighted and daring to take on the project, and fortunately *Running on Empty* did well. When it was released in 1992, only a few books on the subject had been published and these were about personal experiences of illness. I felt that patients needed a book that addressed other facets of CFS, so I wrote a book consisting of three parts: What It Is, What It Does (its effects), and How to Live With It (how to obtain a diagnosis and treatment and how to cope with chronic illness).

I found writing about chronic illness highly gratifying, knowing that I was able to offer information, support, and humor to a broad range of patients with CFS and FM. In addition, I produced five audiotapes and wrote articles for numerous newsletters. I am able to continue my involvement in these areas to a limited degree.

My health is variable, but I remain disabled and quite ill much of the time. I do have fairly good days (those a healthy person would consider merely "average"), but overall my health continues to be quite compromised. I am housebound much of the time. Fortunately, I have a number of sedentary interests and an excellent support system.

I try to practice what I preach: obtaining appropriate medical and adjunctive services, attending to personal needs while recognizing the needs of others, journaling, monitoring self-talk, and recognizing myself as a human being and not simply a human "doing." I attend to simple but good nutrition and try to perform what I call acts of personal hygiene, although I certainly take shortcuts and have more than my share of greasy-hair and same-old-nightgown days.

I maintain frequent contact with friends, my mainstays. I make an effort to maintain friendships with those who are ill and in similar circumstances and who speak a shared language, and with "civilians" and friends who are well and provide a broader perspective.

I resent the hell out of my illness. I can usually live with it or around it; I try to accept what I cannot change, but illness-imposed symptoms and limitations have never become acceptable to me. A few people have said they see illness as a blessing of some sort, and I wonder about them. CFS has offered me some opportunities and learning I would not have experienced otherwise, such as the opportunity to meet some incredible people in similar predicaments, but overall I'd trade in these unwanted learning experiences without hesitation for a life offering fewer growth opportunities.

I am glad that over time chronic fatigue syndrome, the serious illness with the silly name, and fibromyalgia have received more attention and appreciation from the press, the public, and the physicians who diagnose and treat it. Still, we are often dismissed as the unwanted stepchildren of medicine and have a long way to go in disseminating accurate information that

237

reflects the serious nature of these illnesses and their devastating effects on those who are debilitated and often disabled by them. ❖❖❖

❖ ❖ ❖

Diane K. was frustrated that her illness prevented her from volunteering in the community, so she and a friend started a company called "Peter's Garden," through which they give away free dahlia tubers in exchange for a promise that the grower will give the flowers away as random kindness bouquets during their long blooming season. "This gives us a great feeling of spreading good in the world, yet we only need to do a bit of work every other spring or so dividing and giving away the plants," says Diane. "Also, when our new gardeners divide these plants in years to come, they can give the tubers to others who also commit to giving the cut flowers away. Giving and receiving fistfuls of beautiful dahlias makes everyone feel good and Peter's Garden grows exponentially without our direct involvement. This is something we can realistically do."

❖ ❖ ❖

"My work is kind of a funny thing for me," says Jenny G. from Anamosa, Iowa. "I am a housekeeper for a hotel. You wouldn't think I could do it. Although I can only work a couple of times a week, I love it. I get to meet many people, and I don't think about my pain while I work. It is fast paced and hard work, but it is good for me to be able to keep moving. I don't work a lot, and I don't do more than two days in row. I work to pay for my meds."

❖ Getting Your Benefits from Social Security

BY ANNE KYSAR

Anne Kysar graduated from New York University Law School in 1997. Her practice, which is in Seattle, is devoted to representing disabled people in Social Security disability cases. More than half of her clients are people with complicated chronic illnesses such as FM and CFS.

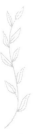

In 1999 the Social Security Administration issued rules that recognize FM and CFS as impairments that can be disabling. As an attorney practicing in this field, I have had gratifying success with FM and CFS cases. In my experience, a person with a good work history and a supportive doctor usually has a very good case.

The Social Security Administration has two different disability benefits programs. One program is Social Security Disability Insurance (SSDI). The other is Supplemental Security Income (SSI). The basic test for disability is whether you have an illness or injury that will keep you from working for at least 12 months.

SSDI is for people who are disabled and have a work history. It is similar to private disability insurance. You can call the Social Security Administration and they will tell you if you have enough work credits to qualify for SSDI. There are no rules about assets for SSDI. You can have a lot of money and still qualify for SSDI.

SSI is a poverty program for disabled people who don't have a work history. This might apply to someone who has been a homemaker, or someone who developed FM or CFS at age 18 before they joined the workforce. You are only eligible for SSI if you have less than $2,000 dollars in assets. Usually when you apply for Social Security, you may also apply for SSI if you don't have significant resources.

If you are on state public assistance or welfare and you are disabled, your welfare worker will encourage you to apply for SSI. This allows the state to shift the cost of supporting you to the federal government. Many state welfare programs require that applicants pay back the money they got from welfare when they are awarded SSI.

If you apply for SSI or SSDI and you are denied benefits, I recommend that you get an attorney. Federal law governs the attorney-client relationship in these cases. The client only pays the attorney fees if they win and does not have to pay the attorney upfront. The fee is statutorily determined; it is 25 percent of the back award, with a maximum fee of $5,300. So if your back award is $10,000, then you pay the attorney $2,500. If your back award is $100,000, you only pay the attorney $5,300. The reason for the cap is because these cases go on so long; it doesn't necessarily mean more work for the attorney, it just means more waiting time.

Recipients of social security benefits are usually reviewed every three years. In my experience, for cases with chronic problems like FM or CFS, people are rarely cut off from benefits. The kind of cases in which people are taken off social security are usually those in which a person is injured and then recovers.

If you are disabled, it is extremely important that you apply for disability benefits instead of just simply waiting for retirement. By obtaining disability benefits, you may increase the amount of your later retirement benefit.

You should apply for disability benefits as soon as you are unable to work. There is no reason to wait. If you are denied benefits, the most important thing to remember is to appeal and not to give up. Most people who do not give up are successful when they appeal.

APPLYING FOR SOCIAL SECURITY

There are several stages to a Social Security case:

✤ The initial application: Most people are denied benefits at this stage. It usually takes 3–6 months to get a decision. If you are denied benefits, you should appeal within 60 days.

✤ Request for reconsideration: Most people are denied benefits at this stage. It usually takes 3–6 months to get a decision. If you are denied benefits, you should appeal within 60 days.

✤ Request for a hearing: It currently takes 18 months to 2 years to get a hearing. Statistically, you have a good chance of success at the hearing stage.

✤ Further appeals: Further appeals are available, including a lawsuit in federal court.

You can re-apply as many times as you want. However, it is much more effective to appeal the denial of benefits than to re-apply.

1. Appeal: Don't give up
2. Be honest: Don't lie about anything and don't minimize or exaggerate
3. Be complete: Tell the Social Security Administration about all medical and mental-health providers you have seen, and include names, phone numbers, and addresses
4. Get treatment: Follow treatment recommendations
5. Stay sober: Don't abuse alcohol or drugs
6. Be sure to document all problems: For example, mental-health issues, learning disabilities, and/or a history of trauma
7. Act soon: Don't wait—the process takes a long time
8. Meet the deadlines: Usually 60 days is allowed in which to appeal or you will have to start the process all over again
9. Get a lawyer: Don't wait; statistics show you have a better chance of winning with a lawyer
10. Get a good doctor: Sometimes people are denied benefits when they are treated exclusively by a naturopathic doctor. Unfortunately, the Social Security Administration gives much more weight to a medical doctor. It is also helpful that you be seen by a doctor who listens to you and understands FM and CFS.

If you follow through with the appeals process, you have a good chance of being awarded benefits. In Washington State (which is a fairly typical example) about 40 percent of people are granted benefits at the initial application stage. At the request for reconsideration stage, only 15 percent of people are granted benefits. However, at the hearing stage, about 60 percent of applicants are awarded benefits. What this means is that if you appeal and do not give up, statistically, there is a good chance that you will be awarded benefits. ❖ ❖ ❖

❖ A Patient's Story: Mary Beth M.

Mary Beth M. is 60, and she worked in the corporate world for many years. She struggled to maintain her fast-paced career while living with CFS and has struggled equally with the benefits process. Mary Beth is now a playwright, working on a children's play, *Three Bugs and a Slug.* She lives in Houston.

In 2000, I began feeling extremely tired and went to my doctor. I had always been a high achiever—I worked full time and went to college or did volunteer work in the evenings and on weekends. I also began studying acting and writing in my spare time. My doctor did a series of blood tests and diagnosed me with a low thyroid condition (hypothyroidism). He started me on thyroid medications. He also diagnosed me with Epstein-Barr virus (EBV). I had had mono in 1968, but at that time, the doctors didn't know it was caused by EBV. He told me to rest as much as possible. So I cut back on acting, writing, and my social life.

A few months later when I was driving home from work one night, a lady ran a red light and totaled my car. My head hurt like the dickens but I wasn't badly injured—just a slight concussion and soft tissue injury. I went through physical therapy and figured I'd slowly improve. Unfortunately, I did not. The fatigue got worse, and I had insomnia more often—as well as memory loss, loss of concentration, and frequent urination. I thought the concussion might have caused some of the symptoms. After more tests, my doctor diagnosed me with CFS and sent me to a specialist here in Houston. She did tests for lupus and Lyme disease, as well as others, but they came back negative. She told me to rest even more—16 hours a day—which is hard to do when you're working.

So I changed my life. I cut out almost all social engagements, began lying down during my lunch hour, and went to bed when I got home from work. I didn't tell many people what I had. I'm single and needed my job,

and I didn't think it would look good in this competitive world to appear "sick." My friends kept telling me they missed seeing me, but I told them I was too exhausted to visit. We talked on the phone instead.

My fatigue began getting even worse. In June 2003 I developed shortness of breath. I went to the ER one day when I was at work. They did tests on my heart, told me it was anxiety, and sent me home. I continued to work for a few months until the breathing problems became so bad I had to use oxygen. I went on medical leave for two months and then went back to work, this time with oxygen. My breathing problems continued to worsen, even with the oxygen, and soon I needed to lie down 20 hours a day.

So I went on medical leave again and applied for short-term disability. The insurance rep didn't believe I was really sick. He called my doctor and told her nurse that I "didn't sound sick on the phone." But with more medical backup, they finally approved my disability benefits. The policy was a small one so my family helped out as well. I also applied for food stamps but I felt like a worm. I'd been working for 40 years. I never thought in my wildest dreams I'd ever be on welfare.

After my short-term disability was used up, I applied for long-term and Social Security disability. Both were denied. While I was gathering medical information for my appeals, I got a letter from my employer. They were laying me off! I couldn't believe it. I was too sick to work but supposedly too healthy for disability. I was terrified. I didn't know what I was going to do.

So I hired an attorney. He sent me for a comprehensive physical and functional capacity test, as well as a neuropsychological test. Armed with these two recommendations for total disability, we won the appeal. I know I never would have won without him. My attorney is now appealing my long-term disability denial, as well as back payments of Social Security disability.

There's other good news as well. My doctor changed one of my medications and my breathing problems improved. They're not entirely gone, but they are somewhat better. On the bad side, this illness has cost me $40,000 in lost wages and medical bills. It also cost me my job. At times I feel so frightened and discouraged it's hard to get out of bed. I worry about my increasing debt. I worry about using up my 401(k) in the next few years. I worry about getting worse. I'm seeing a psychologist but I only talk about my health and financial problems. I know I shouldn't let it, but sometimes my illness defines me, and sometimes I lose hope.

But I'm on the upswing again. Now that I'm getting around better, I've made a new plan. I've begun reading everything I can get my hands on about FM and CFS. I joined a local support group and the national CFIDS organization. I got a massage. I re-committed myself to three light stretching/exercise sessions a week. I started buying organic food, even though it's more expensive. I added magnesium to my daily calcium and multivitamin pills. I watched *My Big Fat Greek Wedding* three times, laughing at the same sight gags every time. And I began meditating. I'm fighting back, and it feels good. ❖❖❖

❖ Protecting Your Legal Rights

BY MORRIS H. ROSENBERG

Morris H. Rosenberg has practiced law in Seattle since 1975. He is a graduate of the University of Virginia School of Law. Morris has been special district counsel for the Washington State Bar Association since 1984. In that capacity, he investigates and makes recommendations regarding complaints of misconduct against attorneys. Morris limits his practice to the representation of injured people, employment discrimination, and family law cases.

I have noticed some trends that might explain why it is so difficult for an injured person to receive a fair resolution of claims when FM or CFS are involved. Insurance companies are for-profit organizations. They take in premium dollars, and their goal is to pay out the smallest awards they can, in order to maximize their profits.

In the cases I handle, which are mostly motor vehicle accidents, the individual often has a history of some medical problems prior to the accident. They may have been treated for nondescript symptoms or depression, and they may have seen a number of doctors. These situations are frequently exploited by insurance companies. They do all they can to make juries believe that the medical difficulties predated the accident.

In contrast, I have had several cases in which a person had a very clean medical history prior to the motor vehicle accident or the trauma that initially triggered FM symptoms. These cases tend to go better for the injured person. When the onset of symptoms can be more clearly traced to a physical trauma, the injured party will generally receive a higher settlement or award.

The situation I often see is one in which a person is injured in a low-impact auto accident and presents with modest soft-tissue damage and whiplash. Over the next four or five months, instead of improving, the injured

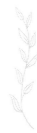

243

person becomes worse. Often they get frustrated with the lack of progress, so they look for another doctor or different kind of care. Then the client has established a history of going to several doctors, not because they're looking for one to help them pull off a scam, but because they're simply not getting any better. Insurance companies will say that person is just trying to work the system and make it look like they've needed a lot of care to get better. They'll say the person is running up big medical bills in an effort to convince a jury or an insurance company that they are in a great deal of pain as a result of the auto accident.

It is important to remember not to tell anyone at the accident site that you are not injured. It is very common for people who are legitimately injured not to feel the effects of the injuries until hours, days, or even months later. Telling a police officer or someone else at the scene that you are not injured can come back to haunt you. We have all had situations in which we have had a strenuous athletic workout and did not feel sore or achy until the next day. This can easily be the situation in an automobile accident, in which there may be injuries to muscles, tendons, and ligaments not visible to the naked eye. If there is any chance that you may be injured, have yourself checked out by a qualified physician at the first opportunity.

If you are injured in a car accident, I urge you to talk to an attorney who is experienced in personal injury law. Almost all lawyers who practice in this arena will meet initially with potential clients, at no charge, to discuss their legal rights. Most are also candid enough to tell you whether it makes sense to hire an attorney. Regrettably, insurance companies will use every means they can to limit their liability. Insurers are adept at finding an "expert" who can be paid to say anything in support of the insurance company. Be wary of insurance representatives who advise you not to seek an attorney or who try to talk you into signing their medical records release forms. This is in their best interest, not yours.

One of my favorite clients in thirty years of practice was a bright, loving, and friendly lady who had a number of serious problems unrelated to FM, some of which predated her accident. However, her ability to be self-supporting was much more seriously impacted by FM than any of these other conditions. The stress of a jury trial would certainly have done nothing good for her and likely would have aggravated her symptoms significantly. The insurance company's attorney treated her with dignity and respect and I believe she saw that. (That did not mean he would not have done his job if the case went to trial, nor did it mean that he would try to talk the insurance company into offering a large settlement.) The case was ultimately settled

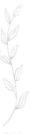

prior to trial in a way that was reasonable in terms of the risk of trial versus the benefit of resolving the claim. However, it was certainly not a fair amount of money for what she had lost and would lose in the future.

My sense is that there is now less disbelief and more willingness on the part of the insurance industry to accept the diagnosis of FM or CFS. However, that does not translate to better results for patients. There has been a continuing trend of jury awards decreasing, particularly in cases in which the physical trauma was not huge. That downward trend also holds true for claims that involve "soft tissue only," which FM is viewed as being, and jurors are quite suspicious of injuries that are not clearly visible to them as they sit in the jury box or that don't show up on imaging. I believe that suspicion is fostered by the large public relations efforts of insurance companies to convince the public that Americans are litigation crazy and hoping for a runaway jury to award them a large windfall. While in fact the data does not support that view, it has been preached so loudly, for so long, that many jurors bring with them a bias against persons who make these kinds of claims. While very few cases go all the way to a jury trial, the cases that do set the marketplace—the precedent—for settlement values. Thus, in general, the value of claims has been on a slow downward slide in many states. The best proof that there are not many runaway juries is that insurance companies, virtually without exception, demand a jury if there is a trial.

It is most critical to give plenty of detail to medical providers about the level of functioning and symptoms, if any, that predate the accident versus the specifics of the pain symptoms and their effects on the activities of daily living and functioning after the accident. The more this can be documented by noninterested persons—for example, health-care providers, co-workers, and friends, rather than out of the mouth of the injured person—the more credible it will be. It is also very important to follow any medical advice given. For example, if an FM patient is told to do an exercise routine, it must be done religiously! Equally important is to find medical providers who are knowledgeable and attuned to FM and CFS. Getting good care and improving as much as possible is always more important than trying to "build the claim."

My sense, anecdotally, is that FM and CFS are now more accepted diagnoses in the medical community. I think that even the doctors working in conjunction with insurance companies will more often agree with the FM and/or CFS diagnosis than they have in the past. Currently, the fight seems to be over the causation of the FM or CFS rather than the diagnosis itself.

❖ ❖ ❖

245

HOW TO OBTAIN A DISABLED PARKING PERMIT

People with invisible illnesses qualify for disabled parking permits, just like people with more obvious disabilities. If you have been diagnosed with FM or CFS, you may be eligible for a disabled person's parking permit. The permit entitles you to park in identified parking spots and to park free at parking meters. Permits are issued for both temporary and long-term disabilities, and it is simple to apply. Your doctor may have a form on hand; if not, forms are available from your local Department of Motor Vehicles. (To save you a trip, you may be able to download the form from your local department's website). The form will require your doctor's signature.

❖ A Patient's Story: Hilary B.

> Hilary B. is 36 years old. Following an accident in her early twenties, she made the difficult decision to give up her ambitious career path and put her health first. Surviving on welfare, social security, and visits to food banks, Hilary continued to hold her head high. She is now a highly successful real estate agent and an associate broker, ranking in the top 15 percent internationally. Hilary lives in Bothell, Washington, with her husband and two young children.

I was a passenger in a three-car collision in December 1993 in New York. We were rear-ended, and I knew immediately that I was injured: My neck and my right arm hurt from bracing against the crash. The police wrote on the accident report that I was injured. We went to the hospital immediately; they diagnosed whiplash, neck sprain, and muscle strain.

I thought I would just go to the chiropractor for a while and eventually recover. I had been seeing a chiropractor prior to the accident due to another car accident several years earlier. I had some minor back problems from that and from being a dancer at an early age. I went through two medical exams (at the request of the insurance company) and passed them both, but the doctors felt I still needed medical treatment. The insurance company paid all of my medical bills related to the car accident. Unfortunately, I was slowly getting worse.

At the time of the accident, I had been actively looking for work and thinking about getting a master's degree. I decided to move to Seattle to continue my job search there. When I finally found a job, I just couldn't do the work. I suddenly became very tired, irritable, and forgetful, and I was constantly in pain. I wasn't sure what was happening to me. I didn't correlate any of my symptoms to any one condition. I thought my pain was due solely to the car accident and that the fatigue was from working long hours in a stressful job. I attributed the forgetfulness to being preoccupied. My sleeping patterns changed; it didn't matter how long I had slept the night before, I always felt tired.

At this point, I still didn't realize that something was seriously wrong with me. I hired an attorney in Seattle to handle my case in New York. The attorney encouraged me to go to an injury rehabilitation doctor he knew. I started seeing him in November 1994. I visited his clinic three or four times a week for massage, biofeedback, TENS therapy, and weight lifting. Whenever I picked up so much as a three-pound weight, I experienced a lot of pain. In fact, I couldn't exercise without having pain. The doctor would say to me, "No pain, no gain." He said, "When you are done here, you will be completely recovered." He never listened to my complaints. Three months later, I was worse off than when I started. I was probably in treatment ten hours a week. The cost all ended up on lien, because my insurance company didn't recognize the fact that FM was related to the car accident. They cut off my benefits.

When I was first diagnosed, I had a major decision to make: Do I quit work, go on welfare, and file for Social Security disability, or do I continue working and suffering, and end up hospitalized? My choice was bittersweet. I chose to stop working because my health meant more to me than anything. If you don't have your health, you have nothing. I thought, "I'm young, I was diagnosed right before my twenty-fifth birthday, and I will get better and get right back to work." I am a very ambitious and motivated person, so I told myself, "I can get past this." Little did I know what kind of journey I was about to go through.

I soon became frightened and full of humility. I couldn't believe this was happening to me. No one in my family has ever been on welfare. My family couldn't help me financially. My parents are divorced and my father didn't help me at all. I was living on $339 a month and $120 in food stamps. At the time, I was living with my boyfriend; he moved with me to Seattle, and although he was working to help supplement the bills, it was really frightening. I had to use my credit card to pay for emergency bills. I would go to food banks when the food stamps ran out. I felt like I was going farther into the ground. I was ill, poor, and unable to work. I had more stress during those months than at any other time in my life. I learned so much about survival in a manner that I never thought I would experience. People treated me differently because I was on welfare. It was awful.

People don't understand what it means to have a chronic illness. They see what you are on the outside, but not inside. Society shuns people with disabilities. I had a hard time getting an apartment because landlords did not like it that the government was paying for it. People looked down upon me because I did not work, and I was ill. I remember my mother's friend asking my mom why I couldn't get a part-time job. For one, I could not get out of bed. It was a very painful time in my life.

The first portion of my settlement came in March 1996. We had mediation against the insurance company of the driver in the second car. And then the rest was settled in October 1996. I feel very fortunate that I got some type of compensation. It certainly made things a little easier. I have paid more than fifty thousand dollars out of pocket for medical bills. The settlement money was put into a special needs irrevocable trust, and my mother is the trustee. It allowed me to stay on state and federal "needy" programs without penalty. The trust can only pay for things that are not paid for by any other means. The trust cannot provide me with personal income. An attorney set this up for me.

I now live a richer life because I cannot afford to sweat the small stuff—I do not have the energy to do everything. I have been a real estate agent since 1998. I got married in 1999, had my first child in 2002, and my second in 2005. I have achieved the ability to have a career I love, a marriage, a family, to give back to society, and to be an active participant in the world.

FM is not a major part of my life anymore. I embrace what it has taught me. It gave me the opportunity to have a healthier sense of self. I have a choice about how I want to live my life. I choose to live abundantly! ❖❖❖

❖ ❖ ❖

As we become more knowledgeable in how to live well with our illnesses, our thoughts turn to the future, and we wonder if there will eventually be effective treatments, perhaps even cures, for FM and CFS. Great strides are being made in that direction. Our next chapter will provide you with an overview of what's going on with FM and CFS research in the United States and around the world.

Chapter 16

The Future of FM and CFS

Each patient carries his own doctor inside him.

— Albert Schweitzer

THE FUTURE OF FM and CFS is changing every day. In this chapter we talk to Drs. Carol Landis and Dennis Turk of the University of Washington. They share their ideas, predictions, and hopes for discovering the cause of these illnesses, treating, and one day curing them. At the end of the chapter, Rich Carson and Dennis Schoen of ProHealth bring us up-to-date on the newest treatments and research.

❖ Sleep Dysfunction and FM

BY CAROL A. LANDIS, PH.D.

Dr. Landis is director of the biobehavioral laboratories in the Center for Women's Health and Gender Research at the University of Washington. Her research focuses on sleep and the health consequences of sleep loss.

Waking up and feeling unrefreshed is a complaint that has long been described as part of the symptomatology of FM. But we don't understand very clearly what is disordered about FM patients' sleep. Some women with FM may have a particular sleep disorder, such as sleep-disordered breathing

249

or sleep apnea. In these cases, treating the sleep apnea can certainly help reduce daytime sleepiness and fatigue. There is also some evidence that the standard treatment for mild sleep disordered breathing reduces pain in women with FM.

Several years ago, we did a study that explored sleep and nighttime hormones in women and how they may impact FM. In our study we carefully screened our control subjects (those without symptoms) to make sure that they were good sleepers. We compared them to women with FM who were recruited from the outpatient department of a large medical center. Both the FM patients and control group of women kept a month-long journal of daily symptoms. We did that because we were interested in tracking how the symptoms fluctuate overtime rather than relying on memory. We also had all subjects record the time they went to bed, the time they got up, how many hours they slept, how well they slept, how stressful their day was, and the types of medications they took. To participate in the study, all of the women with FM had to stop taking analgesics, antidepressants, and sedatives. Getting patients to give up these medications was very difficult. But the only way we can really understand what's happening during sleep is if subjects don't take medications that alter their nighttime sleep patterns, and which probably alter their nighttime hormone patterns as well. All the subjects in the study were also screened for sleep disorders such as sleep disordered breathing and restless legs syndrome.

FM AND HORMONES

Two hormones—growth hormone and prolactin—are secreted in larger amounts during sleep than during the daytime. It has long been known that when you stay up all night and are sleep deprived, the amounts of growth hormone and prolactin in your body go down. In contrast, cortisol is a hormone that is mainly secreted during morning hours and reaches its lowest concentration in the body during the late evening hours and the first few hours of sleep. We found that the women with FM had lower nighttime plasma levels both of growth hormone and prolactin but they had no difference in the amount of cortisol compared to age-matched women without FM. The women with FM also took slightly longer to fall asleep, had lower sleep efficiencies (time asleep/time in bed), and reported poorer sleep quality compared to the control women.

Other investigators have reported reduced amounts of growth hormone, but to our knowledge there have been no other reports of altered levels of nighttime prolactin or cortisol in FM.

❖ Growth hormone and prolactin are considered important growth factors that support anabolism (tissue synthesis) and rebuilding.

❖ Cortisol has many functions and one of them is involved in catabolism (the breakdown of tissues to release energy).

❖ Growth hormone in the brain has been linked to improved cognitive functioning.

❖ Excessive cortisol has been linked with impaired memory.

It is possible that a shift in the balance of the nighttime levels of anabolic versus catabolic hormones might be related to FM symptoms, and we are currently exploring this possibility. Additional research is necessary in order to test this idea further. At this point I don't think we understand enough about the relationship between sleep quality and nighttime hormone levels to predict which therapies would work best.

FM AND IMMUNITY

Pain has been associated with reduced immune function, and prolactin has been linked to increased immune function. So in our study, we also measured how well a certain type of immune cell, the natural killer cell, was capable of inactivating, or "killing," other target cells. This test involves mixing immune cells taken from a blood sample with a standard amount of test or target cells in a test tube. When the immune (natural killer cells) inactivate the target cells, a substance is released that can be measured. The amount of substance released is related to the number of cells that were inactivated. We found that women with FM had slightly more immune cells but a similar level of immune cell function compared to the control women. Thus, although the women with FM had pain and lower levels of prolactin, they did not show evidence of impaired immune function measured by the natural killer cell assay.

FM AND BRAIN WAVE PATTERNS

Much has been written about a particular brain wave pattern of disturbed sleep physiology called "alpha-delta," or "alpha-NREM sleep anomaly." This pattern is considered evidence of "waking" during sleep and it has been linked to increased pain in the morning compared to the previous evening. In our study we did not find that women with FM reported more pain on awakening compared to the previous evening. So we were interested in seeing if this "alpha-delta" pattern was present in the women with FM and absent in our good sleeper control group of women with no sleep

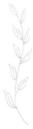

251

problems. However, after completing a visual inspection of their brain waves and using a method to actually quantify the number of "alpha" waves compared to the number of "delta" waves, we found that very few women in our study had any evidence of this alpha-delta pattern.

We decided to see if there was some other abnormality in sleep brain wave patterns of the women with FM. We found that women with FM had fewer "sleep spindles" and reduced spindle activity. Sleep spindles are an important feature of brain wave sleep patterns that are thought to help initiate sleep and to maintain it by keeping environmental noise or other sensations from being perceived during sleep. More importantly, we found that reduced sleep spindles were related to pain. Thus, we think that there is some alteration in the basic mechanisms that are involved with the initiation and maintenance of sleep that is abnormal in FM. Clearly, more research is necessary in order to verify this finding.

Many of the women with FM screened for our study simply refused to stop taking their sleeping pills because they said that if they did not obtain adequate sleep they would not be able to function the next day. Other investigators have shown that pain is increased following a night of poor sleep in patients with FM. Some sleeping pills are known to increase sleep spindles and this may be one mechanism by which these medications help to improve symptoms in FM. ❖❖❖

❖ New Developments in FM Diagnosis

BY DENNIS C. TURK, PH.D.

Dr. Turk is the John and Emma Bonica Professor of Anesthesiology and Pain Research at the University of Washington. He is also director of the university's Fibromyalgia Research Center. He is an adjunct professor of psychiatry at the University of Pittsburgh in Pennsylvania.

Fibromyalgia is a broad term that, in my opinion, probably describes people with different physical and psychological characteristics and symptoms. If we want to understand FM and provide better treatment, we really need to classify subgroups of individuals within this particular diagnosis.

When we look into the literature on treatment options for FM, the confusion we see over and over again is that some treatments seem to be beneficial to some patients, but not to others. Very likely, when we give the same treatment to all individuals, we are providing appropriate treatment for only a small subset of patients. When you try to replicate these findings, what originally looked like promising results don't appear to recur, because we haven't yet identified these subsets of patients. I use the analogy of advising a patient to take multivitamins when they only have a vitamin B deficiency. You would be better off prescribing only vitamin B to that individual rather than giving them a whole range of multivitamins and hoping they are going to get the vitamin B they need.

To truly treat a chronic pain state like FM, we need to consider several areas of assessment.

- ❖ The biomedical or medical domain includes factors associated with physiology, anatomy, and biochemistry.

- ❖ The second domain is psychosocial; that is, how does the presence of these symptoms impact people's lives?

- ❖ The third domain is behavioral, which is how people respond to the presence of this set of symptoms [their coping style].

To date, the research I have been involved with tries to identify subgroups of patients based on how they are coping and adapting to the presence of their symptoms. This taps into the second and third domains, the psychosocial and behavioral aspects. This in no way suggests that I believe psychological factors cause the symptoms of FM, but rather it suggests that when individuals have lived with these symptoms for long periods of time, they develop different responses to their problems.

To treat people appropriately, we must pay attention not only to physical signs, but also psychosocial and behavioral signs. In future research, we hope to subdivide patients based on the physical causal factors that may contribute to their symptoms.

I am optimistic that we will ultimately also have what I call "dual diagnosis." We will then have a medical diagnosis that includes psychosocial factors: the way pain affects people's lives, how they adjust to this, and how it affects their behavior.

We are currently conducting long-term studies demonstrating that there are at least three different subgroups of FM patient coping styles. Patient responses are based on psychosocial and behavioral factors and how individuals adapt to their situation and their set of symptoms. The three subgroups we identified were based on a statistical analysis of patients' responses to a questionnaire. We asked questions about the impact of pain on their lives, how they respond to it, how much control they feel they have over their lives, and how great an impact their illness has had on their actual activities.

These three subgroups consist of the following:

1. The first subgroup we refer to as "dysfunctional." These individuals have high levels of pain and emotional distress. They feel they have little control over their lives and tend to be inactive.

2. The second group we refer to as "interpersonally distressed." These individuals also have high levels of pain and have somewhat higher levels of emotional distress than other patients. What is unique about them is their perception of how their significant others or people in their environment respond to them. Despite the fact that they have pain symptoms like those of the dysfunctional group, they feel they get very little support from the significant people in their lives and many negative responses.

3. The third group we call "adaptive copers." These people, despite the symptoms of FM, appear to be functioning and coping relatively well. Their lives are as impacted as those of other patients, but they tend to remain active.

We hope to be able to identify which patients with what characteristics are most likely to benefit from particular types of interventions. We anticipate that we will then be able to start matching patients with particular characteristics, both physical and psychological, to specific treatments.

The preliminary analyses have demonstrated that, overall, the general rehabilitation treatment has resulted in highly significant improvements in reduction of pain, emotional distress, and functional disability. The treatment protocol consists of informing the patient about FM, aerobic exercises, the use of relaxation techniques and other coping skills, and peer support. Most gratifying was that the results were maintained at six months following treatment termination.

Over time, we will be able to develop better interventions that will be more closely matched to the patient's individual characteristics. The hope is that eventually we will be able to assess groups of FM patients and give each of them a dual diagnosis, which will be a combination of a biomedical diagnosis and a psychosocial behavioral diagnosis.

We received a new grant from the National Institutes of Health in 2005, extending our previous research. The grant has also enabled us to evaluate treatment matched to patients based on their avoidance of physical activities in an effort to prevent exacerbation of pain, fatigue, and exhaustion. We are enthusiastic about the project as it builds on previous re-

search focusing on individual variation and the matching of treatment to characteristics of people who have FM. ❖❖❖

❖ New Directions in FM and CFS Treatment and Research

BY RICH CARSON AND DENNIS SCHOEN
COMPILED BY LEE ANN STIFF, EDITOR, PROHEALTH

Rich Carson was diagnosed with CFS in his early twenties and went on to form ProHealth, Inc., a major vitamin and supplement retailer and resource for patients with FM and CFS. ProHealth provides two websites, immune support.com and fibromyalgiasupport.com, and the newsletter, *Health-watch.* The company has grown to become the largest retailer of specialty FM- and CFS-focused products in the United States, including dietary supplements, the *Cuddle Ewe* line of wool batting bed accessories, and other health products. Dennis Schoen is the CEO of ProHealth. Carson and Schoen raise money for research, and their company has funded FM and CFS studies and provided community support.

NEW MEDICATIONS

Good progress is being made in finding a variety of treatments that work for fibromyalgia-related issues and symptoms. Among the newest promising pharmaceutical drugs for FM pain are Ultracet, Lyrica (Pregabalin), Cymbalta (Duloxetine), and Reboxetine (Edronax, Vestra). For those who prefer over-the-counter products, a new topical pain reliever endorsed by the National Fibromyalgia Association is 024 Fibromyalgia, which showed great results for stopping FM pain in a double-blind, placebo-controlled study with 153 patients. Recently, Neuragen PN, a topical oil, received FDA approval for easing painful conditions including FM, post-shingles pain, and chronic nerve pain.

CURRENT RESEARCH

In terms of new research directions, The Fibromyalgia Treatment Center has underwritten two studies for FM. Both are designed to look at the genetics of the disease. The first study is currently underway at the City of Hope Research Center in Duarte, California. One hundred patients ("probands") and their parents are providing blood samples for a DNA analysis. Researchers are looking at a family of genes associated with prolonged inflammatory conditions.

255

The study will focus on the following:

* White blood cells (neutrophils and monocytes) are being examined for their immune response to inflammatory stimuli.

* Another part of this study involves the analysis of DNA and mRNA for autoinflammatory genes and genetic variations or errors (polymorphisms).

    Gene sequences from the parents will establish the inheritance pattern. If the results show that there is a genetic association, it may be possible to screen people for the risk of FM or to develop a valid blood test for fibromyalgia.

* Colchicine, a medication used for gout attacks, is one of the most effective drugs in treating genetically established autoimmune diseases and will be tested on the white cells in this study.

* Guaifenesin will also be tested in a similar manner.

* Finally, the effect of sex hormones on the inflammatory response will be tested.

This three-year study intends to look at as many genes as funding will allow [ProHealth is one of the supporters of this research].

A second study is in preparation (as of September 2005) at Harbor UCLA to create a protocol that would include DNA analyses, but this time using biopsies obtained from the center of fibromyalgic lesions in the brain. The lead researcher of this study suggests that by analyzing biopsies for affected tissue, and from adjacent normal tissue, he can identify the genes that have been activated and are causing the problem. Microarray technology will be used that allows surveillance of thousands of genes to determine when they are genetically expressed (i.e., they are "turned on," or expressed).

This is the same technique that is frequently used to look at diseases that are thought to be caused by the interaction of defective proteins. Because of the number of symptoms and the great variations in fibromyalgic patients, most researchers now believe that fibromyalgia is not caused just by a single defective gene.

Hopefully, these new directions in treatment and research will contribute significantly to improved quality of life for FM and CFS patients—including better, more targeted treatments and greater respect for patients and the validity of their experience—as we move further down the long road to a cure for these devastating illnesses. ❖ ❖ ❖

❖ ❖ ❖

ProHealth has made it easier than ever to read about the latest research, medicine, and supplements in a new bi-weekly online newsletter. Just sign up by going to wellness@prohealth.com, and the newsletter will show up each week in your e-mail. One week you will be sent the CFSNewsletter @ProHealth.com, and the next week the FM edition will arrive from FM Newsletter@ProHealth.com. Signing up couldn't be easier.

Widen your search for CFS information by using the Google.com search engine. Type in "CFS" and you'll find today's top stories from around the world in "News Results for Chronic Fatigue Syndrome."

It is reassuring to know that the world of FM and CFS research is so dynamic. Gradually, scientific research is lifting the veil of mystery that has shrouded these two illnesses for so long. The rapidly growing body of research suggests that objective tests and, hopefully, cures may be on the horizon. But for now, we must find ways to live rewarding and healthy lives with our illnesses. In our final chapter, we let our respondents have the last word, as we share with you their wonderful tips, comments, and insights into life with FM and CFS.

Chapter 17

Tips from People with FM/CFS

Take incredibly decent and loving care of yourself. Get past your grief and move on with your life. You have to create a new "normal" for yourself, as opposed to trying to get the old you back. You have to find your way back to life in the world instead of getting stuck in life in your illness.

— Diane Kerner, CFS and FM patient

W HEN WE ASKED Christine R. about her "romantic partner" she said, "What romantic partner? :o) Actually, now that I'm feeling better, I am starting to look around more. I may be 55, but I'm not dead yet, and I look better than I have in years." Good for you, Christine!

We could all use a positive attitude like Christine's. In this chapter, we share with you the helpful, practical, inspiring, and sometimes laugh-out-loud-funny tips and observations from the many patients who contacted us. Perhaps the humorous ones can help with your laughter therapy.

Sit down, grab a cup of coffee (or something less stimulating if you've read our nutrition chapter), and think of the ways you have modified your daily life in order to live more easily with your illness. You'll probably have quite a long list—some ideas you've had yourself, strategies that just seem to work, some that friends and physicians have recommended, and some you may have read about in a book or online.

Just consider the many ways you cope with brain fog; for example, Post-it notes on the front door and bathroom mirror, lists everywhere about everything, and reminders such as "two cats are out, two are in" (if you're lucky enough to have four cats, that is). Remember, pre-FM or -CFS, when a list was just a grocery list and not a life list? Then there is the problem of remembering what the post-it notes mean. Always write down the name of who called and not just the number. Our respondents had plenty of tips just like these to share.

❖ Preventing Pain

"Make sure you have a clear path through your home. Move aside anything that might be an obstacle for you to trip over. If you have stairs, make sure they are well lit and you have a sturdy guardrail. There is nothing like taking a tumble down the stairs to aggravate your FM. Also wrap faux lambs wool around the arms of your chair so your elbows don't hit the wood."   — Betty M., Lapwai, Idaho

"If you have trouble balancing in the bathroom and feel slippery floors may be a hazard, consider having grab bars and handrails installed. A medical appliance store can provide you with information on installing and positioning them. Some insurance companies cover this type of equipment. A shower/tub seat is also something to consider. A bath mat should be essential for everyone regardless of whether or not they have a chronic illness!"
                              — Linda J., Phoenix, Arizona

"Your body can perceive cold as pain so make sure you wear adequate clothing for cold weather. Don't forget the hat; you lose up to 70 percent of body heat through your head."
                              — Mari S., Seattle, Washington

"Use an egg timer to keep track of how much time is passing while working on a project. This is very helpful if the project requires prolonged sitting or standing. If the task is enjoyable, it's easy to lose track of time and end up with muscle spasms in your neck or back."
                              — Lois G., Stoughton, Wisconsin

❖ Coping with Pain

"If I'm in pain, I try a nice hot bath or I get into my hot tub. I purchased a hot tub last year, after I found that the only time I was not in pain was when I was in the water. The water therapy helps my sleep, stress, and pain. I'm very fortunate to have the hot tub and manage to find time at least three times a week to use it, either at night before bed or sometimes during the afternoon on a weekend."

— Susan G., Westfield, Massachusetts

"Don't isolate yourself. Save your energy for that evening with the grandkids or go sit in the mall for a half hour, take a book to the local coffee shop, sit in the front yard, just don't let your pain keep you inside four walls all the time."

— Brenda S., Champaign, Illinois

"I think it's important to be involved in an art form, something you feel passionate about that elevates the mind, that puts you on a different plane where pain isn't such a distraction. We all need beauty in our lives, especially when we live with constant pain. I don't notice my pain as much when I dance because dancing makes me happy. Of course, there are other art forms such as painting or enjoying the paintings of others, theatre, or music. The idea is to get involved with an art that is interesting enough to distract you from your pain and give you pleasure."

— Linda M., Seattle, Washington

"I have come to realize that I will be in physical pain no matter where my body is and no matter what I do, so I actively choose to show up for my own life! This realization caused a radical paradigm shift in my being, and although I still have moderate to severe chronic pain, the pain itself moved into the background and my life itself became the central focus."

— Ellen J., Seattle, Washington

❖ Getting the Rest You Need

"Since I live alone, I have made my home a haven for myself. No one gets to disrupt my routine or my 'me time' when I am not feeling good."

— Kim A., Las Vegas, Nevada

"I go to bed at pretty much the same time every day, weekday or weekend. An adequate amount of sleep is a primary concern for me. I have learned to pace myself better. I used to just keep pushing until I was so exhausted I would drop. I no longer do that."
— Christine R., Sault Ste. Marie, Michigan

"I try to plan my FM 'down time' into my schedule each day so it *will* be included!"
— Linda M.

❖ Your Energy Bank

"When I find I've overbooked, I have to back off the scheduling and take some downtime. Deadlines are stressors, so I keep them to a minimum. I try to keep my time frames very flexible. Too many 'Have To Dos' overwhelm me and incapacitate me. I even break easy tasks into small steps and focus on doing just one step, then another, and I may distribute those small steps over more than one day."
— Sally L., Euless, Texas

"I approach tasks a step at a time. I set a goal and then take baby steps—or larger steps if I can—but I try not to pressure myself with deadlines."
— Katrina B., Happy Jack, Arizona

"Be honest with yourself and others about what your strengths and limits are. Remember that you are the only one who really knows how you feel, and that you are the only one who can take care of you. You may not be in control of your body, but you are still in control of your mind."
— Chandy W., Shelbyville, Tennessee

❖ Brain Fog

"I make lists to stay organized. I always try to get the hardest thing done first thing in the morning. I plan meals one week in advance so I don't have to think about them daily."
— Candace Y., Newport Beach, California

"Try writing down what has been going on the day before your flare-up or brain fog. Did you eat pizza or a big pretzel? Are you allergic

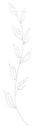

261

to wheat? Has a stressful event happened? With a journal, you may be able to cut down on brain fog if you can find the pattern."

— Mari S.

"Remember your appointments with Post-it notes on the front door. Write them down in your calendar, too. Keep a stack of Post-its everywhere (in the car, in the potting shed). They are invaluable for jotting down impromptu 'To Do' lists."

— Betty M.

"Sticky notes! Seriously, write it down; do not stress yourself by trying to remember."

— Chandy W.

"Use a PDA [personal digital assistant] to keep track of your daily activities. It's useful to remind you not just of appointments, but also chores and fun things you would like to do. For a less high-tech approach, a 3×5 card works great for a short list of your daily activities. Keep your appointments on your main calendar; then jot them down on the card before you go to bed. When you have a particularly busy day, a stack of 3×5 cards by your phone will be a handy way to remind yourself of what's happening."

— Mari S.

♣ Accentuate the Positive

"I love waking every day and looking at my garden and wondering what today will bring. I realize that I am better off than a lot of people. I appreciate everything I can do and see."

— Gaye B., Papakura, New Zealand

"Find humor in yourself. Be realistic but positive about yourself. Laughing is always easier than crying. Besides, no one ever got puffy eyes from laughing."

— Chandy W.

"I deal with my losses and limitations by identifying things I can do, through reading, writing, and communicating with friends."

— Katrina B.

"Life can still be exciting. I may not be able to accomplish all the goals I'd like, but I can accomplish some of them! The wise thing is to be realistic about what I *can* do."

— Linda M.

"Slowly, I've learned to praise myself for the one thing I accomplished that day, instead of berating myself and feeling guilty for the other half dozen I hadn't managed to do."

— Jill M., Burien, Washington.

"I am doing more traveling, and one of my big goals now is to take the master gardener course that is being offered in my community this fall. This is something I have wanted to do for many years. Now it seems possible. It didn't, just four short years ago. At that time, my goals were to stay employed and keep body and soul together."

— Christine R.

❖ Good Ideas

"I organized a number of lunchtime brown-bag presentations at my workplace by local alternative providers—a naturopath, an energy worker, and qigong teacher. This was a wonderful way to get the information I needed."

— Erin P., Seattle, Washington

"If I am able, I turn to my healthy escapes: I read, watch movies on television (the sicker I am, the simpler the plots must be), and try to accomplish small tasks from my endless 'To Do' list for a sense of accomplishment."

— Katrina B.

"Keep your home as tidy as possible. If you can clean up your dishes right after use, or wipe up the bathroom after your shower, it will cut down on bigger jobs later."

— Linda M.

"Find support outside your family and friends. Join a support group, form your own group, get online, start a book club—it doesn't have to be about FM and CFS. Just get involved on some level that forces you to reach out beyond your comfort zone."

— Chandy W.

"Salt baths are my favorite. These have really made a big difference for me, and while I have a basic understanding, I'm looking forward to learning more about how and why it works. I'm also looking forward to my next salt soak!"

— Erin P.

"Remove your clothes from the dryer immediately and hang them up. This will keep them fairly wrinkle-free and cut down on your ironing."   — Mari S.

❖ Journaling

"I use a symptom journal to help me see the progress that I am making on my treatment program."

— Robin N., Carver, Massachusetts

"When I'm having a real bad day, I look back at my journal and think, 'Okay, you've been here before.'"

— Joan H., Victoria, Canada

"Writing about your feelings can be very therapeutic. You don't have to write for publication, you don't have to be an experienced writer, and you don't have to show anyone what you write unless you want to. Try it sometime and see if it helps."   — Linda M.

"I use a 'gratitude journal'—at the end of each day I write five (or more) things I am thankful for that day. It helps shift my focus of attention from all the things to despair about to things I can be grateful for each day, however small they might be."   — Sally L.

❖ Advice for the Soul

"Don't try to be normal. Pace yourself.

"If the housework doesn't get done, so what?

"Get used to the simple things in life, like bird-watching in the garden, watching television, talking on the phone, or reading. If you can't do these things, then daydream. Above all, don't feel sorry for yourself too often; sometimes it can't be helped, but pick yourself up and get on with it. You've been dealt a lousy hand of cards and that's it.

"If you feel angry, be angry, but don't feel too sorry for yourself; that way lies depression."   — Janet L., Falkirk, Scotland

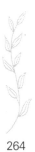

"Acceptance is the door to wider appreciation of what is going on for me. For example, when I wake up sore and have tender points, I

remind myself that there are other 53-year-old females that wake up (without FM), who are having a similar experience."

— Char M., Bellevue, Washington

"When the kids I work with have word-retrieval problems, it helps them not to feel so inadequate when I let them know I've got the same kind of thing happening to me."

— Deborah W. (special education teacher),
North Haverhill, New Hampshire

"Don't feel bad when folks don't understand. Mix with friends who accept you and your limitations. Love yourself as you are and accept yourself."

— Gaye B.

"I read a lot on my own and think of life as my university. I don't think of my life as over or that my future will look just like my present, but remain open to the potential of surprising and exciting possibilities showing up at any moment."

— Erin P.

"I'm finally resigned to the fact that I have to go where this illness is leading me, but I can still do some good and meaningful work."

— Sherril J., Sylvester, Georgia

"I treasure life now and don't want to waste one minute feeling sorry for myself. I missed out on way too much due to this illness and I refuse to let it steal one more second than I can manage."

— Gretchen P., Lexington, South Carolina

"I practice yoga and meditation. I also meditate while walking outdoors and communing with nature. So peaceful and awe-inspiring!"

— Mary R., Mount Forest, Ontario, Canada

"Most people seem to live by rote and do not bother to observe all the little details and joys around us every day. Because my pace has been slowed down to a crawl, everything I do is observable. Every day I take time to sip my herb tea and look at the living, breathing, green, and flowering plants in my apartment. I enjoy washing the dishes and my clothes. I like smelling the fresh, clean, unscented aroma of clean linens while folding the fabrics and putting them

away. I enjoy taking time to answer the phone and giving my full attention to the person on the other end of the line, making intentional connections. I savor the taste of food and the joy of living."

— Ellen J.

"Hope is a strong motivator. Even on my most miserable days, a shred of hope keeps me going. I don't know where it comes from or how I maintain it, but like many others living with chronic illness, I am more resilient than I'd have imagined in my wildest dreams. I don't know how any of us live with chronic illness—but we do. We tap resources we didn't even know were there and we manage to go on."

— Katrina B.

Living As If You Are Well

Do you consider yourself disabled? Or a chronically ill person? Or are you someone who is going to recover your life and get back to doing the things that make you happy? Instead of planning events to enjoy in the future, why not enjoy the time right now? Step out of the shadow of your illness, and live your life as if you are well.

We hope you've enjoyed reading this book and have found plenty of advice to help you. Think of the patients and practitioners in this book as part of your support network—we're not just people in the pages of a book; we're actually out here in the real world, trying our best to live rewarding lives with FM and CFS.

Don't be shy; e-mail us at fmcfsbook@yahoo.com or write to us in care of our publishers at Hunter House. Tell us about your experiences and what has worked best in your situation. It may take us a while to respond, because sometimes we get a little swamped. But we'd love to hear from you.

Appendix A

Medications and Supplements for FM and CFS

The following table lists the pharmacological drugs most often prescribed for FM and CFS. Some of these medications are also available over-the-counter at your local drugstore. We have not listed the recommended dosage since that will vary from patient to patient and will depend on the other medications you are taking.

Some pain relievers are available in ointment form. Zostrix, Icy Hot, Ben Gay, and Flexall can be applied directly to the skin for immediate pain relief. In addition, some medications such as Prozac, Advil, and Aleve are available in liquid form.

Prescription Drugs and Over-the-Counter Medications for FM and CFS

Brand name	Generic name	Class/Indication
Ambien	Zolpidem tartrate	Sleep aid and anti-anxiety
Ativan	Lorazepam	Anti-anxiety
Bentyl	Dicyclomine	Antispasmodic
BuSpar	Buspirone	Anti-anxiety
Celexa	Citalopram	SSRI antidepressant
Cholac	Lactulose	Laxative drink
Correctol	Docuste	Laxative/stool softener
Cymbalta	Duloxetine	SSRI antidepressant and pain reliever
Cytomel	Liothyronine sodium	Thyroid hormone replacement
Darvocet	Propoxyphene with acetaminophen	Narcotic pain reliever
Darvon-N100	Propoxyphene HCL	Narcotic pain reliever

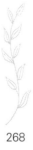

Prescription Drugs and Over-the-Counter Medications for FM and CFS

Brand name	Generic name	Class/Indication
Deltasone	Prednisone	Anti-inflammatory
Desyrel	Trazodone	Tricyclic antidepressant
Dolphine	Methadone	Narcotic pain reliever
Effexor	Venlafaxine	Sleep aid, antidepressant
Elavil	Amitriptyline	Tricyclic antidepressant
EMLA Cream	Lidocaine/Prilocaine	Topical anesthetic
Fentanyl	Duragesic	Narcotic pain-reliever patch
Flexeril	Cyclobenzaprine	Muscle relaxant
Imitrex	Sumatriptan	Migraine relief
Kaopectate	Attapulgite	Relieves diarrhea
Klonopin	Clonazepam	Benzodiazepine used to treat anxiety, insomnia, seizures
Levoxyl	Levothyroxine sodium	Thyroid hormone replacement
Levsinex	Hyoscyamine	Relives the symptoms of irritable bowel syndrome
Lioresal	Baclofen	Muscle relaxant
Lortab	Hydrocodone/Acetaminophen	Pain relief
Marcaine	Bupivacaine HCl	Pain relief
Mirapex	Pramipexole dihydrochloride	Used to treat Parkinson's disease (tremors and rigidity)
Morph Sul	Morphine sulfate	Pain relief
Motrin	Ibuprofen	Pain relief, anti-inflammatory
MS-Contin	Morphine extended release formula	Narcotic pain reliever
Naprosyn	Naproxen	NSAID anti-inflammatory, pain relief
Neurontin	Gabapentin	Neurotransmitter regulation, helps neuropathic pain
Norco	Hydrocodone with acetaminophen	Pain relief

269

(cont'd.)

Prescription Drugs and Over-the-Counter Medications for FM and CFS (cont'd.)

Brand name	Generic name	Class/Indication
Norflex	Orphenadrine citrate	Muscle relaxant
Oxycontin	Oxycodone HCL	Narcotic pain reliever
Pamelor	Nortriptyline HCL	Antidepressant
Paxil	Paroxetine HCL	SSRI Antidepressant
Percocet	Oxycodone and acetaminophen	Narcotic pain reliever
Percodan	Oxycodone with aspirin	Narcotic pain reliever
Procaine	Procaine	Local anesthetic
Prozac	Fluoexetine	Antidepressant, pain relief
Rheumatrex dp	Methotrexate	Autoimmune disease treatment
Robaxin	Methocarbamol	Muscle relaxant
Roxicet	Oxycodone and acetaminophen	Narcotic pain reliever
Roxicodone	Oxycodone	Narcotic pain reliever
Roxiprin	Oxycodone and aspirin	Narcotic pain reliever
Sinemet	Carbidopa-levodopa	Prescribed for Parkinson's disease
Sinequan	Doxepin	Antidepressant, insomnia
Soma	Carisoprodol	Muscle relaxant
Synthroid	Levothyroxine sodium	Thyroid hormone replacement
Toradol	Ketorolac	NSAID, pain relief
Tranzene	Clorazepate dipotassium	Benzodiazepine, muscle relaxant
Tylenol	Acetaminophen	Pain relief
Tylenol 3	Acetaminophen and codeine	Narcotic pain reliever
Tylox	Oxycodone and acetaminophen	Narcotic pain reliever

Prescription Drugs and Over-the-Counter Medications for FM and CFS

Brand name	Generic name	Class/Indication
Ultram	Tramadol	Non-narcotic pain relief
Vicodin	Hydrocodone and acetaminophen	Narcotic pain reliever
Voltaren	Diclofenac	NSAID pain reliever
Wellbutrin	Bupropion	Antidepressant, smoking cessation
Xanax	Alprazolam	Antidepressant and sleep aid
Zanaflex	Tizanidine	Muscle relaxant
Zoloft	Sertraline	SSRI antidepressant

The following table illustrates vitamins, herbs, and other supplements that are commonly recommended for FM and CFS patients:

Vitamins, Herbs, and Supplements Recommended for FM and CFS Patients

Generic or brand name	Scientific or botanical name	Indication
5-HTP	Hydroxytryptophan	Relieves depression, promotes restful sleep
AG Immune	AiE10	Boosts immune response
Acidophilus	*Lactobacillus acidophilus*	Replaces normal bacterial flora, supports digestive health
Alpha lipoic acid		Restores other antioxidants after they have been used by the body
Boswellia	Indian Frankensense	Relieves the symptoms of rheumatoid arthritis and osteoarthritis
Bromelain	(derived from pineapple)	Natural aid to digestion, relieves muscle aches and pains
Burdock	*Arctium lappa*	Blood cleanser
Calcium		Regulates muscle and blood vessel contraction, which helps control headaches
Coenzyme Q10 (CoQ10)	Ubiquinone	Antioxidant, increases energy

271

(cont'd.)

Vitamins, Herbs, and Supplements Recommended for FM and CFS Patients (cont'd.)

Generic or brand name	Scientific or botanical name	Indication
Cysteine	Amino acid	Eliminates toxic chemicals
Dandelion	*Taraxacum officinale*	Liver cleanser
Devil's Claw	*Harpagophytum procumbens*	Anti-inflammatory
Echinacea	Echinacea	Boosts immune response
Evening primrose oil		Anti-inflammatory, eases pain, supports mental function; source of Omega-6 fatty acids
Flaxseed (linseed)		Relieves constipation; source of Omega-3 and -6 fatty acids
Ginger	Ginger	Calms digestive system
Ginkgo	*Ginkgo biloba*	Like aspirin, a mild blood vessel dilator; enhances oxygen availability, aids memory
Glucosamine and chondroitin sulphate		Joint pain repair and relief
Green tea extract		Antioxidant, boosts immune response
Holy basil	*Ocimum sanctum*	Relieves constipation and indigestion
Kava kava	*Piper methysticum*	Relives anxiety and insomnia
Licorice	*Glycyrrhiza glabra*	Adrenal tonic, anti-inflammatory
Magnesium		Energy and muscle relaxation, anti-inflammatory
Malic acid		Energy and muscle relaxation, aids in the absorption of magnesium
Melatonin		Regulates circadian rhythms, initiates sleep
Monolaurin	Lauric acid (from coconut oil)	Anti-microbial, anti-viral

Vitamins, Herbs, and Supplements Recommended for FM and CFS Patients

Generic or brand name	Scientific or botanical name	Indication
MSM	Methyl sulfonyl methane	Muscle pain relief
NK Immune	AiE10	Boosts immune function and natural killer cell production
Oatstraw	Avena	Promotes adrenal health
Olive leaf		Antioxidant, anti-viral agent
Passion flower		Anti-viral, relieves anxiety and insomnia
Potassium		Muscle contractor
Pro-Energy	Magnesium and malic acid	Muscle pain relief
Pynagenol	Grape seed extract	Increases energy
Royal Jelly	Bee pollen	Increases energy
SAM-e	S-Adenosylmethionine	Pain and fatigue, mood elevation, arthritis relief
St. John's wort		Relieves depression, pain relief
Selenium		Antioxidant, stimulates the immune system
Super Blue-Green Algae	Algae	Increases energy
Turmeric		Antioxidant, anti-inflammatory
Valerian root		Sleep aid, calmative herb to reduce anxiety
Vitamin A	Beta-carotene	Antioxidant, decreases free radical damage and muscle inflammation, improves vision and skin
Vitamin B_1	Thiamine	Helps cells produce energy from carbohydrates
Vitamin B_2	Riboflavin	Promotes growth and health of all cells and tissues
Vitamin B_3	Niacin	Aids in the release of energy from food

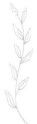

273

(cont'd.)

Vitamins, Herbs, and Supplements Recommended for FM and CFS
Patients (cont'd.)

Generic or brand name	Scientific or botanical name	Indication
Vitamin B_5	Pantothenic acid	Promotes adrenal health
Vitamin B_6	Pyridoxine	Supports the metabolism of nutrients, and the conversion of amino acids from protein into neurotransmitters
Vitamin B_9	Folic acid	Promotes normal red blood cell formation
Vitamin B_{12}	Cobalamin	Works in combination with folate to make red blood cells
Vitamin B complex		Increases energy, supports function of the nervous system
Vitamin C	Ascorbic acid	Antioxidant, supports adrenals and immune system, helps body absorb iron from food, helps repair red blood cells, bones, and tissues
Vitamin D	Calciferol	Promotes absorption of calcium, healing to skin and bone
Vitamin E	Tocopherol	Antioxidant, helps restless legs syndrome and arthritis pain
Vitamin K	Menadiol	Improves circulation, lubricates cells
Zinc	Medizonc orazine	Helps reduce blood clotting; with Vitamin A, enhances immunity via antibody production

Tests You Can Do for Yourself

✤ The Tilt Table Test

The tilt table test is designed to evaluate the body's regulation of blood pressure, through controlled changes in posture. In a clinical setting, the patient is gently tilted on a special table. Physicians monitor the patient's blood pressure as the body responds to various degrees of tilt.

The home variation of this test, often referred to as the "poor man's tilt table test," is quite simple to perform. Be sure to have someone help you with this test since you may feel ill or even lose consciousness. To perform the test, you must attempt to stand in one place for 30 minutes. Normal subjects can often stand for a prolonged period of time without any ill feelings; those with autonomic dysfunctions cannot stand for very long before feeling lightheaded or before fainting due to insufficient blood flow to the brain. If you have a blood pressure cuff, you can monitor your blood pressure during the test for more visible results.

✤ Candida

There is a simple test for candida. First ensure that you have not had anything to eat or drink for at least four hours (testing first thing in the morning may be easiest). Pour a glass of water. Build up as much saliva in your mouth as possible and spit into the glass. Check on the glass periodically over the next hour. If you notice string-like trails of saliva hanging down toward the bottom of the glass, cloudy saliva at the bottom of the glass, or cloudy specks of saliva in the glass, this indicates that there is too much candida in your saliva. If you have a healthy level of candida in your saliva, the saliva will still be floating on top of the water after one hour.

Bibliography

❖ Books

Bell, David S. *The Faces of CFS*. Lyndonville, NY: Self-published, 2002 (Out of print. Available for free: download at www.davidsbell.com).

Berne, Katrina, H. *Chronic Fatigue Syndrome, Fibromyalgia & Other Invisible Illnesses* (completely updated version of *Running on Empty*). Alameda, CA: Hunter House, 2002.

Bingham, John. *The Courage to Start: A Guide to Running for Your Life*. New York: Fireside, 1999.

Byers, Dwight C. *Better Health with Foot Reflexology*. Saint Petersburg, FL: Ingham, 1983.

Carter, Mildred. *Hand Reflexology: Key to Perfect Health*. West Nyack, NY: Parker, 1975.

Cousens, Gabriel. *Conscious Eating*. Berkeley, CA: North Atlantic Books, 2000.

Eden, Donna, and David Feinstein. *Energy Medicine: How to Use Your Body's Energies for Optimum Health and Vitality*. East Rutherford, NJ: Putnam, 1999.

Emoto, Masaru. *The Hidden Messages in Water*. Hillsboro, OR: Beyond Words, 2004.

Englebienne, Patrick, and Kenny De Meirleir (editors). *Chronic Fatigue Syndrome: A Biological Approach*. Boca Raton, FL: CRC Press, 2002.

Findhorn Garden Community, The. *The Findhorn Garden*. New York: Harper-Perennial, 1975.

Fishman, Scott, with Lisa Berger. *The War on Pain*. New York: HarperCollins, 1999.

Gordon, Richard. *Quantum-Touch: Your Power To Heal*. Berkeley, CA: North Atlantic Books, 2002.

Griffin, Susan. *What Her Body Thought*. New York: Anchor Books, 1999.

Haig, Andrew J., and Miles Colwell. *Back Pain: A Guide for the Primary Care Physician*. Philadelphia, PA: American College of Physicians, 2005.

Hall, Carrie, and Lori Thein-Brody (editors). *Therapeutic Exercise: Moving Toward Function*. Philadelphia, PA: Lippincott Williams & Wilkins, 2004.

Holick, Michael. *The UV Advantage*. New York: ibooks, 2004.

Ivons, Maryann. *Homeopathy for Nurses*. Orlando, FL: Bandido, 2004.

Kerner, Diane. *My Own Medicine: The Process of Recovery from Chronic Illness*. Lincoln, NE: iUniverse, 2004.

Khalsa, Dharma Singh. *The Pain Cure*. New York: Warner, 1999.

Kübler-Ross, Elizabeth. *On Death and Dying*. New York: Scribner, 1969.

Lavery, Gerry. *So You've Been Diagnosed with Fibromyalgia* (pamphlet). (To request a copy, e-mail tamingfibro@comcast.net.)

276

Marek, Claudia Craig. *Fibromyalgia: The First Year.* New York: Marlowe & Company, 2003.

Martinson, Linda. *Poetry of Pain.* Lynnwood, WA: Simply Books, 1997.

Norden, Michael J. *Beyond Prozac: Brain-Toxic Lifestyles, Natural Antidotes & New Generation Antidepressants.* New York: HarperCollins, 1996.

Pellegrino, Mark J. *Fibromyalgia: Managing the Pain.* Columbus, OH: Anadem Publishing, 1993.

Pitchford, Paul. *Healing with Whole Foods: Asian Traditions and Modern Nutrition.* Berkeley, CA: North Atlantic Books, 2002.

St. Amand, R. Paul, and Claudia Craig Marek. *What Your Doctor May Not Tell You About Fibromyalgia.* New York: Warner, 2003.

Sarno, John E. *The Mindbody Prescription: Healing the Body, Healing the Pain.* New York, NY: Warner, 1999.

Skelly, Mari A. *Women Living with Fibromyalgia.* Alameda, CA: Hunter House, 2002.

Small Wright, Machaelle. *Behaving as if the God in All Life Mattered: A New Age Ecology.* Warrenton, VA: Perelandra, 1987.

———. *MAP: The Co-Creative White Brotherhood Medical Assistance Program.* Warrenton, VA: Perelandra, 1994.

Starlanyl, Devin, and Mary Ellen Copeland. *Fibromyalgia and Chronic Myofascial Pain: A Survival Manual.* Oakland, CA: New Harbinger, 2001.

Starlanyl, Devin. J. *The Fibromyalgia Advocate: Getting the Support You Need to Cope with Fibromyalgia and Myofascial Pain Syndrome.* Oakland, CA: New Harbinger, 1999.

Teitelbaum, Jacob. *From Fatigued to Fantastic.* New York: Avery, 2001.

Walls, R. Allen. *Magnetic Field Therapy Handbook.* McClean, VA: Inner Search Foundation, 1995.

❖ Periodicals

Aaron, Leslie, et al. "Overlapping Conditions Among Patients with Chronic Fatigue Syndrome, Fibromyalgia, and Temporomandibular Disorder." *Archives of Internal Medicine* 160 (2000): 221–227.

Bell, David S. "The Relationship Between Neurally Mediated Hypotension and CFS." *The Lyndonville News,* July 1999.

Cook, D. B., et al. "Functional Imaging of Pain in Patients with Primary Fibromyalgia." *Journal of Rheumatology* 31(2) (2004): 364–78.

Dayawansa, S., et al. "Autonomic Responses During Inhalation of Natural Fragrance of Cedrol in Humans." *Autonomic Neuroscience* 108(1–2) (2003): 79–86.

Foreman, Judy. "Biology of Chronic Fatigue Gains Focus." *The Boston Globe,* September 5, 2005.

Goldenberg, Don L., et al. "Management of Fibromyalgia Syndrome." *Journal of the American Medical Association* 292 (2004): 2388–2395.

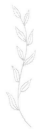

Gracely, R. H., et al. "Functional Magnetic Resonance Imaging Evidence of Augmented Pain Processing in Fibromyalgia." *Arthritis and Rheumatism* 46(5) (2002): 1333–43.

Hokama, Y., et al. "Chronic Phase Lipids in Sera of Chronic Fatigue Syndrome (CFS), Chronic Ciguatera Fish Poisoning (CCFP), Hepatitis B, and Cancer with Antigenic Epitope Resembling Ciguatoxin, as Assessed With MAb-CTX." *Journal of Clinical Laboratory Analysis* 17(4) (2003): 132–9.

Holman, A. J., and R. R. Myers. "A Randomized, Double-Blind, Placebo-Controlled Trial of Pramipexole, a Dopamine Agonist, in Patients with Fibromyalgia Receiving Concomitant Medications." *Arthritis & Rheumatism* 52(8) (2005): 2495–2505.

Holman, A. J., R. A. Neiman, and R. E. Ettlinger. "Preliminary Efficacy of the Dopamine Agonist, Pramipexole, for Fibromyalgia: The First, Open Label Experience." *Journal Musculoskeletal Pain* 12(1) (2004): 69–74.

Holman, A. J. "Fibromyalgia and Pramipexole: Promise and Precaution." [letter] *Journal of Rheumatology* 30(12) (2003): 2733.

Holman, A. J. "Ropinirole, Open Preliminary Observations of a Dopamine Agonist for Refractory Fibromylagia." [letter] *Journal of Clinical Rheumatology* 9(4) (2003): 277–9.

Kerr, J., et al. "Gene Expression in Peripheral Blood Mononuclear Cells from Patients with Chronic Fatigue Syndrome." *Journal of Clinical Pathology* 58 (2005): 826–832.

Martínez-Lavín, M., et al. "Circadian Studies of Autonomic Nervous Tone in Patients with Fibromyalgia: A Heart Rate Variability Analysis." *Arthritis and Rheumatism* 41 (1998): 1966–1971.

Moldofsky, H., et al. "Musculoskeletal Symptoms and Non-REM Sleep Disturbance in Patients with 'Fibrositis Syndrome' and Healthy Subjects." *Psychosomatic Medicine* 37 (1975): 341–351.

Rowe, Peter, et al. "The Relationship Between Neurally Mediated Hypotension and the Chronic Fatigue Syndrome." *Journal of the American Medical Association* 274 (1995): 961–967.

Staud, R., et al. "Maintenance of Windup of Second Pain Requires Less Frequent Stimuli in Fibromyalgia Patients Compared to Normal Controls." *Pain* 110(3) (2004): 689–696.

Sullivan, S., et al. "Assessment of Sun Exposure in Adolescent Girls Using Activity Diaries." *Nutrition Research* 23(5) (2003): 631–644.

Resources and Recommended Reading

❖ FM, CFS, and Related Organizations

The American Association for Chronic Fatigue Syndrome
27 N. Wacker Dr., Suite 416
Chicago IL 60606
(847) 258-7248
www.aacfs.org

American College of Rheumatology
1800 Century Pl., Suite 250
Atlanta GA 30345
(404) 633-3777
www.rheumatology.org

The American Fibromyalgia Syndrome Association
6380 E. Tanque Verde, Suite D
Tucson AZ 85715
(520) 733-1570
www.afsafund.org

The American Sleep Apnea Association
1424 K St. NW
Washington DC 20005
(202) 293-3650
www.sleepapnea.org

Arthritis Foundation
P.O. Box 921907
Norcross GA 30010-9904
(404) 872-7100
Question-and-answer line:
(800) 283-7800
www.arthritis.org

Celiac Disease Foundation
13251 Ventura Blvd., #1
Studio City CA 91604
(818) 990-2354
www.celiac.org

CFIDS Association of America
P.O. Box 220398
Charlotte NC 28222
(704) 365-2343
www.cfids.org

The Depression and Bipolar Support Alliance
730 N. Franklin St., Suite 501
Chicago IL 60610
(800) 826-3632
www.dbsalliance.org

Fibromyalgia Network
P.O. Box 31750
Tucson AZ 85751-1750
(800) 853-2929
www.fmnetnews.com

The Fibromyalgia Treatment Center, Inc.
P.O. Box 7223
Santa Monica CA 90406
(310) 577-7510
www.fibromyalgiatreatment.com

International Foundation for Functional Gastrointestinal Disorders (IFFGD)
P.O. Box 170864
Milwaukee WI 53217-8076
(414) 964-1799
www.iffgd.org

MCS Referral & Resources
618 Wyndhurst Ave., #2
Baltimore MD 21210
(410) 889-6666
www.mcsrr.org
www.mcsurvivors.com

The National CFIDS Foundation
103 Aletha Rd.
Needham MA 02492
(781) 449-3535
www.ncf-net.org

National Fibromyalgia Association
2200 Glassell St., Suite A
Orange CA 92865
(714) 921-0150
www.fmaware.org

National Fibromyalgia Partnership
140 Zinn Way
Linden VA 22642
(866) 725-4404
www.fmpartnership.org

National Fibromyalgia Research Association
P.O. Box 500
Salem OR 97308
www.nfra.net

National Vulvodynia Association
P.O. Box 4491
Silver Spring MD 20914-4491
(301) 299-0775
www.nva.org

ProHealth, Inc.
2040 Alameda Padre Serra, Suite 101
Santa Barbara CA 93103
(805) 564-3064
www.immunesupport.com *or*
www.prohealth.com

Restless Legs Syndrome Foundation
819 Second St., SW
Rochester MN 55902
(507) 287-6465
www.rls.org

The Sarcoidosis Awareness Network
Linda Lanier, President
1031 Farrar Ave.
Cheltenham MD 20623
(301) 372-2885
www.sarcoidosisnetwork.com

SAVE—Suicide Awareness Voices of Education
9001 E. Bloomington Fwy., Suite #150
Bloomington MN 55420
(952) 946-7998
www.save.org

Sjögren's Syndrome Foundation, Inc.
8120 Woodmont Ave.
Bethesda MD 20814
(800) 475-6473
www.sjogrens.org

The Thyroid Foundation of America
One Longfellow Pl., Suite 1518
Boston MA 02114
(800) 832-8321
www.tsh.org

The TMJ Association
P.O. Box 26770
Milwaukee WI 53226
(414) 259-3223
www.tmj.org

❧ Books on FM, CFS, and Overlapping Conditions

Barr, Gilbert. *Me & Sarcoidosis: A Lifetime Partnership.* New York: Writers Club Press, 2002.

Bell, David S. *The Faces of CFS.* Lyndonville, NY: Self-published, 2002 (Out of print. Available for free: download at www.davidsbell.com).

Bell, David S., et al. *A Parent's Guide to CFIDS.* Binghamton, NY: The Haworth Medical Press, 1999.

Bell, David S. *The Doctor's Guide to Chronic Fatigue Syndrome: Understanding, Treating, and Living with CFIDS.* Boston, MA: Addison-Wesley, 1995.

Berkowitz, Jonathan M. *A Victim No More: Overcoming Irritable Bowel Syndrome.* North Bergen, NJ: Basic Health Publications, 2003.

Berne, Katrina, H. *Chronic Fatigue Syndrome, Fibromyalgia and Other Invisible Illnesses* (completely updated version of *Running on Empty*). Alameda, CA: Hunter House, 2002.

Chaudhuri, K. Ray, et al. (eds). *Restless Legs Syndrome.* Philadelphia, PA: Taylor & Francis Group, 2004.

Crook, William G., et al. *The Yeast Connection and Women's Health.* New York: Professional Books/Future Health, 2005.

Duke, Patty. *A Brilliant Madness: Living with Manic Depressive Illness.* New York: Bantam, 1993.

Dyson, Sue. *Positive Options for Sjögren's Syndrome: Self-Help and Treatment.* Alameda, CA: Hunter House, 2005.

Gibson, Pamela Reed. *Multiple Chemical Sensitivity: A Survival Guide.* Oakland, CA: New Harbinger Publishers, 1999.

Glazer, Howard I., and Gay Rodke. *The Vulvodynia Survival Guide: How to Overcome Painful Vaginal Symptoms and Enjoy an Active Lifestyle.* Oakland, CA: New Harbinger, 2002.

Goddard, Greg. *TMJ: The Jaw Connection: The Overlooked Diagnosis: A Self-Care Guide to Diagnosing and Managing This Hidden Ailment.* Santa Fe, NM: Aurora, 1991.

Goldberg, Burton, and Larry Trivieri, Jr. *Chronic Fatigue, Fibromyalgia, and Lyme Disease.* Berkeley, CA: Celestial Arts, 2004.

Goldberg, Burton, et al. *Alternative Medicine Guide to Chronic Fatigue, Fibromyalgia & Environmental Illness.* Boulder, CO: Alternativemedicine.com Books, 1998.

Goldstein, Jay A. *Betrayal by the Brain: The Neurologic Basis of Chronic Fatigue Syndrome, Fibromyalgia Syndrome, and Related Neural Network Disorders.* Binghamton, NY: Haworth Press, 1996.

Gomez, Joan. *Thyroid Problems in Women and Children.* Alameda, CA: Hunter House, 2003.

Griffin, Susan. *What Her Body Thought.* New York: Anchor Books, 1999.

Johnson, Hillary. *Osler's Web: Inside the Labyrinth of the Chronic Fatigue Syndrome Epidemic.* New York, NY: Crown, 1996.

Jamison, Kay Redfield. *An Unquiet Mind: A Memoir of Moods and Madness.* New York: Vintage, 1997.

Kerner, Diane. *My Own Medicine: The Process of Recovery from Chronic Illness.* Lincoln, NE: iUniverse, 2004. (To order a copy, e-mail kdkerner@comcast.net.)

Lavery, Gerry. *So You've Been Diagnosed with Fibromyalgia.* (pamphlet; to request a copy, e-mail tamingfibro@comcast.net.)

Lavie, Peretz. *Restless Nights: Understanding Snoring and Sleep Apnea.* New Haven, CT: Yale University Press, 2003.

Lipski, Elizabeth. *Leaky Gut Syndrome* (Keats Good Health Guide). New York: McGraw-Hill Companies, 1998.

Marek, Claudia Craig. *Fibromyalgia: The First Year.* New York: Marlowe & Company, 2003.

Martinson, Linda. *Poetry of Pain.* Lynnwood, WA: Simply Books, 1997. (To order a copy, visit simplybookspublishing.com.)

Pellegrino, Mark. J. *Fibromyalgia: Up Close & Personal.* Columbus, OH: Anadem, 2005.

St. Amand, R. Paul, and Claudia Craig Marek. *What Your Doctor May Not Tell You about Fibromyalgia Fatigue: The Powerful Program That Helps You Boost Your Energy and Reclaim Your Life.* New York: Warner, 2003.

St. Amand, R. Paul, and Claudia Craig Marek. *What Your Doctor May Not Tell You about Fibromyalgia: The Revolutionary Treatment That Can Reverse the Disease.* New York: Warner, 1999.

Skelly, Mari A. *Women Living With Fibromyalgia.* Alameda, CA: Hunter House, 2002.

Starlanyl, Devin, and Mary Ellen Copeland. *Fibromyalgia and Chronic Myofascial Pain: A Survival Manual.* Oakland, CA: New Harbinger, 2001.

Starlanyl, Devin. J. *The Fibromyalgia Advocate: Getting the Support You Need to Cope with Fibromyalgia and Myofascial Pain Syndrome.* Oakland, CA: New Harbinger, 1999.

Teitelbaum, Jacob. *From Fatigued to Fantastic.* New York: Avery, 2001.

Van Vorous, Heather. *Eating for IBS: 175 Delicious, Nutritious, Low-Fat, Low-Residue Recipes to Stabilize the Touchiest Tummy.* New York: Marlowe & Company, 2000.

Weinberg, Norma Pasekoff. *Natural & Herbal Remedies for Carpal Tunnel Syndrome.* Pownal, VT: Storey, 2000.

Williams, Mary Beth, and Soili Poijula. *The PTSD Workbook: Simple, Effective Techniques for Overcoming Traumatic Stress Symptoms.* Oakland, CA: New Harbinger, 2002.

Wilson, Virginia N. *Sleep Thief: Restless Legs Syndrome.* Orange Park, FL: Galaxy Books, 1996.

❖ Resources for Alternative Treatments

PHYSICAL THERAPY

American Physical Therapy Association
1111 North Fairfax St.
Alexandria VA 22314
(800) 999-2782
www.apta.org

TENS AND CES UNITS

Nancy Stewart Campbell
Distributor, Therapeutic Resources, Inc.
P.O. Box 12608
Mill Creek WA 98082
(800) 488-8492

SLEEP HYGIENE

National Sleep Foundation
1522 K St. NW, Suite 500
Washington DC 20005
(202) 347-3471
www.sleepfoundation.org

Heller, Barbara L. *How to Sleep Soundly Tonight: 250 Simple and Natural Ways to Prevent Sleeplessness.* Pownal, VT: Storey, 2001.
Perl, James. *Sleep Right in Five Nights: A Clear and Effective Guide for Conquering Insomnia.* New York: William Morrow, 1993.

Nirvana Safe Haven
(800) 968-9355
www.nontoxic.com
Certified organic cotton/wool mattresses and organic wool bedding, 100 percent pure rubber mattresses

Comfy Comforter
www.comfycomforter.com
(207) 667-8284

Crescent Moon Duvet and Pillow Company
Alpaca Wool Duvets
(877) 765-2816
www.crescentmoonduvets.com

Certified Organic Products
(800) 542-8888
www.certified-organic.com
Organically grown cotton bed linens

CHIROPRACTIC

The American Chiropractic Association
1701 Clarendon Blvd.
Arlington VA 22209
(800) 986 4636
www.amerchiro.org

Canfield, Jack. *Chicken Soup for the Chiropractic Soul.* New York: HCI, 2002.
Rondberg, Terry. *Chiropractic First: The Fastest Growing Healthcare Choice Before Drugs or Surgery.* New York: Chiropractic Journal, 1996.

OSTEOPATHY

American Academy of Osteopathy
3500 DePauw Blvd., Suite 1080
Indianapolis IN 46268
(317) 879-1881
www.academyofosteopathy.org

Deorra, Tajinder K. *Healing Through Cranial Osteopathy.* London, U.K.: Frances Lincoln, 2004.

MASSAGE

American Massage Therapy Association
500 Davis St., Suite 900
Evanston IL 60201
(877) 905-2700
www.amtamassage.org

Khalsa, Waheguru. *Miracle of Healing Hands: The Complete Guide to Ancient Yogic Healing & Massage Techniques.* New York: Rishi Knot Publishers, 1997.
Lidell, Lucinda. *The Book of Massage: The Complete Step-by-Step Guide to Eastern And Western Technique.* New York: Fireside, 2001.
Prevention Magazine. *Hands-On Healing: Massage Remedies for Hundreds of Health Problems.* New York: Rodale, 1989.
Schatz, Bernard. *Soft Tissue Massage for Pain Relief: How You Can Massage Away the Pain from 37 Health Conditions.* Charlottesville, VA: Hampton Roads Publishing Company, 2001.

TRIGGER POINT THERAPY

Davies, Clair. *The Trigger Point Therapy Workbook: Your Self-Treatment Guide for Pain Relief*, 2nd Edition. Oakland, CA: New Harbinger, 2004.

Gach, Michael Reed. *Acupressure's Potent Points: A Guide to Self-Care for Common Ailments*. New York: Bantam, 1990.

Prudden, Bonnie. *Pain Erasure: The Bonnie Prudden Way*. New York: Ballantine Books, 1985.

REFLEXOLOGY

Byers, Dwight C. *Better Health with Foot Reflexology*. Saint Petersburg, FL: Ingham, 1983.

Carter, Mildred. *Hand Reflexology: Key to Perfect Health*. West Nyack, NY: Parker, 1975.

Rick, Stephanie. *Reflexology Workout: Hand & Foot Massage for Super Health & Rejuvenation*. New York: Crown, 1986.

FELDENKRAIS

Feldenkrais Educational Foundation of North America
3611 SW Hood Ave., Suite 100
Portland OR 97239
(866) 333-6248
www.feldenkrais.com
Audio recordings of Awareness Through Movement Lessons: San Francisco Evening Classes, Volumes 1 through 3, and Lessons for the Elder Citizen are available from the Feldenkrais Educational Foundation of North America.

Alon, Ruthy. *Mindful Spontaneity: Relearning Natural Movement Through Feldenkrais Method*. Berkeley, CA: North Atlantic Books, 1996.

Feldenkrais, Moshe. *Body and Mature Behavior: A Study of Anxiety, Sex, Gravitation, & Learning*. Berkeley, CA: Frog, 2005.

Feldenkrais, Moshe. *The Potent Self: A Study of Spontaneity and Compulsion*. Berkeley, CA: Frog, 2002.

Feldenkrais, Moshe. *Awareness Through Movement*. San Francisco, CA: HarperSanFrancisco, 1991.

Plonka, Lavina. *What Are You Afraid Of? A Body/Mind Guide to Courageous Living*. New York: Jeremy P. Tarcher, 2004.

Shafarman, Steven. *Awareness Heals: The Feldenkrais Method for Dynamic Health*. Boston, MA: Addison-Wesley, 1997.

HANNA SOMATICS

The Association for Hanna Somatic Education, Inc.
925 Golden Gate Dr.
Napa CA 94558

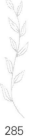

(877) 766-2473
www.hannasomatics.com

Hanna, Thomas. *Somatics: Reawakening the Mind's Control of Movement, Flexibility, and Health.* Cambridge, MA: Da Capo Press, 2004.
Hanna, Thomas. *The Body of Life: Creating New Pathways for Sensory Awareness and Fluid Movement.* Rochester, VT: Healing Arts Press, 1993.

EXERCISE

Anderson, Bob. *Stretching: 20th Anniversary Revised Edition.* Bolinas, CA: Shelter, 2000.
Hall, Carrie, and Lori Thein-Brody (editors). *Therapeutic Exercise: Moving Toward Function.* Philadelphia, PA: Lippincott Williams & Wilkins, 2004.

EASTERN MEDICINE

American Association of Oriental Medicine
PO Box 162340
Sacramento CA 95816
(866) 455-7999
www.aaom.org

www.luminaryhealth.com
Maintained by natural health consultant Wendy Bodin (a contributor to this book)

Joiner, Thomas Richard. *Chinese Herbal Medicine Made Easy.* Alameda, CA: Hunter House, 2001.
Kaptchuk, Ted J. *The Web That Has No Weaver: Understanding Chinese Medicine.* New York: Contemporary, 2000.
Xu, Zong Lan. *Pocket Handbook of Chinese Herbal Medicine.* New York: Wacloin, 2000.

ACUPUNCTURE

American Academy of Medical Acupuncture
4929 Wilshire Blvd., Suite 428
Los Angeles CA 90010
(323) 937-5514
www.medicalacupuncture.org
Provides acupuncture information, medical references with links to other sites, and a practitioner list

Ellis, Andrew, et al. *Fundamentals of Chinese Acupuncture.* Boston, MA: Paradigm Publications, 1991.
Hecker, Hans-Ulrich, et al. *Color Atlas of Acupuncture: Body Points, Ear Points, Trigger Points.* New York: Thieme Medical Publishers, 2001.

AYRUVEDA

Frawley, David, and Vasant Lad. *The Yoga of Herbs: An Ayurvedic Guide to Herbal Medicine.* Twin Lakes, WI: Lotus Light, 1993.

Thirtha, Swami Sada Shiva. *The Ayurveda Encyclopedia—Natural Secrets to Healing, Prevention, and Longevity.* Bayville, NY: Ayurveda Holistic Center Press, 1998.

YOGA

Beeken, Jenny. *Yoga of the Heart.* Liss, Hants, UK: White Eagle Publishing Trust, 1990.

Swami Satchidananda. *Integral Hatha Yoga.* Yogaville, VA: Integral Yoga, 1970.

Sivananda Yoga Center. *The Sivananda Companion to Yoga: A Complete Guide to the Physical Postures, Breathing Exercises, Diet, Relaxation, and Meditation Techniques of Yoga.* New York: Fireside, 2000.

TAI CHI AND QIGONG

www.embracethemoon.com
Website maintained by tai chi and qigong instructor Kim Ivy (a contributor to this book)

Kam-Chuen, Master Lam. *Step-by-Step Tai Chi.* New York: Fireside, 1994.

Kit, Wong Kiew. *The Complete Book of Tai Chi Chuan: A Comprehensive Guide to the Principles and Practice.* North Clarendon, VT: Tuttle, 2002.

ENERGETIC HEALING

Healing Touch International Foundation, Inc.
16211 Clay Rd., Suite 106, Box 215
Houston TX 77084-5478
(281) 856-8340
www.healingtouch.net

The International Center for Reiki Training
21421 Hilltop St., Unit #28
Southfield MI 48034
(800) 332-8112
www.Reiki.org

Association for Comprehensive Energy Psychology
P.O. Box 910244
San Diego CA 92191
(619) 861-ACEP (861-2237)
www.energypsych.org

Callahan Techniques, Ltd.
P.O. Box 1220
La Quinta CA 92253
(800) 359-2873
www.tftrx.com

www.psychicreiki.com
Maintained by Reiki master, teacher, and psychic Maureen Brennan (a contributor to this book)

www.energytherapist.com
Maintained by licensed mental-health practitioner Marti MacEwan (a contributor to this book)

www.cindyrothwell.com
Maintained by Cindy Rothwell, an ordained minister, intuitive counselor, and Quantum-Touch™ practitioner (a contributor to this book)

Brennan, Barbara Ann. *Light Emerging: The Journey of Personal Healing.* Freedom, CA: The Crossing Press, 1993.

Brennan, Barbara Ann. *Hands of Light: A Guide to Healing Through the Human Energy Field.* New York: Bantam, 1988.

Callahan, Roger J. *Tapping the Healer Within: Using Thought Field Therapy to Instantly Conquer Your Fears, Anxieties, and Emotional Distress.* New York: McGraw-Hill Companies, 2002.

Chopra, Deepak. *Quantum Healing: Exploring the Frontiers of Mind/Body Medicine.* New York: Bantam, 1990.

Eden, Donna, and David Feinstein. *Energy Medicine: How to Use Your Body's Energies for Optimum Health and Vitality.* East Rutherford, NJ: Putnam, 1999.

Flint, Garry A. *Emotional Freedom: Techniques for Dealing with Emotional and Physical Distress.* Vernon, BC, Canada: Garry A. Flint, 2001.

Gallo, Fred P. *Energy Tapping: How to Rapidly Eliminate Anxiety, Depression, Cravings & More Using Energy Psychology.* Oakland, CA: New Harbinger, 2000.

Gordon, Richard. *Quantum-Touch: Your Power to Heal.* Berkeley, CA: North Atlantic Books, 2002.

Gordon, Richard. *Your Healing Hands: The Polarity Experience.* Berkeley, CA: North Atlantic Books, 2004.

Murray, Steve. *Reiki: The Ultimate Guide.* Lancaster, UK: Gazelle Drake, 2004.

Rand, William Lee. *Reiki: The Healing Touch.* Southfield, MI: Vision, 2000.

Stein, Diane. *Essential Reiki: A Complete Guide to an Ancient Healing Art.* Freedom, CA: Crossing Press, 1995.

Stein, Diane. *All Women Are Healers: A Comprehensive Guide to Natural Healing.* Freedom, CA: Crossing Press, 1990.

Wright, Machaelle Small. *MAP: The Co-Creative White Brotherhood Medical Assistance Program.* Warrenton, VA: Perelandra, 1994.

MEDITATION AND VISUALIZATION

Schwarz, Jack. *Voluntary Controls: Exercises for Creative Meditation and for Activating the Potential of the Chakras.* New York: E.P. Dutton, 1978.

Amarnick, Claude. *Dr. Amarnick's Mind over Matter Pain Relief Program.* Deerfield Beach, FL: Garrett, 1995.

NUTRITION

Optimum Health Institute of San Diego
6970 Central Ave.
Lemongrove CA 91945
(619) 464-3346
www.optimumhealth.org

Metagenics San Clemente
100 Ave La Pata
San Clemente CA 92673
(800) 692-9400
www.ultrabalance.com

UltraClear Sustain, produced by Metagenics, is a gastrointestinal nutritional supplement only available through licensed health-care providers. To find a distributor in the United States, call (800) 692-9400. To find a distributor outside the United States, call Metagenics at (800) 843-9660 or access the website listed above.

Colbin, Annemarie. *Food and Healing.* New York: Ballantine, 1996.

Cousens, Gabriel. *Conscious Eating.* Berkeley, CA: North Atlantic Books, 2000.

Lipski, Elizabeth. *Digestive Wellness*, 3rd Edition. New York: McGraw-Hill, 2004.

Pitchford, Paul. *Healing with Whole Foods: Asian Traditions and Modern Nutrition.* Berkeley, CA: North Atlantic Books, 2002.

Robbins, John. *May All Be Fed: Diet for a New World.* New York: Avon, 1993.

NATURAL REMEDIES

www.herbweb.com

www.treefrogfarm.com
Website maintained by Diana Pepper (a contributor to this book)

Findhorn Garden Community. *The Findhorn Garden.* New York: HarperPerennial, 1975.

Murray, Michael, and Joseph Pizzorno. *Encyclopedia of Natural Medicine,* 2nd Edition. New York: Prima, 1998.

NATUROPATHY

The American Association of Naturopathic Physicians
4435 Wisconsin Ave. NW, Suite 403
Washington DC 20016
(866) 538-2267
www.naturopathic.org

www.drhuntoon.com
Website of Jenefer Scripps Huntoon, N.D. (a contributor to this book)

Mitchell, Stewart. *Naturopathy: Understanding the Healing Power of Nature*. New York: Element, 1998.
Thiel, Robert J. *Combining Old and New: Naturopathy for the 21st Century*. New York: Whitman, 2001.

HOMEOPATHY

National Center for Homeopathy
801 North Fairfax St., Suite 306
Alexandria VA 22314
(703) 548-7790
www.homeopathic.org

Castro, Miranda. *The Complete Homeopathy Handbook: Safe and Effective Ways to Treat Fevers, Coughs, Colds and Sore Throats, Childhood Ailments, Food Poisoning, Flu, and a Wide Range of Everyday Complaints*. New York: St. Martin's Griffin, 1990.
Ivons, Maryann. *Homeopathy for Nurses*. Orlando, FL: Bandido, 2004.

AROMATHERAPY

Buckle, Jane. *Clinical Aromatherapy: Essential Oils in Practice*. New York: Churchill Livingstone, 2003.
Life Extension Foundation. *Disease Prevention and Treatment*, 4th Edition. Hollywood, FL: Life Extension Media, 2003.
Newmark, Thomas M., and Paul Schulick. *Beyond Aspirin: Nature's Challenge to Arthritis, Cancer & Alzheimer's Disease*. Prescott, AZ: Hohm Press, 2000.
Schnaubelt, Kurt. *Medical Aromatherapy: Healing with Essential Oils*. Berkeley, CA: Frog, 1999.

MENTAL HEALTH

Amen, Daniel G. *Change Your Brain, Change Your Life*. New York: Three Rivers Press, 1998.
Kübler-Ross, Elizabeth. *On Death and Dying*. New York: Scribner, 1969.

SPIRITUALITY

Rest Ministries
P.O. Box 502928
San Diego CA 92150
(888) 751-7378
www.restministries.org

www.CorriesLeapofFaith.siteblast.com
Website maintained by Cornelia Duryeé Moore, a filmmaker and healing prayer minister (a contributor to this book)

Foster, Richard J. *Celebration of Discipline*. San Francisco, CA: HarperSanFrancisco, 1998.
Lawrence, Brother, and Frank Laubach. *Practicing His Presence*. Jacksonville, FL: Seed Sowers, 1985.
Smedes, Lewis B. *Forgive and Forget: Healing the Hurts We Don't Deserve*. San Francisco, CA: HarperSanFrancisco, 1996.
Wagner, James K. *Blessed to Be a Blessing: How to Have an Intentional Healing Ministry in Your Church*. Nashville, TN: Upper Room, 1983.

MAGNET THERAPY

www.5Pillars.com/magneticresearch.cfm
Website maintained by wellness consultant, Carolyn Else (a contributor to this book)

Coghill, Roger. *Book of Magnet Healing: A Holistic Approach to Pain Relief*. New York: Simon & Schuster, 2000.
Lawrence, Ron. *Magnet Therapy: The Pain Cure Alternative*. Rocklin, CA: Prima Publishing, 1998.
Walls, R. Allen. *Magnetic Field Therapy Handbook*. McClean, VA: Inner Search Foundation, 1995.
Whitaker, Julian, and Brenda Adderly. *The Pain Relief Breakthrough*. New York: Little, Brown & Company, 1998.

GOOD ADVICE FOR LIVING WITH A CHRONIC ILLNESS

American Academy of Pain Management
13947 Mono Way #A
Sonora CA 95370
(209) 533-9744
www.aapainmanage.org

American Academy of Pain Medicine
4700 W. Lake

Glenview IL 60025
(847) 375-4731
www.painmed.org

American Pain Foundation
111 S. Calvert St., Suite 2700
Baltimore MD 21202
(888) 615-PAIN (615-7246)
www.painfoundation.org

American Pain Society
4700 W. Lake Ave.
Glenview IL 60025
(847) 375-4715
www.ampainsoc.org

The National Foundation for the Treatment of Pain
P.O. Box 70045
Houston TX 77270
(713) 862-9332
www.paincare.org

Boryseko, Joan. *Minding the Body, Mending the Mind.* New York: Bantam, 1988.
Fishman, Scott, and Lisa Bergman. *The War on Pain.* New York: HarperCollins, 2001.
Kabat-Zinn, Jon. *Full Catastrophe Living: Using the Wisdom of Your Body and Mind to Face Stress, Pain, and Illness.* New York: Delta Trade, 1990.
Khalsa, Dharma Singh. *The Pain Cure.* New York: Warner, 1999.
Sarno, John E. *The Mindbody Prescription: Healing the Body, Healing the Pain.* New York: Warner, 1999.
Spero, David. *The Art of Getting Well: A Five-Step Plan for Maximizing Health When You Have a Chronic Illness.* Alameda, CA: Hunter House Publishers, 2002.

✣ Information for Families, Friends, and Care Givers

Family Caregiver Alliance
180 Montgomery St., Suite 1100
San Francisco CA 94104
(800) 445-8106
www.caregiver.org

The Well Spouse Association
63 West Main St., Suite H

Freehold NJ 07728
(800) 838-0879
www.wellspouse.org

Strong, Maggie Mainstay. *For the Well Spouse of the Chronically Ill.* Boston, MA: Bradford, 1997.
Vanderzalm, Lynn. *Finding Strength in Weakness: Help and Hope for Families Battling Chronic Fatigue Syndrome.* Grand Rapids, MI: Zondervan, 1995

❖ Home Test Kits

Diagnos-Techs, Inc.
6620 South 192nd Pl., Building J
Kent WA 98032
(800) 878-3787
www.diagnostechs.com
Test kits for candida, gastric pH, liver function, adrenal stress, etc.

Doctor's Data, Inc.
P.O. Box 111
West Chicago IL 60186
(800) 323-2784
www.doctorsdata.com
Tests for toxins in hair, blood, and urine

Immunosciences Lab., Inc.
8693 Wilshire Blvd., Suite 200
Beverly Hills CA 90211
(800) 950-4686
www.immuno-sci-lab.com
Comprehensive immune function testing, natural killer-cell activity, chronic fatigue panels, and parasite antibodies

www.heavymetalstest.com/heavymetaltest.php
Provides kits to test yourself and your home for heavy metals and other toxins

❖ Getting Your Benefits from Social Security

Americans With Disabilities Act
Disability Rights Section
U.S. Department of Justice
950 Pennsylvania Ave. NW
Civil Rights Division
Washington DC 20530
www.ada.gov

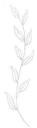

293

Medicare Rights Center
1460 Broadway, 17th Fl.
New York NY 10036
(212) 869-3850
www.medicarerights.org

Social Security Administration
Office of Public Inquiries
Windsor Park Building
6401 Security Blvd.
Baltimore MD 21235
(800) 772-1213
www.socialsecurity.gov
Information on how to apply for benefits; free "Disability Starter Kit" available

Cost Containment Research Institute
www.institute-dc.org
Offers a free booklet with information on programs that can help you obtain free or discounted prescription drugs

Index

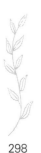

299

303

CHRONIC FATIGUE SYNDROME, FIBROMYALGIA, AND OTHER INVISIBLE ILLNESSES: A Comprehensive and Compassionate Guide
by Katrina Berne, Ph.D.

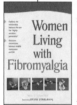

Formerly titled *Running on Empty,* this is an authoritative guide to chronic fatigue syndrome and fibromyalgia written by one of the authorities in the field. This book addresses what we know about the causes of CFS and FMS, and whether they are related; the wide range of symptoms and diagnostic tests; and proven and experimental treatment and self-care options. There is a chapter on CFS and FMS in children, and invaluable advice on dealing with relationship issues and lifestyle changes.

400 pages ... Paperback $16.95 ... Third edition

WOMEN LIVING WITH FIBROMYALGIA
by Mari Skelly

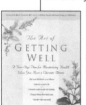

Using interviews, discussions, and personal stories, this book deals with the real-life concerns of women with fibromyalgia. Skelly highlights the strategies and therapies that a broad spectrum of women use to face FM's many challenges — from the student pondering how FM will affect her to the new mother trying to find energy to care for her family.

Topics include possible causes of FM and why it especially affects women; fifty strategies for dealing with pain, fatigue, and sleep disturbances; and exploring spirituality in the face of a disease that is difficult to diagnose and may have no cure.

320 pages ... Paperback $14.95

THE ART OF GETTING WELL: A Five-Step Plan for Maximizing Health When You Have a Chronic Illness *by David Spero, R.N.*

Self-management programs have become a key way for people to deal with chronic illness. In this book, David Spero offers a five-step approach to the medical, psychological, and spiritual aspects of getting well: slow down and use your energy for the things and people that matter — make small, progressive changes that build confidence — get help and nourish your social ties — value your body and treat it with affection and respect — take responsibility for getting the best care that you can.

224 pages ... Paperback $16.95

GET FIT WHILE YOU SIT: Easy Workouts from Your Chair *by Charlene Torkelson*

Here is a total-body workout that can be done right from your chair, anywhere. It is perfect for seniors and those with health limitations. The **One-Hour Chair Program** is a low-impact workout that includes light aerobic exercise. The **5-Day Short Program** features five compact workouts for people who are short on time.

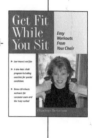

160 pages ... Paperback $14.95 ... Spiral bound $19.95

SELF-HELP FOR HYPERVENTILATION SYNDROME: Recognizing and Correcting Your Breathing-Pattern Disorder *by Dinah Bradley*

Chronic hyperventilation symptoms include breathlessness, chest pains, palpitations, broken sleep, stomach or bowel problems, dizziness, and anxiety. This book explains causes and symptoms, and presents a program that helps readers to break the hyperventilation cycle and breathe freely again.

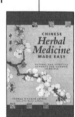

128 pages ... Paperback $12.95 ... Third edition

CHINESE HERBAL MEDICINE MADE EASY: Natural and Effective Remedies for Common Illnesses *by Thomas Richard Joiner*

Chinese herbal medicine is an ancient system for maintaining health and prolonging life. This book has easy-to-read listings of more than 750 herbal remedies for over 250 common complaints ranging from acid reflux to pain, sexual dysfunction, and obesity. A valuable addition to every health library.

432 pages ... Paperback $24.95

I-CAN'T-CHEW COOKBOOK: Delicious Soft-Diet Recipes for People with Chewing, Swallowing and Dry-Mouth Disorders *by J. Randy Wilson*

Over 40 million people in the U.S. need to eat soft foods, including people with TMJ, stroke, cancer, Alzheimer's, AIDS, and lupus. This cookbook features 168 tasty and nutritious soft- or liquid-diet recipes with nutritional analyses and tips on preparation.

Endorsed by medical professionals, it contains an introductory chapter by a registered dietician and is also available in a lie-flat spiral binding.

224 pages ... Paperback $16.95 ... Spiralbound $22.95

ORDER FORM

10% DISCOUNT on orders of $50 or more —
20% DISCOUNT on orders of $150 or more —
30% DISCOUNT on orders of $500 or more —
On cost of books for fully prepaid orders

NAME

ADDRESS

CITY/STATE   ZIP/POSTCODE

PHONE   COUNTRY (outside of U.S.)

TITLE	QTY	PRICE	TOTAL
Alternative Treatments for FM... (2nd ed.)		@ $17.95	
Women Living with Fibromyalgia		@ $14.95	

Prices subject to change without notice

Please list other titles below:

		@ $	
		@ $	
		@ $	
		@ $	
		@ $	

Check here to receive our book catalog ❑   *FREE*

SHIPPING COSTS
*By PRIORITY MAIL, first
  book $5.25, each addi-
  tional book $1.00
By UPS or FEDEX, first
  book $6.00, each addi-
  tional book $1.50
For rush orders and other
  countries call us at
  (510) 865-5282*

TOTAL _____
Less discount @_____% (_____)
TOTAL COST OF BOOKS _____
Calif. residents add 8% sales tax _____
add Shipping & handling _____
TOTAL ENCLOSED _____
Payment accepted in U.S. funds only

❑ Check ❑ Money Order ❑ Visa ❑ MasterCard ❑ Discover

Card # _____ Exp. date _____

Signature _____

Complete and mail to:
Hunter House Inc., Publishers
PO Box 2914, Alameda CA 94501-0914
Phone (510) 865-5282 Fax (510) 865-4295
You can also order by calling **(800) 266-5592**
of from **www.hunterhouse.com**

ATF2-12/2006